NO GRAIN, NO PAIN

A 30-DAY DIET FOR ELIMINATING THE ROOT CAUSE OF CHRONIC PAIN

DR. PETER OSBORNE
WITH OLIVIA BELL BUEHL

Touchstone

New York   London   Toronto   Sydney   New Delhi

Touchstone
An Imprint of Simon & Schuster, Inc.
1230 Avenue of the Americas
New York, NY 10020

First Touchstone hardcover edition January 2016

For information about special discounts for bulk purchases, please contact Simon & Schuster Special Sales at 1-866-506-1949 or business@simonandschuster.com.

The Simon & Schuster Speakers Bureau can bring authors to your live event. For more information or to book an event, contact the Simon & Schuster Speakers Bureau at 1-866-248-3049 or visit our website at www.simonspeakers.com.

Manufactured in the United States of America

10 9 8 7 6 5 4 3 2

Library of Congress Cataloging-in-Publication Data

Osborne, Peter, 1958– author.
    No grain, no pain : a 30-day diet for eliminating the root cause of chronic pain / by Peter Osborne with Olivia Bell Buehl.
        pages   cm
"A Touchstone book."
    1. Chronic pain — Alternative treatment.   2. Pain — Diet therapy.   3. Self-care, Health.   4. HEALTH & FITNESS / Nutrition.   5. HEALTH & FITNESS / Pain Management.   6. HEALTH & FITNESS / Healthy Living.   I. Buehl, Olivia Bell.   II. Title.
    RB127 .O83 2016
    616'.0472   2015028246

ISBN 978-1-5011-2168-5
ISBN 978-1-5011-2170-8 (ebook)

Kate, this book is dedicated to you. You embody the essence of both wife and mother, giving from your heart and soul selflessly, making our children and me better in the process. Without your support, love, and encouragement, *No Grain, No Pain* would not have been possible.

As the saying goes, when you do what you love, you never work a day in your life. It is a gift to be able to help patients from all over the world find hope, health, and happiness. It is a greater gift to have you by my side to share the ride. You are my One.

CONTENTS

FOREWORD

The whole-grain goodness myth reigned supreme when I began training clients a few decades ago. To even question whether cereal or oatmeal could become unhealthy seemed akin to blasphemy within the nutrition world.

Regardless of popular opinion, I often noticed when my clients ate grains and other so-called healthy foods, they felt terrible, became bloated, and struggled to lose fat. It was almost like the very foods they were "supposed" to eat held their weight and health hostage.

Something seemed amiss, and eventually I coined the term "weight loss resistance" to describe people who couldn't consistently lose weight despite their most stalwart efforts.

Later, when I started testing for food intolerances, I found about 70 percent of my clients reacted to gluten and several other highly reactive foods.

Fascinating things happened almost immediately when they eliminated these foods from their diets. Almost overnight, they felt better, suffered less pain, enjoyed more energy, and that stubborn fat finally disappeared.

Gluten-free is hot today, but even a decade ago almost nobody knew what the heck this arcane-sounding protein was or why eating a seemingly healthy food could create such metabolic havoc.

Conventional wisdom is finally catching up. As the movement makes headway, emerging science finds that going and staying gluten-free can do incredible things like reducing inflammation, obesity, and insulin resistance.

Gluten provides a great example about how mainstream medical thinking often falls behind or neglects the underlying roots of disease.

If you constantly struggle with pain, you can bet a dozen pharmaceutical drugs exist to solve this or whatever problem you suffer.

But that fails to address the bigger problem. *What* causes that pain? What if eliminating highly reactive foods like gluten and implementing some simple but powerful lifestyle strategies could radically alter your problem?

As a functional medicine practitioner, Dr. Peter Osborne asks those big, bold questions to address the underlying culprits that become health thieves and contribute to nearly every disease on the planet.

That approach becomes the foundation for *No Grain, No Pain*: Osborne looks at biochemical individuality—in other words, we are all unique; something we all learned at five years old—to show how hidden gluten in foods like corn and rice make you sick, tired, and overweight.

Going gluten-free helps, but manufacturers have become quick to turn this into a profitable industry. A gluten-free, high-sugar cookie ultimately becomes a cookie, period.

Besides, it turns out it isn't just gluten that creates problems. Osborne digs deeper and challenges traditional gluten-free diets to explain why they don't always work.

More important, he finds what *does* work, providing a 30-day grain-free road map that also eliminates soy, dairy, and other potentially problematic foods to help you feel better; relieve pain; and finally attain fast, lasting fat loss.

Osborne's research dives deep into gut, brain, and other areas to show how grains contribute to everything from autoimmunity gut issues to brain health.

Along the way, he blows out some widely circulated myths about grains and also other foods. (Whoa, did you know dairy products could resemble gluten to your immune system?)

His approach becomes comprehensive but not encyclopedic or difficult to understand, allowing you to do the detective work, consult an integrative practitioner if necessary, and determine what might be creating your problems.

Osborne provides a comprehensive list of foods to avoid. He discusses lifestyle strategies like sleep, stress, exercise, and environmental toxins that, taken together, radically shift your health.

Simply put, you've got the tools in this book to become lean, healthy, and finally eliminate pain and other misery that holds you back and stymies your success.

Lest you think this book signals deprivation, simply flip to the delicious, easy-to-prepare recipes that make transforming pain into vitality an absolute breeze.

The plan might be for 30 days, but once you see the improvements—and with many clients, they occur almost immediately—this quickly becomes a plan you'll want to stick with for life.

Beyond creating a groundbreaking understanding about the role grains and other reactive foods play in pain and other illness, Osborne's message centers on self-empowerment.

"With the knowledge you'll gain of functional medicine in general and the deleterious effects of grains specifically," he writes, "I believe that you will be empowered to take an active role in healing yourself."

That becomes the driving force behind functional medicine: *you* have the power to transcend disease and create a pain-free life of health, happiness, and vitality, and it all starts with your fork.

Accept nothing less than that for yourself, because you're worth it.

JJ Virgin, CNS, CHFS,
author of *The Virgin Diet* and *JJ Virgin's Sugar Impact Diet*

HOW TO USE THIS BOOK

Just as my functional medicine practice is different from most medical practices, this book is different from most books, in large part because of its interconnectivity with the Gluten Free Society website (gluten freesociety.org). *No Grain, No Pain* provides a comprehensive introduction to my program as well as the basics of how gluten can produce such a variety of symptoms in different individuals. But understanding that today people read books (and generally gather information) in a variety of ways, I've provided multiple entry points for additional information. It's possible that you (or a family member) are experiencing more than one pain trigger or more than one response to grain, so it's a good idea to read the whole book (even the science-heavy chapters at the beginning). However, at the end of each of the first five chapters, which deal with the various kinds of pain and inflammation, I'll summarize the key points ("What You Need to Know") in case you're in a hurry to get to the program itself. If so, I trust you'll return to these chapters to fully understand why you're hurting and how the changes you'll be making with the No-Grain, No-Pain program help you heal.

Hearing the experiences of others can be highly motivating, so I've included more than a dozen success stories from the thousands of my patients who've resolved their pain (and more), detailing their experiences before and after adopting a *true* gluten-free dietary approach. Once you've read how they escaped the prison of chronic pain, you can "meet" many of them in videos. Look for web links at the end of most stories.

For those wishing to delve deeper into the subject, I've provided a gateway to the "glutenology" community. You'll find links to such "Bonus Features" throughout the text, as well as additional online sources of information. I'm also a great believer in visual aids, so whenever possible, I've used illustrations to simplify sometimes complicated concepts. You'll also find self-tests to track your pain levels and ascertain whether you're apt to have inflammatory conditions. Detailed meal plans with accompanying recipes will make it easy to eliminate *all* gluten from your meals—starting today.

Finally, if you need to find a practitioner who will work with you, I've provided a link to my network of health-care professionals around the country: glutenfreesociety.org/find-doctor. I've trained most of them in my protocols. Welcome to the world of *true* Gluten-Free Warriors.

PART 1

THE PAIN IN THE GRAIN

The Science Behind the Grain-Free Lifestyle

The greatest wealth is health.

—Virgil

Maybe you've been told that your pain is "all in your head." Perhaps you've tried a variety of different therapies and prescription drugs without success. You're tired, you're hurting, and you're fed up.

It's not just you. It happens to countless Americans every year: patients who go to doctors' offices seeking relief and leave with a handful of prescriptions for drugs. Those medications work for a time, then stop—or they may never really work at all. And millions of people may risk becoming dependent on these painkillers, never realizing that the very drugs they are taking to fight pain are actually interfering with their body's own natural healing process, making them feel sicker and more depleted with every passing day.

What if there was a better option to combat pain? What if it didn't involve drugs at all, but rather a way of healing your discomfort and pain from the inside out?

I don't believe that there is a "pill for every ill." This book, *No Grain, No Pain*, offers a different approach for treating pain *and* for promoting overall health and well-being. This alternative approach is known as *functional medicine*, and it's a methodology that's gaining more and more adherents among both doctors and patients alike. Functional medicine focuses on identifying the *root causes* of disease rather than simply treating the symptoms, in order to develop and implement meaningful prevention and treatment methods. This approach encourages a true partnership between patient and doctor. The goal is not just to return the patient to health, but also to teach him or her how to remain healthy and prevent disease, in the process becoming less dependent on the doctor.

It's obvious that *something* new is needed. Americans spend billions of dollars a year on medical treatments and medications. Why, then, do we remain among the world's sickest people?

- The number of people suffering from cancer and heart disease continues to grow every year, despite mainstream medicine's massive efforts to treat them.
- Prescription medications are overprescribed, and often their effectiveness is underwhelming.
- A multitude of adverse effects from taking "properly" prescribed drugs is the fourth leading cause of death in this country. Millions of other people experience serious or disabling side effects.

How can this be? Some of it is due to the fact that most doctors spend very little time with patients. Medical schools don't train physicians how to ascertain the origin of disease; instead, they are taught to eliminate symptoms with drugs that manipulate the body's chemistry. I'm not saying that this kind of medicine (and doctors who practice it) isn't well intentioned. But I do think there's a different, better way.

Each person has a unique set of genetics and biochemistry, and an equally unique set of environmental and lifestyle factors, all of which interact with one another. This means that you could potentially have the same disease as a friend, but with a completely different set of causes. Likewise, the same factors could result in different disease states in different individuals. Instead of relying on synthetic drugs, functional medicine seeks to understand a patient's overall medical history, lifestyle, and environmental factors, using specialized lab tests as well as a comprehensive physical evaluation.

A book, too, can convey the principles of health from a functional medicine viewpoint, which I do with *No Grain, No Pain.* Of course, while I can describe the health-restoring experiences of a number of my patients in the pages that follow, as well as explain how I was able to heal them of an array of painful conditions, without getting to know you as an individual and running specialized tests on you, I obviously cannot treat you. But with the knowledge you'll gain of functional medicine in general and the deleterious effects of grain specifically, I believe that you will be empowered to take an active role in healing yourself. Initially, that will take the form of giving the Grain-Free, Pain-Free program a 30-day test drive. Assuming you feel better at that point—and I know you will—I hope that will spark your decision to seek out a practitioner of functional medicine or initiate a discussion on functional medicine with your doctor.

But back to why you picked up this book: to find a solution to your pain. I'm going to offer that, and so much more, in *No Grain, No Pain.* In part 1, I'll simplify the science of why grain causes pain. We'll discuss how inflammation is at the root of all pain and puncture the myth that only wheat, barley, and rye contain glutens. You'll learn how to escape what I call the "cycle of pain" and avoid "gluten-free whiplash." You'll also come to understand the link between your brain and your gut, as well as the role that grain plays in obesity and other metabolic diseases. Along the way, you'll meet many of my patients who've gone from pain ridden to pain free once they changed their diet. Then, in part 2, we'll move on to the actual 30-day program, which will help you rid your diet of grain and other problematic foods and make other lifestyle changes, so you, too, can start feeling better and living pain free. Read on!

CHAPTER 1

WHAT'S THE GRAIN-PAIN CONNECTION?

Why "Healthy" Foods Make Us Feel So Bad

All truth passes through three stages. First, it is ridiculed. Second, it is violently opposed. Third, it is accepted as being self-evident.

—Paraphrased from the writings of Arthur Schopenhauer, nineteenth-century German philosopher

The gluten-free diet has been all the rage these past few years. Lots of plans show you how to cut sugar, wheat, and other empty carbs out of your diet to lose weight—and those approaches generally work, very successfully. Other diet books argue that eliminating grain will improve your memory and brain function, both today and tomorrow. There is solid research backing this thesis: improved memory now, and memory protection in the future, is a clear side effect of a grain-free diet.

Many of the people who come to my clinic in Sugar Land, Texas, come through the doors because they are in pain: the kind of debilitating pain that infiltrates every aspect of life and makes each day a little darker and a lot more challenging. For them, changing their diet isn't just a lifestyle choice; it's the difference between relief and chronic pain. Sometimes it's even the difference between life and death.

If you're in such pain, you've probably tried many ways to deal with it, including physical therapy and massage, as well as the use of over-the-counter and prescription painkillers. None of these "solutions" likely worked for long. Quite possibly, you've experimented with some form of a so-called gluten-free diet, again without any lasting improvement. You may be at your wits' end.

Hold on. Help is at hand.

In *No Grain, No Pain*, I'm going to offer you something revolutionary: a 30-day, step-by-step plan that will get at the real root cause of your pain. You'll learn:

- Why foods you've always been told were "healthy" may actually be making and keeping you sick

- How painkillers and other drugs deplete your body of vitamins and minerals vital to healing, actually aggravating the root cause of the pain

- That just because you don't test positive for celiac disease doesn't mean you aren't sensitive to gluten

- Because glutens are present in *all* grains, not just wheat, barley, and rye, why following a traditional gluten-free diet rarely results in a cure

- Why removing all grains (and often certain other foods) can eliminate chronic pain once and for all

- Why other health problems you may never have associated with grain may also be caused by gluten sensitivity

- How to detect hidden grains in processed foods and even personal care products

- How to replace the nutrients of which your body has been robbed with the right food and targeted supplementation

- How intermittent fasting can help speed your return to pain-free health and vitality
- Why eliminating grains can help you achieve and maintain a healthy weight

Finally, you will receive reinforcement that your pain is not just in your head, but instead arises from a physical cause, one that you have the power to change.

SENT HOME TO DIE

A little girl I worked with once desperately needed just such help. Ginger was only 9 years old when her mother brought her to my office. She had been diagnosed with a debilitating disease called juvenile rheumatoid arthritis, and her doctors didn't know if she would make it. In fact, her situation was so dire that the Make-A-Wish Foundation stepped in and granted Ginger her wish to go to Alaska to see whales off the coast with her family.

Ginger's condition wracked her body with headaches, muscle pain, joint pain, indigestion, and stomach pain. She had been suffering since her introduction to normal foods at 20 months of age. She was in and out of the hospital so frequently that she had to have a permanent stent placed in her arm so that whenever she was hospitalized, it was easier to give her an IV.

Imagine going through years of hospital trips, doctors' visits, and horrible pain all before you reach the age of 10. This was Ginger's daily reality—until I saw her. After an extensive exam and laboratory testing, I identified Ginger as having non-celiac gluten sensitivity. We changed her diet—not just cutting out wheat, but overhauling even the hidden sources of gluten that I'll tell you more about shortly. Today, Ginger is gluten free and very much alive. She no longer has a plastic stent in her arm. She is growing normally. She doesn't need to take any medications. She plays on her school volleyball team and has a new lease on life. As long as she avoids all grains, Ginger is symptom free, but if she does eat food that contains gluten, her joints swell. Despite her youth, Ginger is able to stick with her diet because the correlation between what she eats and the swelling and pain is undeniable.

There is no question that Ginger is alive today because she is grain free. Does this sound like a fad diet?

GETTING TO THE ROOT

This youngster was an extreme case, but she is only one of the thousands of success stories I've treated in my practice in the past fifteen years. You'll meet lots more of them throughout this book—people who have suffered from ailments as diverse as depression, vertigo, irritable bowel syndrome (IBS), osteoarthritis, and eczema. Some of them have overcome debilitating pain and illness. Others have improved their lives in more subtle ways, exchanging discomfort after every meal and sore joints after every physical exertion with energy and exuberance. All of them share one thing in common: by identifying and eliminating the *root cause* of their pain, they have been able to get on with their (pain-free) lives.

So what is the root cause of their pain? As you'll soon see, so often it's the *hidden* sources of gluten in our diets. Many of us think that if we cut out bread and pasta and buy the official "gluten-free" bread, pasta, cookies, crackers, and other products available at every major health-food store (and increasingly in every supermarket), we're eating a gluten-free diet. That's just not the case. I'm going to show you why those so-called gluten-free processed foods (usually made with rice, corn, sorghum, or other grains—as well as soy) can be just as much of a trigger to gluten-sensitive people as a bowl of Wheaties or an English muffin. And you'll learn how to make smarter choices, ones that will utterly revolutionize the way you feel every day.

Yes, many of my patients lose some weight on a grain-free diet, sometimes a substantial amount. Meanwhile, those who are malnourished as a result of intestinal issues stemming from the grain in their diet are able to *add* crucially needed pounds. And yes, many of them also report feeling "sharper," more mentally clear, and more able to focus. But when I see a patient whose joints have bothered her for years enjoy walking again, then resume jogging, and then finally run a 5K, I know I've made a measurable difference in her quality of life. When I see another patient who was in too much agony to get off the couch unassisted now able to plop down on the carpet and roughhouse with his grandkids without wincing, that's a real measure of success.

In addition to their remarkable physical transformations, I like to think that I also offer my patients something else: hope. Hope that there *is* a solution to their physical and emotional suffering. This book will offer you the same. Follow my Grain-Free, Pain-Free program, and you'll feel dramatically better within 30 days.

Did You Know?

The suffix *itis*, derived from Greek and Latin, means "inflammation." So arthritis is inflammation of a joint; colitis is inflammation of the colon; bronchitis is inflammation of the bronchial tubes; hepatitis is inflammation of the liver. When you see any word ending in *itis*, it's describing inflammation. We tend to think of inflammation as swelling, a blister, or redness. However, it can also occur internally without symptoms and, over time, lead to painful diseases. And guess which is one of the common causes? Right, grain consumption.

WHAT DOES GLUTEN HAVE TO DO WITH PAIN?

This book focuses on chronic pain in the joints, muscles, and nerves, appearing as hypothyroidism, fibromyalgia, arthritis, hormonal changes that lead to pain, and migraine headaches. And that's just for starters. Pain can also take the form of emotional pain—depression, for example. When you get used to living with constant pain, you may fool yourself into thinking that it's normal to get headaches, feel joint pain, or have a persistent backache, even though you may regard yourself as perfectly healthy.

It is vital that you understand that pain is *never* normal; rather, it is a signal from your body that something is wrong. Likewise, the older you get, the more likely you are to assume that aches and pains are a normal part of aging. Your doctor probably tells you to just accept the discomfort. In my experience, most doctors prescribe a pain pill, espousing the old "it's just normal arthritis" line. But that's crazy! This lie has only become "truth" because most doctors reinforce it over and over again. Having seen thousands of people escape the prison of pain—at any age—when they change their eating habits, I refuse to accept this as true—and so should you.[1] I can assure you that a pain-free future awaits you.

As we're now learning, there's a clear connection between the inflammation caused by certain foods containing gluten (and similar substances) and the pain that manifests itself in our joints and other parts of our body. We'll talk more about inflammation later, but first: what exactly is gluten, anyway?

The traditional use of the word *gluten* implies that it is a *single* protein found in wheat, barley, and rye—and sometimes oats. (All four are grains, which are the seeds of a grass.) End of story. But as you'll soon see, that definition is overly simplistic. The true definition of gluten is that it is a large family of storage proteins found in *all* forms of grain, including rice, corn, and many others.[2] The word comes from the Latin for *glue*. Each grain contains different forms of gluten. (The primary gluten in wheat, for example, is gliadin—see "How Much Gluten Is in Different Grains?" on page 17.) But for the sake of simplicity, I'll use the singular *gluten* when talking about the family or the glutens in more than one grain.

If you are gluten sensitive, you will likely react to any form of gluten in a similar way, regardless of its source. Individual responses can vary greatly, although inflammation and pain are common denominators. Gluten may trigger migraines and gut pain in one person, for example, while another presents with psoriasis and arthritis. I created the term *glutenology*, meaning the science of gluten, to help people understand that the effect of this family of proteins is more comprehensive than the one currently held by the mainstream gluten community. The celiac disease support network, patients, most doctors, and the food industry still narrowly define gluten and its impact on health.

THE HIDDEN SOURCES OF GLUTEN IN OUR DIETS

Some people—an estimated 1 in 133 people—suffer from celiac disease, a chronic intestinal condition resulting from a genetic predisposition (meaning it is inherited) in combination with exposure to forms of gluten found in wheat, barley, and rye. Consuming any of these foods triggers an immune response in celiac patients, which damages the mucosal lining of the intestine. Celiac disease causes pain, bloating, diarrhea, and constipation, as well as bone loss, anemia, and malabsorption of minerals and vitamins. If not diagnosed early, celiac disease can be life threatening. The ancients described the symptoms of celiac disease more than two thousand years ago, but its cause was unknown until the 1950s. A few years ago, when an archeological excavation of a site that dated back to the first century BCE in what is now Tuscany, Italy, unearthed the skeleton of a young woman, it revealed typical damage from celiac disease: failure to thrive and malnutrition.[3] Her remains also contained the positive gene marker for gluten sensitivity. Writing about a hundred and fifty years after her death in a treatise on disease, the Greek physician Aretaeus of Cappadocia described the symptoms ("suffering in the bowels") now known as celiac disease. It has been around a long time.

During World War II, wheat, barley, and rye were rationed in Europe. Dr. Willem Dicke, a Dutch pediatrician who cared for children hospitalized with celiac disease, noticed that the change in their diet (no bread) had eliminated or alleviated their painful symptoms.[4] He also observed that after the war ended and the three grains were once again available, the kids relapsed. Bingo! This was the first conclusive evidence that grains trigger celiac disease. But which component in grains was to blame? Initially, researchers targeted the carbohydrates in the grains,[5] but soon after, another study concluded that the protein components, the glutens,[6] were the culprit.

An unintended consequence of finding the cause of celiac disease was that it mistakenly established the "truth" that these three grains—wheat, barley, and rye—were the sole sources of gluten. (Later oats were added to the list.[7] Some studies have found that the gluten in oats does provoke a gluten reaction; others have not.[8] For this reason, most celiac centers warn of the potential for a reaction without declaring, "go oat free.") But here's the thing: these kids lived in the Netherlands, where wheat, barley, and rye are staple grains. Rice and corn weren't really a part of the traditional diet in that part of the world, so no one thought to remove them or test their bodies' reaction to these foods. And for decades after, conventional wisdom said that rice and corn were "safer" grains to consume for people with celiac disease and gluten sensitivity.

Fact is, rice and corn have both been shown to provoke inflammatory responses.[9] But sixty years later this flawed assumption still holds among many physicians. According to Mintel, a market research company, annual sales of "gluten-free" processed foods are expected to hit $15 billion in 2016.[10] Products such as crackers, breakfast cereals, and bread made with corn or rice are purported to be acceptable for people with celiac disease or gluten sensitivity to consume. In fact, the (supposedly) gluten-free industry is largely responsible for the persistent suffering of the vast proportion of people eating these products. Yes, read that sentence again. The very products being hawked as gluten free are contributing to the poor health of those trying to avoid all gluten.

How do we know that there is gluten in many "gluten-free" products? In one study, 82 percent of patients who had previously strictly followed a traditional gluten-free diet without relief of their symptoms were put on a three-to-six-month diet of whole, unprocessed foods. This meant no so-called gluten-free processed foods. The gluten contamination elimination diet succeeded in eliminating symptoms for most of the subjects.[11] In another study, eating such products and avoiding only wheat, barley, rye, and oats did *not* result in complete recovery (meaning reversal of intestinal damage) for 92 percent of adults with celiac disease.[12]

The bottom line is this: the majority of gluten-sensitive people who eliminate only wheat, barley, rye, and oats but continue to consume other grains don't get better!

Discovering the cause of celiac disease was a huge medical break-through. To this day, it is the only autoimmune condition for which we know the cause with 100 percent certainty. But the 1 in 133 people who have celiac disease aren't the only ones who can benefit from a gluten-free diet. Whether non-celiac gluten sensitivity (NCGS) exists was hotly contested for years, but recent research has confirmed that it is possible to be sensitive to gluten without having celiac disease.[13] In fact, a much larger number of people have this related condition, known simply as gluten sensitivity. Although the research community is excited about this groundbreaking work, most of the medical establishment is either unaware of or unwilling to accept its implications. Most doctors still confuse gluten sensitivity with celiac disease. But gluten sensitivity clearly activates other autoimmune diseases and other manifestations of pain. We know this both from the large body of scientific research and because when patients with diverse autoimmune diseases remove all grains from their diet, they also eliminate the pain and quell other symptoms.

CELIAC DISEASE AND GLUTEN SENSITIVITY AREN'T SYNONYMOUS

Imagine that you told ten thousand individuals who regularly took aspirin to report their side effects over time. Some would develop ulcers or gastric bleeding, others would have an allergic response, some would experience relief of their symptoms, and a few would vomit blood.[14] This single drug provides a variety of responses. It's the same thing with gluten sensitivity: when gluten-sensitive individuals consume grains, they experience numerous responses.

Gluten sensitivity is not a disease. It is a genetic predisposition, meaning not that the genes are bad, but rather that they activate an inflammatory cascade within the body, triggered by grain consumption. Enough inflammation over time contributes to autoimmunity, meaning your body becomes confused and your immune system starts attacking your own tissues. We know that celiac disease is one of the autoimmune diseases gluten causes. Therefore, we could say everyone with celiac disease is gluten sensitive; however, we cannot say that everyone with gluten sensitivity will develop celiac disease. To date, gluten has been shown to cause or contribute to more than a hundred symptoms and medical conditions.[15] If you're gluten sensitive and continue to eat grains, you'll eventually develop inflammation, which over time is likely to lead to an autoimmune disease. The most commonly studied gluten-induced disease is celiac disease.

Gluten sensitivity can be elusive, because most people wait to see a doctor until they have a gluten-induced disease or symptoms they can no longer ignore. As of 2012, it was estimated that 18 million Americans have gluten sensitivity.[16] That's 20 to 30 percent of the population! And that number could be considerably higher. Compare that to the less than 1 percent of the population with diagnosed celiac disease.

THE DIFFERENCE BETWEEN
GLUTEN SENSITIVITY AND CELIAC DISEASE

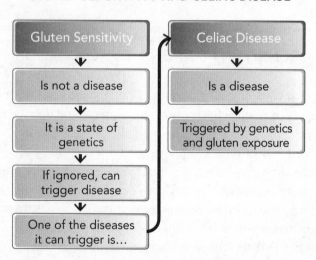

Celiac disease is caused by gluten sensitivity, but celiac is only one of many autoimmune diseases also triggered by gluten sensitivity.

If you or a family member is genetically predisposed to be sensitive to gluten, the sooner you confirm that and begin to proactively deal with it, the better. Gluten-induced damage can begin at conception and continue through the gluten in breast milk (assuming Mom is eating foods with gluten in them).[17] A family history of gluten sensitivity increases the likelihood that you share this predisposition.

EIGHT MYTHS ABOUT GLUTEN

All progress starts with the unvarnished truth, but until you deal with the truth right in front of your nose, you cannot move forward. My mission is to shine a big light on the myths perpetuated about gluten (out of ignorance, an unwillingness to acknowledge error, or for mercenary reasons), reveal the truth based on the latest research and the experiences of thousands of people, and change the message. That message is based on a definition of gluten that hasn't evolved over more than sixty years! Only when you understand and accept that truth will you be able to rid yourself of pain and restore your health.

Let's look at the eight myths and eight truths that underlie the No-Grain, No-Pain program.

Myth 1: **Gluten is found only in wheat, barley, and rye—and sometimes oats.**
Not true! Gluten is not a single protein found in a few grains; rather, it refers to a huge family of proteins. And only one protein, gliadin, found in wheat, barley, and rye, has been extensively studied. Each grain has one or more types of gluten proteins. A recent study identified four hundred new forms of gluten, forty of which were more damaging than the form of gluten for which doctors most commonly test.[18]

Myth 2: **If you are gluten-sensitive, you can safely eat whole grain substitutes such as corn and rice.**
Not true! All grains contain some form of gluten. Research shows that corn (and corn oil) also produces numerous intestinal and health problems for the gluten sensitive.[19] Remember, corn is a grain, not a

vegetable—and it is in thousands of "Frankenfoods," aka junk-food products. (We'll discuss this in greater detail in part 2.) For a list of hidden corn–based ingredients, visit glutenfreesociety.org/hidden -corn-based-ingredients.

Myth 3: **Eating dairy products is safe because they are gluten free.**
Not true! It has been found that milk "looks" like gluten to your immune system, so if you're gluten sensitive your immune system may react to it.[20]

Myth 4: **If you don't have celiac disease, you can eat all the gluten you want.**
Not true! Celiac disease is just the tip of the gluten-sensitivity iceberg and only one of many autoimmune and other conditions it can cause.[21]

Myth 5: **Gluten sensitivity is the same thing as celiac disease.**
Not true! Most people (and most health professionals) think gluten affects just the gut. They don't realize that gluten sensitivity is in fact indicated by a host of other symptoms, from headaches to muscle pain, arthritis, and hypothyroidism. Celiac disease is only one manifestation of gluten sensitivity, which is a genetic state that can express itself through multiple painful disorders when triggered by gluten.

Myth 6: **Lab testing for gluten sensitivity is accurate.**
Not true! There is no lab test for all of the different forms of gluten. When doctors test blood for gluten reactions, the test measures only one type of gluten found in wheat, barley, and rye, creating a potential false sense of security. Even the most progressive lab in the world only looks at a dozen distinct gluten proteins.

Myth 7: **Eating a gluten-free diet is dangerous if you're not gluten sensitive.**
Not true! In fact, if one member of the household is gluten sensitive, getting (and keeping) that family member on a gluten-free diet works best if the whole family supports him/her by eating the same way. There is no scientific evidence that humans need to eat grains.

Myth 8: **Gluten-free processed foods are safe.**

Not true! These foods are usually full of grains (and soy) to which gluten-sensitive people are likely to react.[22] Don't eat these foods if you value your health.

HOW MUCH GLUTEN IS IN DIFFERENT GRAINS?

GRAIN	PRIMARY FORM OF GLUTEN	PERCENTAGE OF TOTAL PROTEIN
Wheat	Gliadin	69
Rye	Secalin	30–50
Barley	Hordein	46–52
Oats	Avenin	12–16
Millet	Panicin	40
Corn	Zein	55
Rice	Oryzenin	5
Sorghum	Kafirin	52
Teff	Penniseiten	11

SYMPTOMS APLENTY

When Ginger became my patient, her condition was a matter of life and death. Fortunately, not all grain-induced conditions are life threatening, but chronic pain certainly does threaten the quality of life. Such as the case with Lynette, who came to see me initially suffering from migraine headaches, stomach pain, insomnia, severe fatigue, sinus congestion, and blurred vision. She had been hospitalized for almost a week due to intestinal inflammation, but her traditional medical treatment had not led to satisfactory improvement. And her debilitating headaches and fatigue made her unable to take care of her family.

What had made her so sick?

You guessed it: grain. Lynette was gluten sensitive, but in combination with the inflammation from her intestinal infection, she was experiencing a one-two punch. Her intestines were so badly damaged that she was severely malnourished, deficient in ten different nutrients including iron; carnitine; vitamins B_{12}, B_6, D, and E; glutamine, gluta-thione, chromium, and overall antioxidants. Although deficiencies of vitamin B_{12} and iron are known to cause migraine headaches, unfortu-nately most doctors don't measure them. They are also the two most common deficiencies caused by grain consumption.

Within a month of changing her diet and correcting her nutritional deficiencies, Lynette's symptoms were dramatically improved. She had more energy. The headaches had dramatically subsided in intensity and frequency. She was sleeping well. Within two months, her symptoms were completely resolved. All of them!

HOW *MUCH* DO YOU HURT?

Here is the first thing I want you to do before you start the No-Grain, No-Pain program. Just as you would weigh yourself before beginning a weight-loss program, measure your pain level, using the simple chart, opposite, as well as in the self-test; below. That way you can establish a baseline for both the intensity and the frequency of pain. This will enable you to quantify your improvement over the next 30 days and beyond. After all, you need to know your starting point to get where you're going.

Pain is relative. My tolerance of pain may be very different from yours. That makes pain difficult to quantify. Also, we tend to forget the actual experience of pain over time. This explains why research on pain can be so confusing and so subjective. But perform this quick pain test now so you can track how *your* pain level diminishes over time.

ARE YOU GLUTEN SENSITIVE? A SELF-TEST

As the title of this book promises, if you think you are gluten sensitive you may simply stop eating grains to see if you feel better within 30 days. After reading this chapter, you probably have a pretty good idea whether or not you are indeed gluten sensitive. Nonetheless, it could be motivating to take the following self-test. You may well see that something you never connected to the source of your pain is actually a

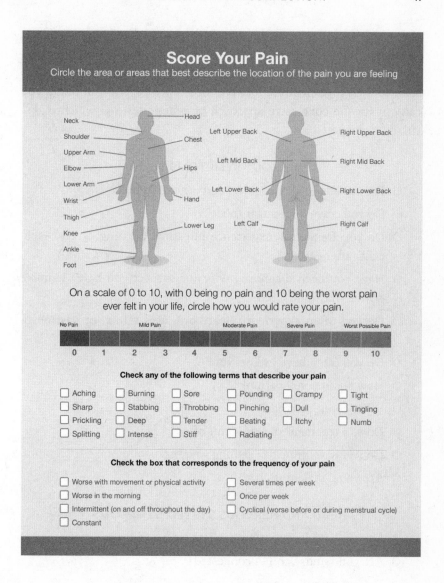

Score Your Pain

Circle the area or areas that best describe the location of the pain you are feeling

Neck — Head
Shoulder — Chest
Upper Arm
Elbow
Lower Arm
Wrist — Hand
Thigh
Knee — Lower Leg
Ankle
Foot
Hips

Left Upper Back — Right Upper Back
Left Mid Back — Right Mid Back
Left Lower Back — Right Lower Back
Left Calf — Right Calf

On a scale of 0 to 10, with 0 being no pain and 10 being the worst pain ever felt in your life, circle how you would rate your pain.

No Pain	Mild Pain	Moderate Pain	Severe Pain	Worst Possible Pain

0   1   2   3   4   5   6   7   8   9   10

Check any of the following terms that describe your pain

☐ Aching   ☐ Burning   ☐ Sore   ☐ Pounding   ☐ Crampy   ☐ Tight
☐ Sharp   ☐ Stabbing   ☐ Throbbing ☐ Pinching   ☐ Dull   ☐ Tingling
☐ Prickling ☐ Deep   ☐ Tender   ☐ Beating   ☐ Itchy   ☐ Numb
☐ Splitting ☐ Intense   ☐ Stiff   ☐ Radiating

Check the box that corresponds to the frequency of your pain

☐ Worse with movement or physical activity   ☐ Several times per week
☐ Worse in the morning   ☐ Once per week
☐ Intermittent (on and off throughout the day) ☐ Cyclical (worse before or during menstrual cycle)
☐ Constant

factor, or that two separate conditions may share a common cause you hadn't previously associated.

Are you experiencing any of the following symptoms, or have you been diagnosed with any of these conditions? If you answer yes to two or more of these questions, you may be gluten sensitive. If so, the sooner you stop eating grains—even small amounts can cause damage—the better. If you see improvement after 30 days, you may decide to forgo any testing and just continue to follow the Grain-Free, Pain-Free program. However, if you need confirmation to motivate you to stick to the program going forward, or simply for peace of mind, you can opt for the conclusive approach of genetic testing, which is discussed in chapter 11.

GUT SYMPTOMS

- Do you crave cake, cookies, and other baked goods?
- Do you crave high-sugar foods?
- Do you frequently experience intestinal bloating or gas, especially after eating?
- Have you been diagnosed with (or suspect you have) irritable bowel syndrome (IBS)?
- Do you often experience heartburn, acid reflux, or gastroesophageal reflux disease (GERD)?
- Do you often have indigestion?
- How about constipation?
- What about diarrhea?
- Do you feel nauseous or vomit often?
- Do you have difficulty gaining weight?
- Are you deficient in iron?

HEAD AND NERVOUS SYSTEM SYMPTOMS

- Do you have frequent headaches?
- Are your sinuses often congested?
- Do you get migraine headaches?
- Do you suffer with frequent vertigo (dizziness)?
- Is your memory poor?
- Do you have difficulty recalling words?
- Do you experience brain fog?
- Do you find it hard to concentrate?

O Have you been diagnosed with ADD or ADHD?

O Are you depressed?

O Are you often anxious?

O Do you have neuropathy in your arms and legs (numbness, pins and needles, sensations of heat and cold, or dull pain)?

O Are you irritable for no reason?

O Do your moods swing back and forth?

O Do you have restless leg syndrome?

O Have you been diagnosed with chronic fatigue syndrome?

O Have you been diagnosed with multiple sclerosis or Parkinson's?

MUSCLE AND JOINT SYMPTOMS

O Do you have frequent joint pain with or without activity?

O Do your muscles ache chronically?

O Do you have migrating joint pain (without injury)?

O Do you have frequent muscle spasms (especially in the legs)?

O Have you been diagnosed with fibromyalgia?

O Have you been diagnosed with autoimmune arthritis, rheumatoid arthritis, lupus, psoriatic arthritis, reactive arthritis, ankylosing spondylitis, or Sjögren's?

O Do your bones hurt?

O Are you feeling growing pains?

O Do you have osteoporosis or osteopenia?

HORMONAL SYMPTOMS

O Are you always fatigued?

O Are you unable to lose weight?

O Do you have difficulty falling asleep or staying asleep?

O Are you unable to conceive?

O Do you have a history of miscarriage or spontaneous abortion?

O Do you have menstrual problems or PMS?

- O Do you have thyroid disease?
- O Have you been diagnosed with hyperprolactinemia?
- O Have you been diagnosed with type 1 or type 2 diabetes?
- O Are you hypoglycemic?
- O Do you have polycystic ovary syndrome?
- O Do you have endometriosis?

IMMUNE SYMPTOMS

- O Do you get chronic urinary tract infections?
- O Do you have chronic respiratory infections?
- O Do you have asthma?
- O Do you have vaginal, oral, or nail bed yeast infections?

SKIN PROBLEMS

- O Do you get fever blisters or mouth ulcers?
- O Do you have a skin rash?
- O Do you have eczema?
- O Do you have psoriasis?
- O Have you been diagnosed with dermatitis herpetiformis? (This skin condition is caused by gluten consumption. If you have been diagnosed with this disease, you are gluten sensitive.)
- O Do you have vitiligo?

OTHER INTERNAL DISEASES/PROBLEMS

- O Do you have gallbladder problems?
- O Are your liver enzymes elevated?
- O Do you have non-alcoholic fatty liver disease?
- O Do you have autoimmune hepatitis?
- O Do you have lymphoma?
- O Do you have platelet disorders?

Once you test your pain level and your sensitivity to grains, your answers will give you a good idea of whether this program is going to work for you (or a family member) or not. (Of course, I know it's going to work, but what's important is that you know it, too.) To fully understand *how* pain and grain are entwined, you'll want to read this whole book. You'll learn the sources of your pain and, of course, *how* to banish that pain once and for all. Pain is such a huge and varied subject that I devote the following four chapters to the *whys*, *hows*, and *wheres* of grain-induced pain. In part 2, we'll get into the specifics of the *true* gluten-free diet.

WHAT YOU NEED TO KNOW

○ Gluten is a kind of protein found in all grains.

○ Celiac disease was initially identified as an immune system response to three (and later four) grains.

○ Eliminating the classic three or four gluten grains—barley, rye, oats, and wheat (BROW)—from the diet does not remedy all symptoms in the vast majority of people with celiac disease.

○ Celiac disease is only one example of gluten sensitivity.

○ Gluten sensitivity leads to a hyperimmune response, which results in inflammation and pain and can appear in almost any part of the body.

○ People with gluten sensitivity respond well when they remove all grains from their diet.

○ Pain is never normal and signals that something is wrong that needs to be addressed.

○ Each gluten-sensitive individual may respond differently to eating grains.

BONUS FEATURE

Video on gluten sensitivity: What Is It?: glutenfreesociety.org/video -tutorial/gluten-sensitivity-what-is-it.

CHAPTER 2

WHERE DOES IT HURT?

Escaping the Pain-Futility
Cycle for Good

That which does not kill us makes us stronger.

—Friedrich Nietzsche

Chronic pain is the number one reason people visit a doctor's office. I realize that knowing that millions of others are also experiencing rampant pain provides no solace. (Whoever came up with the saying *misery loves company* clearly wasn't experiencing chronic pain!) You want a *real* solution, not just a prescription for drugs that merely treat the symptoms without resolving the underlying cause. The idea that anyone needs to be dependent upon painkillers is yet another myth I want to dispel. In many cases, the key to becoming pain free is to completely eliminate grains from your diet. I can't wait to share more of that solution with you, but first let me explain how freeing my patients of pain became my mission in life.

As an intern in a VA hospital, where I trained in rheumatology (autoimmune diseases that cause chronic pain), I saw that the approach to treating patients with painful inflammatory autoimmune diseases was always the same: dose after dose of toxic drugs. It didn't matter whether the person had rheumatoid arthritis, fibromyalgia, migraine headaches, or a host of other painful conditions. Drugs did temporarily relieve their pain, but never resulted in a cure. For many patients, drug treatment actually created a variety of additional problems, including side effects that often were as bad as the symptoms they were supposedly treating. Additionally, these very same drugs were responsible for robbing the body of the vitamins and minerals it needs to naturally heal painful conditions.

DIET INSTEAD OF DRUGS

When I suggested that the VA hospital try another approach, I was told there was nothing else we could do to help these patients. But when I looked for research on pain and autoimmune diseases, I discovered this simply wasn't true. (Once again, a myth was posing as the truth.) Study after study linked numerous diseases to:

- Gluten sensitivity
- Food allergies to corn, dairy products, and other foods
- Dietary deficiencies of vitamins, minerals, and other nutrients

And the most compelling evidence of all pointed to the fact that people with pain symptoms show dramatic improvement when fasting. If removing a certain food solves a problem, then that food is clearly the cause. This is especially true of the glutens found in grains. Moreover, if drugs can target inflammation as a treatment, it only makes sense that food can do the same. After all, isn't food a drug of sorts? That logic led me away from drugs and toward diet as the key to relieving chronic pain. Over and over again I see patients get better after eliminating grain and other inflammatory foods from their diets. *No Grain, No Pain* will help you do so, as well.

I continued my research after my internship and spent a year developing nutritional treatment protocols before setting up my practice. In the fifteen years since, I've helped thousands of patients recover from chronic and debilitating conditions. As a chiropractor and nutritionist, my goal is to find the origin of a disease, instead of simply treating the symptoms. I am intimately familiar with the types of pain that send patients to my clinic seeking relief, as well as the most effective ways to alleviate different kinds of pain. Many of my patients come to me after trying other approaches to minimize or eliminate chronic pain associated with rheumatoid arthritis, migraine headaches, fibromyalgia, irritable bowel syndrome, osteoarthritis, and other muscle and joint problems resulting from hormone imbalance.

My reputation for successfully treating patients with supposedly incurable pain-based diseases quickly spread through word of mouth, abetted by my online presence. Soon people from all over the world were flying in to meet with me. Realizing that I couldn't help everyone with pain myself, I created educational programs for other health practitioners. I've also organized local and online seminars for laypersons. But as part of my mission to shine a light on the connection between pain and grain to those most in need of it—people like you—I decided to write *No Grain, No Pain*. My hope is that it will not only help you understand the source of your pain and the permanent solution to living pain free, but also enable you to open an informed dialogue with your doctor. Unfortunately, the case study on the following page is an all-too-familiar example of how most doctors simply prescribe painkillers and antidepressants rather than explore the root causes of pain and other autoimmune symptoms.

Doctors Aren't Trained in Nutrition

Why are most doctors so unwilling to accept that nutrition plays a role in good health and the restoration of health? Most of them simply have had little or no training in nutrition. A 2010 study that polled medical schools about their nutritional curriculum found:[1]

- Only 25 percent of schools require a dedicated nutrition class.
- Medical students receive less than twenty hours of nutrition instruction during their whole education.

- Only 27 percent of medical schools meet the minimum twenty-five hours in nutrition required by the National Academy of Sciences. The average number is only seven hours.

This lack of respect for the science of nutrition has created a national health disaster. The reality is that the average person knows more about nutrition than the doctors from whom they are seeking nutritional advice. In contrast, I have more than five hundred hours of formal nutritional training, and closer to ten thousand hours if you include my postgraduate internship and private study. I'm not saying this to boast, but simply to make it clear that nutrition is a fundamental science of its own, and most medical schools offer no meaningful nutritional training.

MULTIPLE PAIN POINTS, MULTIPLE DRUGS, BUT ZERO RELIEF

Tim came to see me with severe back pain and an interstitial cystitis, an autoimmune condition that causes severe bladder pain and inflammation. He also had an inflamed prostate, headaches, and high blood pressure. Both urination and intercourse were so painful that he developed severe anxiety. Tim was under the care of three different doctors and taking seven medications, including the pain-blocking opiate tramadol, two blood pressure medications, an antibiotic, two medications for his bladder and prostate, and Xanax for his anxiety. Tim was understandably frustrated that despite five years of medical treatment, nothing had really helped. He was on the verge of a complete breakdown.

Genetic testing revealed that Tim had a gluten-sensitive gene pattern. Other tests revealed that he was allergic to several different forms of pesticides as well as several common food additives and dyes. In addition, Tim was deficient in vitamins D, B_6, B_8, and K, as well as the mineral manganese, due undoubtedly to depletion from the multiple medications he was on.

My protocol included changing Tim's diet, as well as avoidance of allergens, and nutritional supplementation to target his deficiencies. I also put him on high doses of probiotics to restore his good bacteria and offset the various antibiotics he had taken. Within three weeks of changing his diet, Tim was able to cut the dosage of his opiate medication for pain relief in half. Within two months, his blood pressure had normalized so he no longer needed those medications. His back and bladder pain were controlled with the diet and regular exercise. After five years of visits to many physicians (some of them specialists), multiple medicines, and untold amounts of pain and frustration, all his complaints were resolved within just two months of removing grain from his diet.

THE HOWS OF GRAIN PAIN

There are multiple ways eating grains contributes to pain.

- *If you're gluten sensitive, the direct effect is inflammation and damage.* Eating grain causes the production of immune chemicals, which the body experiences as pain and other symptoms. Grains cause the immune system to attack the body, in the process creating damage to virtually any tissue in the body. Think of inflammation as a high-speed train and your bloodstream as the train tracks. Inflammation comes barreling along, delivering pain to various stations along the way. It may visit some of your joints, muscles, or nerves. It may go express to your GI tract. Or it may head to your liver. Inflammation tends to seek out the body's weakest areas, which are most subject to pain.

- *Grain consumption also leads to vitamin and/or mineral deficiencies.* A deficiency in essential nutrients promotes inflammation and inhibits the body's ability to properly heal. This can lead to a breakdown in muscles, joints, bones, and other body tissues, with the side effect of pain.

- *Grain causes leaky gut, which is a precursor to autoimmune diseases.* Microscopic holes in the gut lining allow bacteria, chemicals, toxins, and other ne'er-do-wells to enter the bloodstream, confusing the immune system and leading to internal warfare. The collateral damage includes such painful autoimmune conditions as migraines, rheumatoid arthritis, fibromyalgia, and IBS.

- *Grain is extremely difficult to digest.* The proteins in grain are resistant to enzymatic breakdown, taxing the gut's ability to digest food.

THE REAL DEAL ON INFLAMMATION AND VEGETABLE OILS

Time to shine that bright light of truth on some more myths. Here are two more to add to the inventory that began on page 15:

Myth 9: **Inflammation is a bad thing.**

Not true! Inflammation actually initiates the body's natural healing process by clearing out damaged cells or tissue, so they can be replaced or repaired. I like to think of inflammation as the body's live-in housekeeper, always on the alert for things that need tidying up. This process is ongoing. But excessive inflammation or inflammation that goes unchecked is problematic.

Myth 10: **Vegetable oils are healthy.**

Not true—for two reasons. First of all, the oil labeled *vegetable oil* you'll find on your supermarket shelf is made from some combination of corn, canola, soy, peanut, safflower, sunflower, and cottonseed oil. None of these is a vegetable. Corn is a grain. Canola oil is made from rapeseed, which in its natural state is poisonous to humans. The Canadian oil industry genetically altered it, hence the more appealing name. Soy and peanuts are both legumes. Safflower and sunflower are seeds. Cotton, of course, belongs in your sheets and towels, not in your tummy. These relatively low-cost ingredients are then subjected to heat and chemical solvents to extract the oil and render it tasteless and odorless. To make things worse, these ingredients all have a highly inflammatory concentration of omega-6 fats, which add fuel to the fire of chronic inflammation. Remember, grain equals pain. (Coldwater fish like sardines, salmon, and mackerel, as well as walnuts and other tree nuts, are good sources of omega-3 fatty acids, which are anti-inflammatory.)

Celiac Disease Is Rarely Found Alone

As you now know, everyone with celiac disease is gluten sensitive, but it is also highly likely that anyone with celiac disease also has at least one other painful autoimmune disease, and quite possibly several. Evidence now points to the fact that people who develop celiac disease also turn up with other autoimmune diseases.[2] Unfortunately these conditions are often blamed on other causes such as family history. The celiac disease gets all the attention and the patient never makes the connection that grain is also the trigger for the other problems. On the other side of the coin, many people who react to grain have not received a diagnosis of celiac disease (or have not tested positive for it), and therefore never suspect that grains may be the problem.

Pain Here, There, and Everywhere

Location	Common Conditions
Head	Migraine headaches (see "Nerves," below)
	Tension headaches
	Cluster headaches
Skin	Eczema
	Psoriasis
	Vitiligo
	Urticaria
Gut	Irritable bowel syndrome (IBS)
	Celiac disease
	Crohn's disease
	Ulcerative colitis
	Gut migraines
	Leaky gut

Location	Common Conditions
Muscles	Pain and weakness
	Fibromyalgia
	Polymyalgia
	Dermatomyositis
Joints	Osteoarthritis
	Rheumatoid arthritis
	Lupus
	Ankylosing spondylitis
Nerves	Migraine headaches
	Dysautonomia
	Restless leg syndrome
	Reflex sympathetic dystrophy syndrome
	Peripheral neuropathy
	Cerebellar ataxia
	Vertigo
	Multiple sclerosis

For many people, chronic pain is part of an autoimmune disease. Tim's pain surfaced in his back, but that is only one of many places and ways in which grain-induced pain can appear. Typically the name is specific to the pain's location. For example, Crohn's disease refers to the right side of the large intestine, ulcerative colitis to the left side. Celiac disease affects the small intestine.

Even if you have not yet been diagnosed with an autoimmune disease, you may well be suffering chronic pain in one (or several) of the following parts of your body. There are actually about 140 autoimmune diseases that can be triggered by eating grain and have been linked to gluten sensitivity.[3] (For a complete list, see aarda.org/autoimmune-information/list-of-diseases.) People diagnosed with these conditions may benefit tremendously by being genetically tested for gluten sensitivity, although I hasten to add that other triggers can also initiate the autoimmune response. We'll look at some of these conditions on the following pages, and the others in the next three chapters.

MY ACHING HEAD

• *Migraine headaches,* a very common side effect of grain consumption, may be either neurological or vascular, resulting from a nerve triggering a response within the brain, or from the rapid contraction and expansion of blood vessels, respectively.

• *Tension headaches* are caused by inflammation, which can be brought on by chronic stress and tension, as well as generally tighter muscles in the neck and back, although jaw clenching can also stimulate them. A variation is a *vertebrogenic headache,* which occurs when the vertebrae in the neck and back don't glide and move properly, resulting in tension in the neck, which leads to a tension headache.

• *Cluster headaches* are generally thought to be caused by hypothalamic dysfunction in the brain—the hypothalamus part of the brain, among other functions, releases hormones. But I have also seen cluster headaches disappear with a grain-free diet. The name refers to the recurrent pattern of occurrence at a certain time of day or certain time of year. So, for example, every day at six p.m., boom, your headache might reappear. What is the connection between grain and cluster headaches? Glutens disrupt the hypothalamus and thus the timing and release of the hormones that help regulate circadian rhythm (your internal clock).[4]

PAINFUL, ITCHY SKIN CONDITIONS

The four most common grain-induced skin conditions are:

• *Eczema,* or atopic dermatitis, is a chronic autoimmune condition in which the skin becomes inflamed, red, and thickened, accompanied by itching. There are a number of subsets of eczema specific to body location.

- *Psoriasis* is an itchy and often painful rash characterized by thick, scaly, red skin on the face and/or the palms of the hands or the soles of the feet. It can also occur in other parts of the body such as the armpits, buttocks, and under a woman's breasts.

- *Vitiligo* is characterized by lack of skin pigmentation overall, or in patches.

- *Urticaria*, or hives, are swollen reddish bumps that itch, burn, or sting, and can appear anywhere on the body. They usually last no longer than a day, but may last considerably longer. They are often the result of an allergic reaction to a food or food additive.

MUSCLE AND JOINT PAIN

One of the most common side effects I see in people sensitive to gluten is muscle and joint inflammation, with accompanying pain. This can lead to a certain pattern of weight gain (belly fat), loss of mobility, and increased risk for injury when exercising. Furthermore, the inflammation can cause muscle atrophy and stimulate the immune system to attack the muscles and joints, further degrading muscle and joint integrity. When you artificially block pain with NSAIDs (non-steroidal anti-inflammatory drugs) and other pain medication, you hinder the natural ability of the body to initiate and control healing. This sets the stage for osteoarthritis, rheumatoid arthritis, and lupus, which will be discussed in chapter 3.

Meanwhile, having less muscle mass makes it harder to exercise, and because a smaller muscle is tighter, it is more prone to injury. It also accelerates cartilage wear and tear. Lack of exercise leads to even less muscle tone and more body fat, and if the cycle continues for years we don't just gain weight; our health also deteriorates. This is why so many Americans are sick. Muscle loss weakens the immune system,[5] limits our ability to move, wrecks our quality of life, and in the end kills us twenty years early. Many of my patients discover that when they eliminate grains from their diet, they experience a dramatic reduction in muscle and joint pain. Pains that were once considered a consequence of aging often completely resolve. Chapter 3 is devoted to inflammation, where we'll address muscle and joint pain in greater detail.

RIGHT TO THE GUT

The most common painful diseases of the GI tract include leaky gut, irritable bowel syndrome (IBS), celiac disease, Crohn's disease, ulcerative colitis, and gut migraines. Some of these conditions are caused by grain-induced inflammation. Some are caused by grains' ability to alter gut bacteria, others from the inability to digest grains in general, both of which will be discussed in chapter 4.

A Brief History of Bread Madness

From the 1500s to the 1700s in Europe, madness was often associated with witchcraft and referred to as bread madness. Such unfortunates may well have eaten rye bread contaminated with a fungus called ergot, which is akin to LSD. Fifty years ago, schizophrenia was sometimes called bread madness because symptoms might disappear when schizophrenics stopped eating foods made with wheat. At that time, several researchers speculated that wheat gluten triggered or promoted schizophrenia. Although it's not generally accepted in the mental health field, there is evidence that people with celiac disease who also have psychiatric and neurological disorders such as schizophrenia, ADHD, depression, and bipolar syndrome tend to produce more antibodies to components in wheat than most people.[6] Several studies on people with schizophrenia have found that removing grain and dairy products—the casein in milk "looks" like gluten and can cause the same kind of reaction—from the diet improves their condition, but they relapse when they reintroduce grain and dairy products into their diet.[7]

Over the past twenty years, evidence that schizophrenia is a biologically based brain disease has grown stronger, supported by brain-imaging techniques that show the destruction of brain tissue in people with schizophrenia. People with this condition, as well as with autism and some other mental disorders, seem to improve or even recover on a gluten-free diet, even if they don't have celiac disease. Although schizophrenics don't make the antibodies that define celiac disease, they do have an inflammatory reaction to gluten.[8] Some more provocative findings:

- There is roughly the same prevalence of celiac disease and schizophrenia in the population, but there is more celiac disease among schizophrenia patients.[9]

- Schizophrenia patients who have a higher level of antibodies to wheat gluten may share some immunologic features of celiac disease.[10]

- A wheat protein other than gliadin may prompt an autoimmune reaction in most people with schizophrenia.[11]

About 1 percent of the population suffers from schizophrenia, a strong argument for further research on this association.[12] Bread madness may *not* be a thing of the past.

NERVE PAIN

Gluten is a known neurotoxin.[13] Grain in general and glutens in specific have been shown to stimulate neuronal antibodies. If you're sensitive to grain but continue to consume it, your body makes antibodies against its own nerve tissue, just as it does with other tissue, which leads to inflammation and ultimately autoimmune nerve diseases. Depending upon which nerves are attacked, the inflammation can appear in a myriad of forms. If it's the nerves in the brain, it could create a migraine headache. If it's the nerves in the extremities, it could create painful neuropathy; nerves in the wrist could create carpal tunnel syndrome. Think of nerves as wires that conduct electricity. A short in the wires leads to miscommunication, which could manifest as pain or muscle spasms. The brain communicates with every other part of the body along the nerves, with reciprocal communications to the brain via the same paths. Some of the more common ways nerve pain may present include:

- *Restless leg syndrome* (RLS) is a serious medical condition. Some people who suffer from RLS find their legs jumping up and down; others experience numbness and tingling, or even shooting nerve pains, making it extremely difficult to sleep. RLS appears to be linked to bacterial overgrowth in the intestine resulting from gluten sensitivity,[14] which in turn leads to an autoimmune response in peripheral nerves.

- *Peripheral neuropathy* leads to numbness, tingling, burning, and pain in the arms, legs, hands, and feet. Over time it can lead to muscle degeneration. Peripheral neuropathy can be triggered by a diabetic infection, physical trauma to nerves exiting the spinal cord, a herniated disc, exposure to toxic metals, or vitamin B deficiencies, as well as gluten sensitivity. Going gluten free has reversed neuropathy symptoms in many people.[15]

- *Cerebellar ataxia:* When the brain's cerebellum is inflamed, it creates a problem with your balance control center. You become dizzy, find it harder to maintain your equilibrium, and have difficulty walking. Gluten has been directly linked to cerebellar ataxia.[16] In addition, in effort to maintain balance, you may strain muscles, creating muscle pain.

- *Vertigo:* As with cerebellar ataxia, vertigo can be the result of damage to the vestibulocochlear nerve that feeds the inner ear. The role of the vestibulocochlear nerve is to allow proper functioning as you move your head from side to side. When all is well, small canals in the ear send messages to that nerve so that you don't get dizzy and fall over. When the nerve is inflamed, it can get confused, resulting in dizziness and loss of balance.

- *Multiple sclerosis (MS):* In this condition, the autoimmune reaction against the nervous system skews the way in which nerve messages are sent. Again, there is evidence linking gluten to MS.[17] (The same is true for reflex sympathetic dystrophy syndrome and dysautonomia, discussed below. All are very painful conditions, which can appear on one side of the body or can inflict pain all over.) In MS, the spinal cord and nerves, including the optic nerves, are impacted, creating vision and balance-control problems, muscle weakness, and spasms as well as numbness and pain. Nerve fibers are normally protected by myelin, a fatty substance that wraps around them. When an immune system attack destroys the myelin, the nerves are damaged, interfering with signal transmission throughout the body. Some people experience only mild symptoms. For others, MS interferes with basic mobility and the normal functions of daily life.

• *Reflex sympathetic dystrophy syndrome* refers to a collection of symptoms that include pain (often described as "burning"), tenderness, and swelling of an arm or leg, along with excessive sweating, warmth and/or coolness, flushing, discoloration, irritation, and shiny skin.[18]

• *Dysautonomia:* This is a collection of conditions in which the autonomic nervous system, which controls such involuntary actions as digestion, breathing, and sweating, malfunctions. Consuming gluten can play a role, manifesting in many ways, including difficulty in changing posture and digestive symptoms, accompanied by pain.[19]

Grain has been shown to cause or contribute to all these conditions; however, it is not the only possible agent. Nonetheless, when people stop eating grain, such symptoms tend to disappear or vastly improve. Because most doctors specializing in the treatment of arthritis, joint pain, muscle pain, nerve pain, gastric distress, and other autoimmune diseases never even consider the composition of a patient's diet as a contributing factor to pain and inflammation, it is always important to consult with a functional medicine doctor who is knowledgeable in these areas and will provide the best guidance. Just as diabetes, a chronic disease of blood sugar disruption, can be caused by diet, the chronic condition of pain is usually related to diet. Most specifically, the cause of inflammation and autoimmune conditions that result in pain is usually one form or another of gluten—and according to voluminous research, the only proven cure for such grain-induced pain is dietary change.

The True Cost of Pain

Consider these facts:

- More than 100 million adults suffer from chronic pain.[20]
- Pain is the most common reason why people visit a doctor's office.
- Pain is also the most common reason employees miss work.
- 5 percent of American women aged 18 to 65 experience headaches at least every other day.[21]
- Acute headaches account for more than 2 million annual visits to emergency rooms.
- 62 percent of nursing home residents report pain, most commonly from arthritis.[22]
- 26.4 percent of Americans report having had low back pain lasting at least a day in the past three months.[23]
- Pain medications are the most commonly prescribed drugs.[24]
- In 2012 U.S. physicians wrote 259 million prescriptions for opioid painkillers.[25] Compare that to our estimated adult population in 2014 of 245 million.[26] Obviously, not every adult is using opiates, but some are using a great deal of them.
- Hydrocodone and acetaminophen, a combination narcotic analgesic sold under the brand name Vicodin, is the most commonly prescribed prescription drug, with 136 million prescriptions written annually.
- Prescription drugs are a multibillion-dollar industry, with almost 4 billion prescriptions written in 2011.[27]
- The top-selling category of over-the-counter medication is painkillers for muscle and joint pain, headaches, and more.
- The estimated annual cost of dealing with chronic pain in this country is at least $560 billion and up to $635 billion.

TREAT THE SYMPTOM, NOT THE CAUSE

The fact that millions of people continue to suffer from chronic and often debilitating pain despite the wide use (and huge cost) of medication is powerful evidence that the pharmacological approach simply isn't solving the problem. I mentioned it before, but it is worth repeating: properly prescribed medication is the fourth leading cause of death in the United States.[28] Yes, *properly* prescribed! This creates a circular paradigm: The very thing that is supposed to help you might kill you. And even if they don't kill, narcotics obviously create the opportunity for abuse and accidental overdoses, which have become an epidemic in the past two decades. Legally prescribed oxycodone and similar drugs are increasingly becoming "gateway" drugs to narcotic abuse.[29] Narcotics can be effective to get past a painful incident and encourage healing; however, they are not a long-term solution.[30] And over time the same dosage may no longer mute pain, necessitating a higher dose.

And then there are the unintended consequences of using pain medication long term. It's not just opiates that are the problem. Steroids can also induce lupus, a chronic, painful form of autoimmune arthritis, as well as osteoporosis. Nonsteroidals can produce gastric bleeding. And again, painkilling drugs can actually aggravate the very cause of pain they are supposedly treating. They can also exacerbate the inflammatory effects of grains by destroying the intestinal barrier, causing gastric bleeding, which leads to leaky gut, which we'll discuss in chapter 4. This allows grains and other materials access to the bloodstream and ultimately tissues and organs.

I call this the Pain-Futility Cycle—you feel pain, you take more pain medication, and that causes more pain . . . repeat ad infinitum. But you can break out of this negative feedback loop. Rather than pop NSAIDs to mask the pain, the real objective is to normalize our body's inflammation process once we identify its source.

THE DRUG ROUTE

There are four types of drugs used to relieve pain and inflammation. After analgesics prove ineffective, most physicians prescribe nonsteroidal anti-inflammatory medications (NSAIDs) and then move to a steroid if necessary. If that brings inadequate relief, they often refer the patient to a pain management specialist, who may prescribe opiates. Let's take a quick look at how each works, as well as its side effects and the names under which it is marketed.

GENERAL ANALGESICS

How they work: Block pain but do not address inflammation.

Side effects: Overuse or high doses can create glutathione deficiency, which can impede the liver's ability to remove toxins, eventually causing liver damage.[31] An overburden of toxins can contribute to long-term pain and inflammation.

Sold as: Acetaminophen; brand names: Excedrin, Tylenol, and Panadol.

NSAIDs

How they work: Temporarily block the perception of pain and reduce fever, but also block the natural chemicals that promote the inflammation necessary to initiate healing. (There are two subsets of inflammatory chemicals and two subsets of NSAIDs, known as COX-1 and COX-2 inhibitors.)

Side effects: Gastric distress, intestinal bleeding, leaky gut, and more. Regular use of salicylates such as aspirin can deplete stores of vitamin C, folate (a B vitamin), and iron, or interfere with their absorption. Sulfasalazine causes folate loss, as does indomethacin, which also depletes iron. Wheat gluten consumption in concert with indomethacin may induce intestinal lesions associated with celiac disease.[32] (Yes, a drug prescribed to alleviate the pain of celiac disease may actually help cause it.)

Sold over the counter as: Salicylates (aspirin) such as Anacin, Bufferin, and Ecotrin; ibuprofen (Motrin, Advil), and naproxen (Aleve, Anaprox, Naprelan, and Naprosyn), and ketoprofen (Orudis KT).

Prescribed as: Celecoxib (Celebrex), diclofenac (Cambia, Cataflam, Voltaren XR, Zipsor, and Zorvolex), indomethacin (Indocin), oxaprozin (Daypro), piroxicam (Feldene), and salsalate (Disalcid). Sulfasalazine (Azulfidine) for ulcerative colitis and rheumatoid arthritis is also used off label for Crohn's disease and ankylosing spondylitis.

STEROIDS

How they work: Mimic the action of cortisol,[33] produced by the adrenal glands to fight stress and inflammation and reduce pain. (Synthetic corticosteroids are not to be confused with anabolic steroids used by body builders.) May be taken by mouth, inhaled, applied as creams, or injected.

Side effects: Long-term use, even at low dosages, can suppress natural cortisol production. Also weight gain and bone loss[34] and diminished absorption of calcium, magnesium, selenium, potassium, and vitamins A, C, and D, which interfere with the body's own arsenal of nutrients to counter inflammation, which causes the pain in the first place.[35]

Sold as: Prednisone, marketed under numerous brand names.

NARCOTICS

How they work: Much the way heroin does, bonding to the same receptors in the brain. Both natural opiates and narcotic drugs downregulate our receptors, and over time may actually cause us to feel pain more intensely, a process called hyperalgesia.

Side effects: Physical dependency, increased pain, and withdrawal symptoms.

Prescribed as: Codeine (Tylenol No. 3), hydrocodone (Vicodin), and oxycodone (Percocet and OxyContin).

HOW PAIN-RELIEF DRUGS CAN INDUCE PAIN

Now, the reason you take any painkiller is to block or reduce pain, right? But ironically, many drugs have side effects that actually induce deficiencies of the very nutrients that naturally help relieve the inflammation and pain. For example:

- *Folate* helps make the components of energy and enables the formation of cartilage, which lines your joints and is essential for joint integrity. If cartilage is malnourished because of insufficient folate, it becomes painful, and you're back to the starting point. But NSAIDs inhibit our body's absorption of folate. Why take a drug to relieve pain when that drug can interfere with your body's uptake of a natural component that protects you from pain?

- *Iron* has multiple purposes, including helping to make hemoglobin for red blood cells, which carry the oxygen necessary to produce energy. NSAIDs can cause iron-deficiency anemia, leading to depriving your tissues of oxygen, resulting in fatigue, muscle spasms, and pain. Once more, a drug you are taking for pain induces a mineral deficiency that leads to the problem you were trying to treat in the first place. I call it chasing your tail!

- *Collagen* is the backbone protein your body uses to make muscles, tendons, ligaments, cartilage, and joints. When collagen is weakened, it interferes with joint healing, which predisposes you to injury. However, because your pain receptors are blocked by NSAIDs, you may be more active than you would otherwise be, and therefore more prone to injury. If you suffer an injury, you will need more painkillers. It's that dreaded pain-feedback loop again.

THE VICIOUS CYCLE OF PRESCRIPTION PAIN MEDS

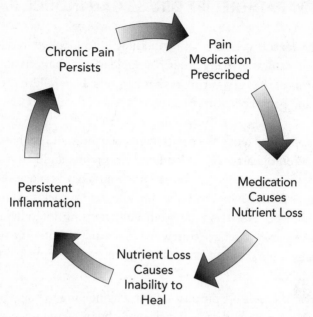

Drugs only mask inflammation; they do nothing to correct the underlying cause. Many pain medications also cause vitamin and mineral deficiencies, which in turn interfere with long-term healing.

UNNECESSARY SURGERY THANKS TO IBUPROFEN

James came to see me after having 5 inches of his small intestine removed. His problems had begun a few years earlier, after a back injury when his doctor prescribed high doses of ibuprofen to allevi-ate the pain. The ibuprofen damaged the mucosal lining of his stom-ach and intestine, resulting in leaky gut, and he started to have large amounts of blood in his stool. This prompted him to visit his gastroen-terologist who diagnosed him with *H. pylori* (a bacterial infection) and a gastric ulcer. James was treated with strong antibiotics and antacid medications. Although there was no follow-up testing after this treat-ment, he did experience some small relief from pain.

However, a few months later James experienced severe abdominal pain and wound up in the ER, where the doctor on call diagnosed him with Crohn's disease. He then proceeded to remove 5 inches of James's intestine. The surgery was probably unnecessary, because James was not in an acutely life-threatening situation. Unfortunately, the long-term effect of this surgery created a lifelong risk of nutritional deficiency problems, especially of B_{12} and iron.

The sad part of this whole story is that none of the doctors James had seen earlier asked about his ibuprofen use. Why is this important? A common and well-known consequence of taking ibuprofen is intestinal damage, evidenced by bloody stools. James could have avoided this medical horror story had his doctors told him about the dangers of overusing this NSAID.

After a full nutritional investigation, I found James to have several issues:

- Glutamine deficiency
- B_1 and B_3 deficiencies
- Gluten sensitivity
- A host of other food allergies, including potatoes and bananas
- An intestinal yeast overgrowth

A year after giving up ibuprofen and making diet changes, James has made a full recovery. His back pain is gone, along with his intestinal bleeding. He is able to work full time and exercise without pain or flare-ups. Unfortunately, he will never get back the 5 inches of his intestine, and he has a lifetime risk of the nutritional problems associated with that loss.

PAIN AND THE BRAIN

Pain itself can change the way the nerve chemicals in the mind communicate. Pain in and of itself creates a neurological stimulation that perpetuates inflammation, which can suppress natural pain-reducing chemicals such as dopamine and serotonin. So here we have another vicious cycle: being in pain produces brain chemicals that make it harder to overcome pain. Moreover, if you are in pain, you are probably not inclined to exercise, which means you don't produce happy brain chemicals. So now you are in pain, depressed, and gaining weight. Not good. At this point, many people give up and gravitate toward foods like cake, cookies, bread, chips, crackers, and other junk foods that provide a temporary high.

Like morphine, a protein in grain called gluteomorphin or gliadorphin sedates pain and enhances mood. Dairy products contain a similar protein called casomorphin.[36] Both these compounds provide temporary relief but perpetuate the primary issue. And like morphine, this protein in grains can make such foods addictive.

Your neurons are plastic, so they can change over time just as your muscles can either bulk up or atrophy. The things that you exercise, neurologically speaking, will get better, but if you don't regularly secrete happy hormones and produce only painful ones, then you'll actually promote those pathways. Unfortunately, the cascade of effects doesn't end there. Avoiding exercise due to pain and depression also interferes with proper regulation of insulin and blood glucose. Excessive glucose that's not being turned into energy has a fatiguing effect. So now one is in pain, depressed, and tired, sapping the motivation to exercise.

WHAT YOU NEED TO KNOW

O Pain is one of our most common medical problems and costs billions of dollars in doctor's bills, drugs, and other treatments, all too often without resolution.

O The conventional approach has been to prescribe drugs to mask the pain, rather than address the real cause. Drugs can also cause nutritional deficiencies that interfere with body's natural healing process.

O The real cause is often an immune response to grain or other foods, leading over time to chronic inflammation and pain.

O Grain consumption also leads to vitamin and/or mineral deficiencies, which weaken the body's innate healing abilities.

O After years of releasing antibodies against grain, the immune system overreacts and starts to attack itself.

O Inflammatory pain can show up anywhere in the body and encompass dozens of autoimmune diseases.

O Removing all grains from the diet is more effective and safer than prescribing drugs, whether NSAIDs, steroids, or opiates.

In the next chapter, we will get to the heart of the matter: how the perfectly normal and essential process of inflammation can be put into overdrive with disastrous consequences when you ignore certain signals and continue to eat foods to which your body reacts poorly.

BONUS FEATURE

Video on different mechanisms that produce pain: glutenfreesociety .org/no-grain-no-pain-pain-mechanisms.

CHAPTER 3

PAIN CAUSED BY GRAINFLAMMATION

Building Strong Muscles and Avoiding Gluten-Free Whiplash

The doctor of the future will give no medicine, but will instruct his patients in the care of the human frame, in diet and in the cause and prevention of disease.

—Thomas Edison

Inflammation gets a bad rap, but as you now know, it's the normal and ongoing process by which the body repairs damaged tissue. New tissue is constantly replacing old tissue. I referred to inflammation earlier as a conscientious housekeeper, but when necessary, it acts like a wrecking ball. When a building is so full of toxic mold, termites, or another problem that cannot be remediated, the damaged sections must be removed to restore the building and create an overall healthy environment. If we "criminalize" inflammation by blocking it, as most pain medicines do, we never allow for the removal of damaged tissue. In this case, the body can never fully repair itself and damaged tissue remains susceptible to a chronic inflammatory process. The body is stuck in breakdown mode, with no chance to rebuild.

Grainflammation is my word for inflammation stemming from an overconsumption of grain. This occurs via multiple mechanisms that have rarely been discussed. In this chapter, we'll delve into these various pathways.

A PAIR OF IMMUNE SYSTEMS

Basically, an allergy to a food or another factor is the equivalent of an immune response. And all immune responses lead to inflammation, so the final common denominator is excessive inflammation. However, there are many different ways in which the immune system creates inflammation. You probably think of your immune system as a single entity. You never refer to your immune *systems* when talking about battling a cold or the flu. But this is another myth. You actually have *two* immune systems, which wage war against anything that threatens your health. Let me explain.

You come into the world with your *innate immune system*, but it is not fully developed until you are about three years old. Until then, your immunity is boosted by your mom's breast milk, which contains antibodies, probiotics, and immune-supporting compounds like colostrum.[1] (Children who are not breast-fed lose out on this advantage, putting them at greater risk for multiple diseases.[2] Likewise, a baby delivered by C-section isn't exposed to protective bacteria in the birth canal and is more likely to have problems with allergens.[3]) The innate system relies on physical barriers and the body's production of non-specific chemicals that operate like scatter bombs. They simply destroy anything they don't "like" in their path. For example, if you inhale something noxious, your body creates mucus in your nose and throat (physical barrier) full of chemicals ("scatter bombs") to protect you. That's your innate immune system in action.

Over time the *humoral immune system* evolves. It adapts to your individual environment, and its battle approach is to develop specific antibodies to protect you from particular dangers. Like drones or guided missiles, these antibodies are targeted, going after a certain bad guy, whether a childhood disease, tobacco smoke in the home, emissions from a chemical factory, or pesticides sprayed by a crop duster—and, of course, the foods you eat. If it's a temporary environmental threat, like a virus or bacteria, your humoral system usually makes the specific antibodies, kills and defeats the virus or the bacteria, and then moves on when the threat is gone. However, if the same threat recurs, memory cells re-create those same defensive antibodies. When your body produces antibodies to a specific virus, such as influenza, that's your humoral immune system at work.

Once both immune systems are fully functional, the innate is always your first line of defense. But when its generalized defense strategy is not enough to rout the invader, the humoral system sends in the snipers. An easy way to distinguish between the two is that the innate system relies on physical barriers and chemical "bombs," while the humoral relies on specific antibodies to attack. Have a look at Shanna's story below to see how these two immune systems went rogue, sabotaging her health, and how a dietary change was able to turn them around.

FIVE DECADES OF PAIN AND SHAME GONE IN THREE WEEKS

From early childhood, Shanna had a history of severe eczema, allergies, and gastric problems. Her visits to different doctors only led to prescriptions for steroid creams, antibiotics, allergy shots, and antidepressants. Her eczema was so severe that it covered her entire face. She was so anxious about her condition and her appearance that she told me she had become "scared of living." She tried changing her skin care and makeup products to no avail. Her doctors told her that despite the fact that long-term steroid use causes bone loss, hormone disruption, and other health issues, she must stay on them permanently or she would become crippled.

Shortly before coming to see me at age 50, Shanna was diagnosed with polymyalgia, an autoimmune condition that creates such pain and stiffness that she was unable to climb stairs, lift her arms, or turn the steering wheel of her car. Her rheumatologist's solution: even higher doses of steroids to control the inflammation. The pain and stiffness were somewhat under control with medications, but she still had physical limitations, irritable bowel syndrome (IBS), and eczema outbreaks on her face, and knew that the drug side effects would eventually catch up with her.

Shanna tested positive for gluten sensitivity, and had additional food allergies to bananas, rosemary, honey, olives, cabbage, and artificial sweeteners. On top of that she was deficient in zinc, selenium, vitamin E, and glutamine, and had a parasite infection and low levels of healthy bacteria in her GI tract. Additionally, she had high levels of mercury and lead in her blood.

Within three weeks of removing all glutens and the other foods to which she was allergic, in concert with a supplement program, Shanna was able to discontinue her pain medications. She also responded well to oral chelation and supplements for heavy metal toxicity. After two months, she no longer had IBS symptoms and reported improved energy and mental clarity. Today, Shanna is free from stiffness and the grip of pain. The eczema that has plagued her since girlhood is gone. She can run, jump on her trampoline, work out, drive, and travel to visit her daughters. (You'll meet one of them in the next chapter.) She feels better at sixty than she ever did before.

For more of Shanna's story, visit glutenfreesociety.org/pain-in-the -grain.

How were both immune systems at work? Shanna's innate immune response accounted for her eczema. Her liver was so overwhelmed by the drugs she had been prescribed that toxins were escaping through her skin. Her humoral immune response produced antibodies against her muscles, causing the polymyalgia.

GLUTEN AND THE INFLAMMATORY RESPONSE

Both immune systems come into play with gluten, which is why there is so much confusion about how it can affect different people differently.

Gluten sensitivity, which most people associate with celiac disease, is an innate response and the reaction is the production of nonspecific chemicals. In contrast, a humoral response to gluten involves the production of antibodies, which are specific. That's the difference. But whatever the cause, the result is the same: inflammation.

"So," you may be muttering, "why do I care whether my immune response is innate or humoral?" I'm glad you asked. The biggest problem in diagnosing gluten sensitivity is that most doctors only measure the broadest humoral response, using lab tests for celiac disease, which measure either IgG or IgA antibodies to one or two forms of gluten. But some of those thousands of different proteins in the gluten family trigger your humoral immune response and others your innate immune response. If you're testing for a reaction to only one or two forms of gluten, and only for a humoral response, you're going to miss some (or many) of the possible immune responses. The truth is, most people with gluten problems fail to get an accurate diagnosis when using conventional testing.

Redefining gluten sensitivity as a state of genetics is much more accurate. That's because it tells us that when your immune systems confront gluten, you're going to have either a humoral or an innate response to it—or potentially both, as Shanna did. In contrast, the standard (and often inaccurate) lab tests may lead to a completely wrong diagnosis. That's why it takes nine years, on average, to get an accurate diagnosis of gluten sensitivity. You don't want you to go through years of suffering before you get the answer. Now that you understand the roles of the two immune systems, you should realize why saying that you don't have a gluten issue because you don't react to two tests for just two chemicals out of thousands is absurd, or at the very least not definitive. The outcome of an immune reaction is always inflammation, but not knowing the cause delays resolution of the problem.

In theory, to know if you *are* gluten sensitive, we would have to be able to measure every one of the thousands of different glutens in every way that we know the immune system can respond. But that technology doesn't exist. That's why the gold standard for gluten sensitivity is still trial by diet: eliminate it for six months. However, few people are willing to commit for that length of time without a definitive answer.

Nonetheless, going completely grain free for 30 days should give you a pretty good idea.

Just to be clear, an autoimmune response to grain doesn't always result from a week or two of exposure; it's more like ten years in the form of your breakfast bagel, lunchtime sandwich, and pizza dinner. Chronic inflammation means there's no opportunity to rebuild damaged tissue, by which time the collateral damage is enormous. Despite their arsenal of weapons, when your immune systems get overwhelmed from multiple inflammatory factors or even chronic exposure to one or more factors, you're likely to suffer from general malaise. It's like having a perpetual infection, but the source of the "infection" is your diet.

To date, scientists haven't figured out all of the mechanisms for how gluten sensitivity works, but they do know that it is part of the innate immune system response, meaning that your body sees the gluten, doesn't like it, and goes into automatic attack mode. There are several ways grain has been shown to cause an immune response:

- The grain triggers the innate immune system response directly.
- Eating grain triggers leaky gut, which overstimulates the immune system.
- The immune response is actually caused by the pesticide within the grain.
- Genetic hybridization and manipulation of the genes in grains are to blame.
- Mycotoxins—chemicals created by mold on grain, as well as on peanuts and other foods, and equipped with immune-suppressing qualities—may also be a factor.
- Finally, other proteins found in grains, such as amylase trypsin inhibitors (ATIs), which we'll also discuss later, and Glo-3A, a non-gluten protein, also trigger immune inflammation.

And, of course, it is possible that two or more of these factors are in cahoots, working in different ways as allies in the war against your body. The final common denominator is the message I keep reiterating: when a person who is gluten sensitive removes the grain from his or her diet, the pain and other symptoms alleviate because the origin of the inflammation has been removed.

GLUTEN-FREE WHIPLASH

As you now know, the simplistic definition of gluten offers just a lick and a promise—and an empty promise at that. If you've already tried to eliminate gluten from your diet, you may have had a certain experience. You faithfully avoided the "traditional" gluten grains and instead ate specialty products that claim to be gluten free, but you didn't notice much of a change in how you felt. Or perhaps you actually *did* feel better for a short time. But then the pain and other unpleasant symptoms returned. How come that blessed relief was so fleeting?

Welcome to gluten-free whiplash, which usually occurs three to six months after eliminating gluten. Let me explain. When people are initially diagnosed with gluten sensitivity or celiac disease, most of them begin to feel better soon after they remove the "traditional" BROW (barley, rye, oats, and wheat) grains from their diet. However, all too soon, many discover the gluten-free food aisle, with its beckoning array of bread, crackers, cereals, cookies, and more. *Aha*, they think, *I can have my proverbial cake and eat it, too. I'll replace my wheat bread with gluten-free bread and my Oreos with gluten-free cookies. That will make it so much easier to follow my doctor or nutritionist's orders.*

But as they start to incorporate these corn-, rice-, and other grain-rich (plus soy-rich) foods (made with GMO crops) in their diet, the old painful symptoms that led to their avoidance of BROW often pay a return visit. Gluten-free whiplash is proof that it's not just those three or four grains that contain gluten. A traditional "gluten-free" diet promotes the use of processed packaged foods made with grains such as millet, corn, rice, and sorghum. To add insult to injury, such foods usually contain genetically modified (GMO) grain-based pesticides, heavy metals, added sugars, and preservatives, all of which create additional problems, as we'll discuss in chapter 10.

Regardless of gluten content, a diet full of packaged convenience foods is not conducive to healing. It has been known since the early

1950s that when people with celiac disease switched to a totally grain-free diet they recovered completely.[4] Fifty years ago, when practitioners had their celiac patients remove just the three grains from their diets, they, too, recovered. Today, that advice doesn't hold true. So what is so different today? I think you know the answer. Processed food—what I call "frood"—now dominates most people's diets. And the supposedly gluten-free products are among the worst. A significant percentage of celiac patients who use products containing rice, millet, corn, and buckwheat don't recover from intestinal damage.

The good news is that when people with persistent celiac disease stop eating "gluten-free" processed food, their recovery vastly improves.[5] These findings align with fifty years of other studies. They also reflect what other functional medicine doctors and I see with our patients. That signals loud and clear that our society's changes in eating habits, especially the increased use of processed foods, requires a new approach to celiac disease. The same goes for those of us suffering from other gluten-sensitive conditions. Unfortunately, it can take twenty years or more for research to filter down to the public and even to conventional health practitioners.

More Food, Less Nutrition

Cultivation of wheat in the Fertile Crescent, now Iraq, Kuwait, Syria, Jordan, Israel, Egypt, and other Middle Eastern countries, as well as parts of Turkey and Iran, began about ten thousand years ago. Raising crops instead of relying on hunting and gathering gave people time for activities other than feeding themselves. By the fifth century BCE, grain had become a dietary staple in Greece and in the Roman Empire. In the next few centuries, the Greeks practiced crop rotation and the Romans improved crop yield with irrigation made possible by a vast aqueduct system, mechanized the harvesting process with automatic reapers, and used water wheels to grind flour. While the agricultural revolution allowed a population explosion and technological and cultural advances, there was a huge trade-off: people did not enjoy better health. Skeletal remains show that people were smaller after grain became a staple of the diet. The Book of Exodus,

written in the sixth or fifth century BCE, alludes to digestive symptoms related to eating bread and grains. See glutenfreesociety.org
/history-gluten-grain-free-diet for more on the human implications
in the history of grain.

WHY GLUTEN-FREE WHIPLASH ISN'T ALWAYS APPARENT

What if you never experience an outward and obvious whiplash phenomenon? Are you just one of the lucky ones who can continue to
eat processed "gluten-free" products because you react poorly only to
wheat, barley, rye, and perhaps oats? I hate to break it to you, but this
may well not be an occasion to celebrate. Continuing to eat processed
food guarantees that you are creating inflammation, but it may as yet
be "silent," meaning it is not yet provoking any symptoms. It can take
decades for responses to the demon gluten to surface.

Then there are people who have multiple autoimmune problems or
have been diagnosed with celiac disease. They eliminate the traditional
gluten sources, but continue to eat other grains. Their gut pain and
other intestinal symptoms abate, but other issues persist. For example,
someone with recurring migraine headaches may simply not realize
that they are a response to the corn and rice in her diet. Her gastroen-
terologist may have never mentioned migraines to her, so she never
makes the connection that she is experiencing gluten-free whiplash.
The good news is that once you say good-bye to all grains and so-called
gluten-free products, whiplash will be a thing of the past.

MUSCULAR BREAKDOWN SHOWS UP AS PAIN

Now let's get into some of the more common conditions caused by
grainflammation, specifically those that manifest as joint and muscle
pain. We tend to think of muscles as the group of tissues that moves

our bones so that we can walk, climb stairs, pick up a child, use a pencil or a computer, and so forth. But we're not just talking about muscles in our arms, legs, shoulders, and fingers. The job of your heart is to pump blood throughout your body and reoxygenate it. The last thing you want is for your heart muscle to be in meltdown mode. Your blood vessels are also muscles, albeit tiny ones. Your muscles help pump cerebrospinal fluid around the brain and lymphatic fluids through the immune system. Both are critical to healthy immune function. The vital proteins in your muscles also serve as a reserve bank for your immune system. Remember, those protective chemicals are largely made from proteins, and muscle breakdown occurs when the immune system lacks sufficient protein to do its job.

Preserving muscle mass as we age is the number one factor in predicting life span.[6] The term *sarcopenia* refers to age-related muscle loss, which is a predictor of early death. A number of different disease conditions can create muscular breakdown, including fibromyalgia and rheumatoid arthritis. Someone already living a sedentary lifestyle tends to have very little muscle tone. If she is also gluten sensitive, and you

THE GLUTEN MUSCLE-WASTING CYCLE

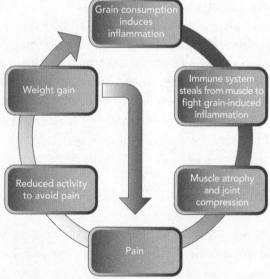

throw grain into the mix, it aggravates the situation. Her immune system goes crazy because day after day she eats something that creates more inflammation instead of helping heal, repair, and maintain her body.

Over time, protein is withdrawn from the muscle bank to feed the immune system so it can combat the food's inflammatory effects. Meanwhile, the muscle becomes progressively weaker and less dense. As it shrinks and shortens, muscle atrophies, which compresses joints, producing pain. Here we have another one of those vicious cycles: the muscle shrinks to feed the immune system, in the process causing joint compression, which leads to friction, irritation, and more inflammation, in turn creating pain. Of course, this is likely to make you more sedentary, so you pack on extra pounds. Added weight increases pressure on the joints still more. Welcome to yet another of your body's battle sites in the immune system's war against grain.

MUSCLES PAY THE PRICE

One way to understand inflammatory muscle breakdown is that it is akin to what could happen were you to work out to excess without consuming adequate protein: your body instead turns to muscle for energy. By its very nature, exercise tears and inflames the muscle fibers so that they will rebuild in a stronger form. And that's a good thing, just as inflammation is good when it isn't chronic. But not taking in enough of the raw ingredients necessary to rebuild muscle adversely impacts muscle growth. Instead of building muscle mass that makes you look trim and shapely, you could be depleting existing muscle, making you look flabby.

Just as you can damage muscle through extreme workouts, an autoimmune disease can degrade it. It's why cancer patients waste away, as do people who regularly come down with colds and the flu, run high fevers, and stay in bed for days on end. It's a sign that their immune system is losing the battle, and the only way it can prevail is to tap into the protein in the muscle reserve, which makes the muscles ache and also depletes the body of pounds of fluid. Therein lies the most important message about muscle: regardless of which painful auto-immune condition a person develops, the muscles are going to pay a price. And the muscle thief doesn't discriminate. It steals from any muscle it can find to fuel its war against inflammation. As long as you remain unaware of the cause and don't make changes in your diet, your muscle bank account will continue to show withdrawals.

MUSCLE AND FAT OUT OF WHACK

The toxic combination of glutens and other proteins in grains, which contributes to muscle inflammation, weakness, and loss, prevents your system from properly maintaining your normal body weight. But just removing grain from your diet isn't enough to restore good muscle health. There are two prescriptions for longevity on which all research-ers agree: eating foods low in calories but high in nutrients, and build-ing and maintaining good-quality muscle mass. Diet and exercise are two sides of the same healthy coin.

The more grain we eat, the more glucose hits our bloodstream. The more blood sugar, the more insulin we release. The more insulin we release, the more tummy fat (fat around our vital organs) we produce, giving the body a distinctive apple shape. Meanwhile, elevated blood sugar also increases cortisol production, which also leads to fat stor-age, along with bloating. (One of the side effects of taking steroids is bloating.) Elevated insulin and cortisol deliver a double whammy. The more fat we store, the less muscle mass we have relative to our total body weight. The hormonal effects of a diet high in grain, what I call *grainbesity*, is the subject of chapter 5.

A MISDIAGNOSED HEART CONDITION

Al's experience is a great example of how medical advice to stop exer-cising and take drugs caused weight gain and depletion of the very nutrients that fight inflammation. He noticed that he was short of breath during his morning runs, and over time developed intense pain and pressure in his chest, at which point he was hospitalized. A follow-up visit to a cardiologist identified an inflammatory condition called pericarditis (swelling around the heart). The doctor couldn't tell him why this was happening, but prescribed both blood pressure– and cholesterol-lowering meds "just to be safe," even though Al had neither high blood pressure nor high cholesterol. He was also put on aspirin to thin his blood. Despite taking the medications, Al continued to experience chest pain. At this point, his doctor told him to stop exercising because it might prompt a heart attack. Al soon gained 15 pounds, and his chest pain persisted. His doctor then prescribed a medicine to block pain and inflammation.

At this point Al came to see me. He didn't want to continue his pharmaceutical cocktail, to which he attributed the fatigue and brain fog he had recently developed. He was also frustrated by his weight gain, and it made no sense to him to abandon his exercise regimen since the objective was to prevent heart disease.

After an in-depth conversation with Al, I performed a detailed physical exam and ordered several functional medicine lab tests. You guessed it: he had a gluten-sensitive gene pattern. In addition, he had high levels of an inflammatory substance called C-reactive protein and was deficient in vitamins C and B_2, along with zinc, all three of which naturally help control inflammation but were being blocked by the drugs. Within three weeks of starting a supplementation program and eliminating grains from his diet, Al no longer had chest pain or shortness of breath, and was able to resume running. A year later at a nutritional checkup, he confessed that consuming lots of beer at a recent guys' night on the town had led to a recurrence of his chest pain. Since then he hasn't been tempted to deviate from his diet. No grain, no pain.

MORE MYTHS TO PUNCTURE

Myth 11: **Pain is inherent in aging, and aching joints are a normal result of aging.**

Not true! You can either aggravate aches and pains or take steps to prevent them. And even if you're already experiencing aches and pain, it is possible to reverse that process. Aging is not synonymous with a natural degradation process; in reality, aging is just the function of time. On the other hand, damage over time leads to loss of function. So it is not aging per se that's the enemy; rather, it's aging with a lifetime accumulation of poor eating habits and insufficient activity, with resultant damage.

Myth 12: **Your genes determine your metabolic rate.**

Not true! You've probably heard friends say (or maybe *you* have), "I have difficulty losing weight because I was born with a slow metabolism." In reality, the more muscle mass you have and the more toned your muscles, the higher your metabolism. A sedentary lifestyle produces a low metabolic rate. Muscle plays another enormously important role, setting your basal metabolic rate.

Myth 13: **Your metabolism naturally slows as you age.**

Not true! The reality is that metabolism slows over the years only because inflammation and pain lead to inactivity, diminishing muscle mass. (Simply being sedentary can do the same.) This makes it more difficult to lose weight, but not because you have a slower metabolism or because you are getting on in years. Instead, habits you are capable of reversing, namely sitting on your butt and not moving around, have slowed your metabolism. The good news is that once you're motivated and empowered, you *can* change your behavior—and you can lose weight, no matter what your age.

ARTHRITIS IN ALL ITS FORMS

Remember I told you that *itis* means "inflammation." Well, arthritis is inflammation of the joints. *Osteoarthritis,* the most common form of arthritis, refers to the damage to bone and cartilage from wear and tear over the years. It can appear in any bone or joint from a finger to the spine, although weight-bearing joints, such as the hips and the knees, are often the most vulnerable. I've seen thousands of patients recover from what they thought was age-related arthritis after ditching grain. Following are some of the other types of arthritis I see most often in my practice. As you'll see below and throughout this book, these chronic painful conditions follow a pattern: they're autoimmune diseases linked to grain consumption.

- *Rheumatoid arthritis* (RA) is only one of several forms of systemic autoimmune arthritis, all of which affect the muscles or joints, and sometimes other parts of the body. A disordered immune response produces antibodies, which typically attack tissues in the body's weakest areas. Rheumatoid arthritis primarily affects joints, which may become deformed and painful, even leading to loss of function, but can also involve muscles. About 1 percent of the adult population has RA, which is more common in old age, but can also strike earlier.

- About 12 to 15 percent of people with psoriasis develop *psoriatic arthritis*, which involves both skin and joint inflammation. People with this condition have been shown to have high levels of antibodies to gluten.[7]

- Other common forms of arthritis associated with gluten and autoimmunity include *ankylosing spondylitis*,[8] *spondyloarthritis* (spinal fusion), *reactive arthritis, Reiter's syndrome*,[9] and *dermatomyositis*.[10] Dermatomyositis is characterized by muscle weakness and a violet or dusky red rash that usually appears on the face, eyelids, nails, elbows, knees, chest, or back. The rash may precede muscle weakness.

FIBROMYALGIA, LUPUS, AND OTHER SOFT-TISSUE PROBLEMS

Fibromyalgia is second only to osteoarthritis as the most common painful musculoskeletal condition. Typically, it involves muscle and joint pain throughout the body, and is often paired with chronic fatigue syndrome. Multiple studies illustrate the benefits of a gluten-free diet for patients with fibromyalgia.[11]

The full name of *lupus* is *systemic lupus erythematosus* (SLE), which sometimes occurs in those with gluten sensitivity.[12] SLE often presents with a "malar rash" across the cheekbones and the bridge of the nose, but also causes rashes elsewhere on the body, along with joint and muscle pain. Lupus is often confused with rheumatoid arthritis because the symptoms are similar.

Tendon disorders are another common manifestation of the need for sensitive individuals to avoid grain.[13] Often referred to as enthesopathies, these inflammatory tendon conditions commonly occur in the elbows and ankles. Ever heard of Achilles tendinitis?

If you've been diagnosed with any of the painful conditions listed above and don't know why, you should rule out gluten sensitivity before embarking on a course of steroids, painkillers, and antirheumatic drugs.

On average, patients with celiac disease will be diagnosed with an additional seven autoimmune diseases, including type 1 diabetes, rheumatoid arthritis, and vitiligo, in their lifetime. Unfortunately, many rheumatologists persist in ignoring these facts and continue to prescribe steroids, painkillers, and DMARDs (disease modifying antirheumatic drugs). Research continues to link the autoimmune spectrum of diseases to gluten sensitivity.

JOINTS: USE 'EM OR LOSE 'EM

Unlike other tissues in the body, joints have no direct blood supply. Instead, they're nourished through motion. So if you're sedentary, your joints actually don't receive sufficient oxygen, nor do they get the vitamins and minerals they need. Joints are bathed in synovial fluid, which, as you move, nourishes the cartilage and prevents further deterioration.

Decades ago, doctors would recommend an extended period of bed rest for patients with back pain. The result was that their muscles would atrophy and their joints remain immobile, which led to further deterioration of vertebrae. When the patient did finally get out of bed, he or she would find it difficult and painful to move around.

Nowadays, doctors generally recommend rehabilitation after a brief period of rest. The therapeutic benefit of movement and exercise during rehab includes the release of endorphins, your body's natural pain relievers.

Rapid rehab has another benefit. It changes the way that scar tissue forms. When you injure a tendon, ligament, or muscle, little microfibers get torn and replaced by scar tissue. The scar tissue doesn't necessarily form in the orientation of the muscle; instead, it can lay down in a crosswise direction. As a result, when you extend or contract the muscle, it can tear through the newly formed scar tissue. If you're not active in the first few weeks after an injury, the scar tissue will be thick, which could lead to aggressive tearing and more chronic pain and inflammation. By moving around as soon as possible after an injury, you force the scar tissue to properly align with the orientation of the muscle fibers, tendons, and ligaments.

Understand that we are not just talking about physical injuries, such as spraining your ankle. A biochemical injury also creates chronic pain and inflammation. What if the "injury" was eating a huge piece of cake, which created all kinds of inflammatory mediators that barged in and destroyed some muscle tissue? Now we're talking about a biochemical injury, which requires the same motion and movement to rehab it. (Movement is an active process, while motion can be either active or passive.) People don't realize that aspect of injury to the body. Because they didn't injure themselves physically although they feel lousy, they default to bed rest. The kind of rehab recommended for a physical injury simply doesn't come to mind.

Bottom line: Whether the insult to the joints (or another part of the body) is a physical trauma or a biochemical one, the prescription for healing is motion. (And in the case of the cake, you know you're better off just avoiding that trauma!) If you are gluten sensitive and continue to eat grains, you're going to lose further muscle, have persistent inflammatory pain, and start or continue to gain weight. You'll become part of the grainbesity crowd.

Now let's talk about another assault to your joints. They are made out of a fibrous material known as collagen, which is the main protein in connective tissue. (Cartilage is one kind of collagen.) For collagen to be strong, resilient, and elastic, it needs vitamin C, iron, and folate. When these nutrients are blocked, as happens with chronic use of NSAIDs and some other painkillers, cartilage synthesis is inhibited. That's why pain drugs never work long term. They can be great to banish the occasional ache or pain, but they never allow the joint to heal. Without those nutrients, the collagen is more vulnerable, even under a normal load and with day-to-day wear and tear, leaving joints more prone to injury, inflammation, and pain.

NERVES AND THE GUT

When we chronically inflame our bodies with problematic foods, the sympathetic part of the nervous system—our fight-or-flight instinct—gets turned on, just as when we are facing an obvious danger such as a stranger acting in a threatening fashion. We make lots of adrenaline or epinephrine in case we need to leap into action, either to run or to fight like the dickens. Our hormones divert blood into the tissues necessary for either action, diverting blood away from the gut and the digestive process. Why is that important? Remember, the gut is the largest nervous system in the body, second only to the brain, so it, too, can be impacted by nerve damage from inflammation.

If every time you eat you overactivate your sympathetic nervous system, it stimulates your fight-or-flight instinct. Meanwhile, your parasympathetic nervous system, which is all about healing, digestion, sleep, and relaxation, gets shunted aside and suppressed. People who are chronically inflamed as a result of their diet have their fight-or-flight radar always dialed up to high and their parasympathetic nervous system turned down really low. That combination means that food is not digested properly, and before long, leaky gut may present itself as well.[14] When the gut is damaged and incapable of processing food, and the nervous system is incapable of stimulating proper peristalsis (the automatic contractions that move along the contents of the intestine) and hormone and digestive enzyme release, the mere act of eating becomes dangerous. Instead of digesting food, we ferment it. The rotting food becomes a further source of inflammation that feeds the existing inflammation.

In the following chapter, we'll look more closely at the gut and its relationship with grains, but I'll give you something to chew on before you turn the page. The reason fasting can work so well when a person has severe digestive issues is that it takes away the external source of inflammation while giving the gut a rest.

WHAT YOU NEED TO KNOW

O Inflammation is the normal and ongoing process by which the body repairs and replaces damaged tissue, but it can go haywire if it is constantly challenged.

O When we block inflammation with pain medications, it interferes with the body's normal repair process.

O Overconsumption of grain can lead to chronic inflammation the body cannot cope with.

O Our innate immune and humoral immune systems protect us. One or both of them may react to grain, but the outcome is the same: inflammation.

O Eating grains other than the BROW grains or supposedly gluten-free processed foods produces gluten-free whiplash, in which pain and other symptoms that had initially resolved return. This is scientific evidence that gluten or gluten-like proteins are in all these foods.

O Inflammation caused by grain consumption (or other autoimmune responses) weakens muscles, which contributes to more joint pain, an increasingly sedentary lifestyle, and ultimately muscle wasting.

O Muscle sets the metabolism, meaning we can maintain a high metabolism and a lean, muscular body by being physically active and eating a nutrient-rich diet.

O Chronic inflammation can manifest in conditions involving the muscles, joints, and cartilage, such as many forms of arthritis, as well as lupus, fibromyalgia, and numerous other autoimmune diseases.

BONUS FEATURE

Update on the different elements in grain that cause inflammation: glutenfreesociety.org/is-it-gluten-sensitivity-or-grain-induced-inflammation-research-update/.

CHAPTER 4

PAIN CAUSED BY IMBALANCES IN THE GUT

The Truth about "Leaky Gut" and How Diet Can Heal (or Aggravate) It

When there is pain, there are no words. All pain is the same.

—Toni Morrison

The poor scarecrow in _The Wizard of Oz_ didn't have a brain in his hollow body. You, on the other hand, have two brains. In addition to one in your head, you have another one in your gut. Say what?

You've no doubt heard the phrase _gut instinct_. Well, just as your brain is a complex nervous system, scientists refer to the estimated 500 million neurons that make up your gut (which extends roughly 30 feet from your esophagus to your anus) as the second brain. Until now you may not have thought much about what happens to your food once you eat it. Think again. This other brain rules you in ways just as important and complex as your main brain. As you'll learn, your gut may not "think" the way your brain does, but it's sentient in its own way, sending messages to the brain along neural pathways.

Complementary Brains

The brain in your gut is as essential to life as the one in your head. The gut brain plays a major role in the production of dopamine and serotonin, nerve chemicals that relieve pain. If their production is compromised, you'll experience more pain. In fact, a class of drugs called selective serotonin reuptake inhibitors (SSRIs) is sometimes prescribed for chronic pain.

Brain	Second (Gut) Brain
85 billon neurons	500 million neurons
100 neurotransmitters identified	40 neurotransmitters identified
Produces 50 percent of dopamine	Produces 50 percent of dopamine
Produces 5 percent of serotonin	Produces 95 percent of serotonin
Barrier restricts blood flow to brain	Barrier restricts blood flow to gut

FOOD FIGHT

Food is clearly essential for life and can be pleasurable for both gustatory and social reasons, but the mere act of eating can set up a battle within your body. The gut is not just breaking down food, metabolizing nutrients, and expelling waste; it also must protect you from bacteria, viruses, and other enemies invading the rest of your body. The gut has five barriers, as we'll discuss shortly. In the event that those enemies smash through all the barriers and penetrate your gut lining, your immune system—specifically the immune cells in the gut wall—go on the offensive. They secrete histamine and other inflammatory chemicals, which send messages to the gut brain to get rid of the invader. One defensive maneuver triggers diarrhea. Or the gut brain may send an IM to the main brain to expel the invader by vomiting it out. Or, as a fail-safe method, the two brains may work in concert, triggering both responses.

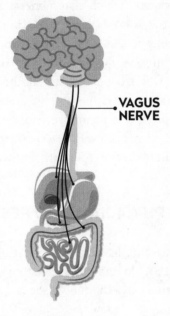

The vagus nerve links the brain and the gut.

THE BRAIN-GUT CONNECTION

In ancient times medical practitioners believed the brain and the gut interacted to influence health and disease states. In the early 1900s, researchers began to revisit this alliance when they realized that the enteric nervous system (ENS), which is embedded in the gut wall, could act independently of the brain. Still, it wasn't until the 1990s that the study of the brain-gut connection, known as neurogastroenterology, was born. We now know that roughly 90 percent of signals between the vagus nerve, which runs from the brain to the colon, originate with the ENS.[1]

Back to gut instinct. When you're stressed, the sensation of having butterflies in your stomach is the result of your fight-or-flight response, which originates in your brain, diverting blood away from your stomach to your muscles. The stress connection goes both ways. Stress stimulates the intestines to ramp up the production of ghrelin, aka the hunger hormone, which also moderates anxiety and depression. The message travels from the gut to the brain via the vagus nerve. There's a reason your gut asks for food when you're stressed.

Take a few minutes to digest this information (pun intended). Meanwhile, I want to introduce you to another one of my patients, Jessica. You've already met her mother, Shanna, who had some of the same symptoms, but each woman also had her own distinct painful conditions. Treating them both was a fascinating lesson in how gluten sensitivity can manifest in numerous different ways.

SIX PHYSICIANS, NO RESULTS

Before coming to see me, Jessica had been diagnosed with irritable bowel syndrome (IBS), thyroid disease, asthma, and eczema, among other conditions. From early childhood, she had suffered from chronic headaches and muscle pain in her neck and back, plus fatigue and recurring infections. When we met, she was under the care of six different doctors, including a GP, allergists, an endocrinologist, and several gastroenterologists. She was losing her hair, fighting a fungal infection, had stopped menstruating, and at only 86 pounds was wasting away. One of her prior doctors had actually accused her of being anorexic. Jessica was also experiencing severe burning nerve pain (neuropathy) on the soles of her feet, making it difficult to walk. Although she was being pumped full of steroids, antibiotics, antifungals, and anti-inflammatories, she was not responding to this barrage of medications.

I discovered that not only was Jessica gluten sensitive, but she also had allergic reactions to eggs, sugar, dairy, and many other foods, which contributed to her overall inflammation burden. Her iron levels were so low that she couldn't make enough red blood cells to deliver oxygen to her tissues. She was deficient in vitamins C, B_5, and D. Chronic prescription drug use and vitamin deficiencies had weakened her immune system and damaged her liver, making her skin jaundiced. Her compromised immune system was incapable of fighting off the three types of parasitic worms identified by lab work, which was why she couldn't keep weight on and her hair was falling out.

Within two months of eliminating grain and other foods to which she was allergic, as well as correcting her nutritional deficiencies, Jessica experienced a dramatic increase in energy. Her headaches subsided significantly, both in intensity and frequency; her nerve pain was cut in half; and she started to gain weight. Her bowel movements also started to normalize as her stomach pain and bloating diminished. The asthma symptoms vanished and Jessica was able to discontinue her breathing medications. Today, she is off all drugs and the pain and headaches are history, along with her IBS, neuropathy, chronic infections, and skin rashes. She is now a normal weight and enjoys boundless energy.

The sad part about Jessica's story is that not a single one of her six other doctors called me to ask how we were able to accomplish so much without drugs. For a video: glutenfreesociety.org/no-grain-no -pain-jessicas-story.

FOUR PATHS TO THE SAME DESTINATION

In this chapter, we'll delve into the four ways that grain wages war on the gut, inducing pain and damage.

1. Direct inflammation can change the nature of the intestinal bacteria and the balance between friendly and unfriendly types.[2]

2. Grain itself can cause intestinal permeability, known as leaky gut.[3]

3. Grain is itself hard to digest, but it also contains proteins that inhibit digestion of other foods,[4] leading to fermentation in the gut, which creates gas, bloating, pain, and other symptoms of IBS.

4. Finally, grain can alter healthy bacteria, which can, in turn, contribute to a host of problems including leaky gut, yeast overgrowth, and disrupted digestion and absorption.[5]

GRAIN—4 MECHANISMS OF DAMAGE

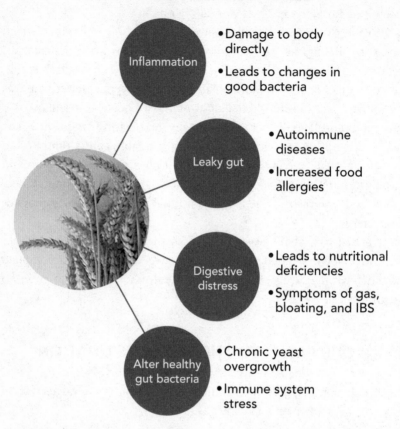

Inflammation
- Damage to body directly
- Leads to changes in good bacteria

Leaky gut
- Autoimmune diseases
- Increased food allergies

Digestive distress
- Leads to nutritional deficiencies
- Symptoms of gas, bloating, and IBS

Alter healthy gut bacteria
- Chronic yeast overgrowth
- Immune system stress

All these mechanisms can destroy the gut. This process leads to the development of additional food allergies, which put the immune system on high alert, creating inflammation and ultimately contributing to autoimmune disease. Guess what triggers this cascade? Recent research has confirmed that grain can be the direct cause.[6]

LEAKY GUT: THE BATTLE WITHIN

One of the ways that grain wages war on our digestive system is by promoting the condition known as *leaky gut*. Leaky gut—a nasty situation that occurs when the protective barrier that keeps waste and bacteria in the intestine is breached, allowing these substances, along with partially digested food, to escape into the bloodstream—was originally discovered as a side effect of gluten sensitivity. This condition is extremely dangerous for several reasons. Let me lead you through the process:

- Due to permeability, the gut wall becomes compromised, allowing a barrage of foreign substances to flood the immune system, leading to systemic inflammation as well as the development of multiple food-based allergies.
- The body creates antibodies that attack these foreign substances.
- Some of these foreign substances resemble tissues in the body, in what is called molecular mimicry. Over time, the immune system turns on its own tissues, including muscles, tendons, ligaments, bone, cartilage, and nerves, leading to an all-out autoimmune assault on the body.
- The inflammatory damage caused by leaky gut results in inhibited digestion, compromised nutrition, and loss of vitamins and minerals.
- Chronic gut inflammation changes the ratio of healthy gut bacteria, contributing to yeast overgrowth and small intestinal bacteria overgrowth (SIBO).
- The breakdown in the intestinal barrier leads to persistent and chronic pain and inflammation.

Grain Robs Vitamins and Minerals

Gluten and other grain proteins have been shown to impact intestinal absorption, but they can also damage other organs integral to the digestive process. The stomach, liver, gallbladder, and pancreas all help break down nutrients in food, but gluten-induced damage to these organs can create vitamin and mineral deficiencies. Vitamin B_{12} plays a major role in the repair and healing of the intestine, but many patients with gluten sensitivity are deficient in it, creating a catch-22 scenario. The gluten-damaged gut needs vitamins and minerals to aid in its repair, but the existing damage is preventing their absorption. As with the regular use of NSAIDs and other pain-killers and anti-inflammatory drugs, continuing to eat grains sets up a vicious cycle that impedes the body's natural healing capacity.

WHAT ARE GUT MIGRAINES?

If you have any doubt that the brain and the gut are intimately connected, you have probably never had a gut headache. That's a head-splitting migraine combined with stomach pain, which can vary in intensity, along with nausea, vomiting, and the inability to eat. Gut migraines may be preceded by the aura that migraine sufferers often experience, signaling that a headache is imminent. The abdominal symptoms can last for days, although they may also be quite brief. Glutens[7] and other foreign proteins[8] that have leaked into the bloodstream appear to trigger the migraine. Taking NSAIDs, which are a major cause of leaky gut, only fuels the fire.[9]

FIVE FIRE WALLS

The gastrointestinal (GI) tract is a marvel of defensive mechanical engineering. But just as the walls of a fortress equipped with moats, ramparts, and other defensive structures can be breached if the enemy is wily enough and the sentries guarding the fortress are not on constant high alert, so, too, can your GI tract be penetrated. Let's look at each of its five main barriers.

Barrier 1: **GALT** (gastro-associated lymphoid tissue) sits immediately behind the cells of your gut wall, and is home to about 70 to 80 percent of your entire immune system. To understand how GALT works, think about the role of tonsils. Like a pair of sentries protecting an army of white blood cells, they stand guard at the back of your throat, ready to spring into action. If you eat or inhale something that you should avoid, your tonsils take on the invader. So when doctors remove swollen tonsils, they're actually doing more damage than good. Instead of figuring out what has caused the swelling—usually a certain food—most doctors simply cut them out. Fortunately, this doesn't leave you completely undefended. If the intruder makes it past your tonsils, it confronts a second barrier, which acts much the way tonsils do.

The GALT looks nothing like your tonsils—it wraps around the small intestine—but it is tasked with the same job. Like tonsils, it is lymph tissue that houses immune cells and immune proteins. The GALT protects the bloodstream from anything that might seep through a leaky gut and into the body. The lymphatic system is an interconnected complex of tubes that run throughout the body, removing waste products and toxins and transporting white blood cells to different areas. Your blood system's job is to get oxygen and nutrients to your tissues, via the pump known as your heart. The lymphatic system's job is to distribute antibodies and immune cells to the different tissues. Instead of a single pump like the heart, the lymphatic system relies on the body's muscles, movement, and motion.

Barrier 2: **Tight junctions** are tiny anchor-like proteins that "snap" intestinal cells together, much like Lego pieces. If they're not clicked together, the whole Lego tower falls apart. We know for certain that gluten can disrupt tight junctions. Bacterial infections can also break apart tight junctions. Other suspected agents of disruption include chemicals such as glyphosate, the active ingredient in the weed killer Roundup, as well as atrazine, another herbicide. Yeast overgrowth and chronic inflammation in the gut are other disruptive factors. For example, if somebody is popping 800 milligrams of Advil daily to deal with pain, the NSAID erodes the mucosal layer (see page 83), and as it dissipates, the tight junctions are exposed and become more vulnerable to damage. Imagine chipping away mortar between the pieces of masonry that make up that fortress. Remove enough mortar over time, and you can loosen the stones and break through the wall. It's the same with the tight junctions.[10]

KNOWN CAUSES OF LEAKY GUT

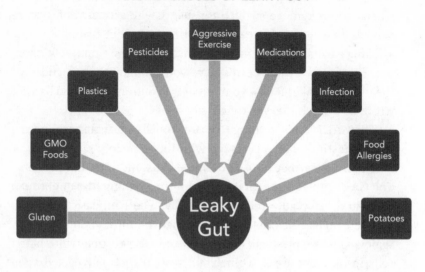

Barrier 3: **The mucosal layer.** Think of mucus as a barrier that provides physical protection. Inside that mucus is an important antibody called secretory IgA. Comparable to the handcuffs with which
a policeman restrains a suspect while checking his background, the
secretory IgA "analyzes" the threat level before acting. The surface
of the gut's mucosal lining contains millions of column-shaped cells.
On their surface are minute finger-like tendrils, which in turn are
covered with even tinier tendrils called villi and microvilli, respectively. When the gut becomes inflamed because of an immune reaction, these tiny projections are flattened or destroyed, producing
what is known as villous flattening or villous atrophy. Why are the
villi and microvilli so important? They enhance the GI surface area
of the intestine, which if flattened and spread out would be the size
of a tennis court. For every fold, every bend, and every twist, there
is more surface area to absorb and to digest nutrients.

Patients with celiac disease are often severely malnourished
because villous atrophy has significantly reduced the area that can
absorb nutrients. (The most common deficiencies are iron, B_{12}, and
zinc, in that order.) Once the villi are destroyed, you can no longer
absorb iron. There are also certain areas in your intestine that are

responsible for the absorption of B vitamins, vitamin C, and other nutrients. Depending on which area(s) get(s) destroyed, there may be particular nutritional losses or deficits. This is not because someone isn't eating enough, but because the area of the small intestine responsible for digesting that particular nutrient has become dysfunctional.

Barrier 4: **Good bacteria,** which live on the surface of the mucosal barrier, help the body synthesize cells, make vitamins, enable immune cells to communicate with one another, and aid in regulating energy metabolism. The food you eat can impact the types of bacteria in your system. The wrong types of bacteria can promote inflammation and yeast overgrowth. Certain diseases are linked to certain types of bacterial flora, such as peptic, gastric, and duodenal ulcers;[11] chronic diarrhea; Crohn's disease;[12] and ulcerative colitis.[13] Bacterial imbalance, aka dysbiosis, can cause the immune system to attack its host.[14] That's you! If bacteria that spew out chemical toxins invade your body, the imbalance is called a bacterial overgrowth. A bacterial infection such as dysentery is passed along when somebody drinks water polluted with human or animal waste. The infection creates a bacterial imbalance within the gut, resulting in an acute reaction: diarrhea, stomach cramping, and possible dehydration. However, chronic changes in bacterial flora can also evoke a response. Eating grain can alter some of the bacteria within the gut within thirty minutes. A couple of different species of bacteria likely to be altered are what we call good-neighbor species.[15]

Good bacteria species are protective, just as good neighbors are. They care for their own their home and help out their neighbors when necessary. We want these good neighbors in our GI tract. When you reduce the number of friendly bacteria, it's like having a rental house next door filled with tenants who trash the place. If you have enough bad renters, the neighborhood changes, property values drop, and the good neighbors may move out. Good bacteria facilitate the production of both B vitamins and vitamin K. They also enable your immune system to keep the normal inflammation process on track.

The good guys also help prevent the overgrowth of disease-causing agents such as yeast, parasites, and *H. pylori*.[16] One reason why so many people benefit from a good-quality probiotic is that their gut neighborhood has been compromised, often by overuse of antibiotics. However, bacteria that cause disease aren't the only problem. So-called commensal bacteria aren't bad bacteria; they're normally present in the gut, but when their numbers explode, they change the chemical nature of how the gut digests and processes food. Small intestine bacterial overgrowth (SIBO) is not a true infection, but can produce gastric or intestinal bloating, inflammation, discomfort, and irritable bowel–like symptoms.[17] Gluten and especially grains that have been genetically modified can create imbalances in gut bacteria, leading not just to SIBO, but also to IBS, ulcerative colitis, and Crohn's disease, among other GI conditions. In a recent review of more than one hundred earlier studies, researchers found that abnormal commensal bacteria change immune messaging in the gut, which can lead to overactive immune responses.[18]

Sometimes redressing low levels of good bacteria is just a matter of adding good bacteria and lots of omega-3 fats. Or the issue may not necessarily be a paucity of good guys, but the dominance of too many bad guys. In that case, the protocol becomes a matter of how to get rid of the overgrowth of the bad guys without damaging the helpful guys. That's why how I treat different patients varies. In part 2, we will talk about ways to enhance the good bacteria in your gut.

Gut Bacteria and Weight

Two of the good bacteria in your GI tract, known as Bacteroidetes and Firmicutes, work hard to keep you healthy. But an overgrowth of bad bacteria can damage not just your health but also make the difference between being slim or overweight. In one fascinating study, overweight diabetic men took antibiotics to destroy their own gut bacteria, which were then replaced with transplanted bacteria from men who were slim and in good health.[19] After this treatment, the heavy men followed one of two weight-loss diets. In both cases, they slimmed down. But here's the surprising part: when their gut bacteria were analyzed, it was similar to that of the donors. The relative ratio of Bacteroidetes to Firmicutes had increased, which matches the pattern in lean people. (Heavy people tend to have a smaller proportion of Bacteroidetes.) This suggests that obesity has a microbial component.[20]

Barrier 5: **Stomach acid** plays an important role in digesting protein and neutralizing such bad bacteria as *H. pylori* and *E. coli*. It is also necessary for proper absorption of vitamins, minerals, and other nutrients essential to health. Sales of acid-inhibiting over-the-counter and prescription drugs to address chest tightness, hoarseness, burning in the stomach or throat, and indigestion are enormous, meaning millions of people are experiencing acid reflux. Rolaids, Tums, Maalox, Alka-Seltzer, Nexium, Tagamet, Zantac, Prilosec, and Protonix all block the production of stomach acid. Nexium is the most frequently prescribed medication for Medicare patients, at a total annual cost of $2.5 billion.[21] Unfortunately, doctors rarely tell their patients that taking these drugs can create a host of additional problems, including vitamin B_{12} deficiency, which is the most common nutritional problem for those who take drugs that interfere with production of stomach acid.[22]

Now let's bring gluten sensitivity into the equation. Gluten causes both acid reflux and vitamin B_{12} deficiency.[23] Do you see where I am heading? This combination of gluten-induced problems sets up the stage for another vicious cycle of vitamin B_{12} loss. Many of the symptoms linked to gluten sensitivity are caused by a deficiency of this crucial vitamin, including neuropathy, anemia (which leads to fatigue, depression, shortness of breath, irritability, headaches, and exercise intolerance), and delayed gut healing. The epithelial cells lining the intestine have a life span of about two to seven days, and vitamin B_{12} is essential for them to regenerate adequately. This nutritional deficit is one of the most common reasons why people who switch to a "traditional" gluten-free diet continue to experience delayed healing and persistent GI symptoms. Stomach acid is a critical factor in our immune system balance. Medications that block or hinder stomach acid can contribute to leaky gut, incomplete protein digestion, vitamin and mineral deficiencies, and increased risk of infections.

IF THE BARRIERS ARE BREACHED

So what happens if the enemy gets through all five of the firewalls? The contents of the gut leak through into the GALT, but the damage doesn't stop there. It overstimulates the immune system—remember, 70 to 80 percent of it is in your gut—creating collateral damage by providing access to your bloodstream. Just to be clear, let's run through the sequence again: gluten causes gut damage in those sensitive to it, which leads to leaky gut, which leads indirectly to autoimmunity by overstimulating the immune system over time.

If you have a stable gut, a single layer of cells with a coating of mucus is its first line of defense. But if and when you're exposed to some type of environmental chemical or grain, the wrong food, certain bacteria, or an infection, the invader can stimulate the production of the protein zonulin, which disrupts the tight junctions that seal your gut lining. If the invader penetrates the cell walls or if your immune system recognizes it as a bad guy, the immune cells in the gut trigger an inflammatory response. If the mucous layer remains intact, then the inflammation will blow over and not poke holes in the gut. However, if inflammation persists, because you continue to eat the same inflammatory food, for example, the mucosal layer will continue to leak and erode over time. The body's normal response is to heal up these tiny erosions, and all is well and good. But when we increase the workload beyond the gut's natural capacity for ongoing repair, it becomes overwhelmed and creates defensive antibodies, which then exacerbate the damage.

Even working out too aggressively on a regular basis can cause leaky gut. If you've ever seen somebody vomiting after exercising excessively or completing a long run, it's because he's created gut leakage and his body is reflexively emptying the stomach and intestine contents to avoid dumping chemical toxins (and what he has just eaten) into the bloodstream. That's one reason it's not a good idea to eat a big meal before running a marathon or starting a CrossFit workout.

LEAKY GUT AND BEYOND

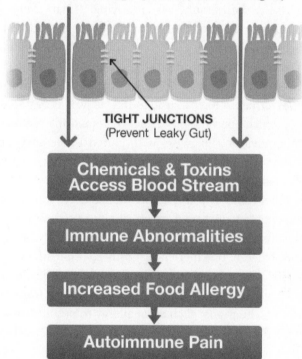

LEAKY GUT
(Occurs when tight junctions are damaged)

TIGHT JUNCTIONS
(Prevent Leaky Gut)

Chemicals & Toxins Access Blood Stream

Immune Abnormalities

Increased Food Allergy

Autoimmune Pain

THE DIFFERENCE BETWEEN
INTOLERANCE AND ALLERGY

Although the two terms are often used interchangeably, there is a significant difference between gluten intolerance and gluten allergy. Let me clarify using the dairy analogy. Most people understand that lactose intolerance refers to difficulty in digesting milk and other dairy products. (Lactose is a sugar in dairy products.) It is *not* an immune response. It's *not* the immune system saying, "I hate dairy." Instead, it's the gut saying, "We don't have enough enzymes to digest that lactose." When the gut cannot do the job, bacteria in the gut take on the task. Instead of supplying nutrients, the dairy rots in your gut, producing by-products of gas and diarrhea, with resultant bloating and pain. The bacterial fermentation can lead to IBS, as well as bacterial or yeast overgrowth, which open the proverbial can of worms, leading to leaky gut and inflammation. Likewise, with gluten intolerance, your body similarly can't tolerate gluten because it doesn't make enough enzymes capable of breaking it down, with similar results.

On the other hand, if you have a gluten allergy, your immune system will make targeted weapons to attack the gluten. We tend to think of an allergic reaction as something acute. You quickly break out into hives, vomit, wheeze, or experience shortness of breath or a migraine. Cause and effect are clear. This is the classic, dramatic situation with your body relaying a clear message to cease and desist from eating gluten. In extreme situations, such as an allergy to peanuts or bee stings, without immediate medical care, you could go into anaphylactic shock and die.

In the case of a delayed reaction to gluten, there is no immediate signal of trouble; instead, the reaction gradually builds over time and with continued exposure, making it difficult to connect the dots between the trigger and the result. In such a case, you might not realize for years that you are allergic to gluten. You could also have both an acute and a delayed gluten allergy. For example, your response to wheat could occur immediately, while your response to an oat allergy is delayed.

WHAT IS GLUTEN SENSITIVITY?

Some doctors continue to claim that non-celiac gluten sensitivity doesn't exist. However, current research leads most doctors and scientists to think that it is an innate (remember the two systems?) immune system reaction to multiple properties within the grain (not just gluten). The outcome of chronic exposure to these elements contributes to acute and delayed inflammation as well as leaky gut and digestive distress. This is one reason why people who are gluten sensitive have such a variety of reactions and symptoms when exposed to it.

As I have mentioned before, most laboratories measure only one kind of immunoglobulin (or antibody) response to just a few different types of gluten when testing for celiac disease (or gluten sensitivity). With thousands of specific types of gluten, no wonder so many tests come back negative despite the fact that countless people have found that cutting out gluten results in dramatic health improvements. This form of testing is clearly flawed.

Many doctors are aware of this problem and are concerned that current methodology is inadequate, missing many people who have a problem with gluten. (In chapter 11, we'll look at more accurate tests.) The proof is in the results—not just in your mind!

GRAINS ARE HARD TO DIGEST

Even absent any genetic predisposition to respond poorly to gluten, anyone can experience a bad reaction to the inherent qualities of grains, plus the proteins in them are a challenge to digest, as we just discussed. Although you may not have an immune system reaction to them, grains can create a digestive overload, which burdens the gut. Imagine asking an 8-year-old, whose muscles aren't developed, to carry a 50-pound bag of concrete across the yard. Someone of his age and size is simply incapable of handling the job. When you eat too much of any hard-to-digest food, the gut simply cannot handle it, and if you are already intolerant of the food, bacterial abnormalities can set in. Your bacteria set to work processing the grain, but those that thrive on it typically aren't the good neighbors. So you are feeding the bad bacteria and neglecting the good bacteria.

Regardless of whether you are gluten intolerant or allergic to gluten, there are a number of painful—sometimes excruciatingly painful—diseases of the GI tract. They can also destroy your gut, your lymphatic system, and your life. Many of them end in *itis*. Remember, that suffix derives from a Greek word for "inflammation."

Your Brain Can Also Spring a Leak

Now that you are familiar with leaky gut and understand the interconnected relationship of your brain and your GI tract, let me introduce the concept of leaky brain. Research on gluten sensitivity has identified this syndrome and revealed a connection between gluten-induced leaky gut and leaky brain, confirming the far-reaching effects of gluten on many diseases.[24] Leaky brain means that the blood-brain barrier is breached, just as the gut walls can be breached by damage inflicted by grain. The blood-brain barrier is designed to keep toxic compounds out of the brain's blood supply, so its disruption could lead to a battery of different neurological and mental symptoms. In addition to schizophrenia, gluten-induced damage can create other neurological problems, including depression,[25] bipolar disease,[26] seizure disorders (epilepsy),[27] facial palsies such as Bell's palsy,[28] ADD/ADHD,[29] and autism[30] and others. You could be gluten sensitive *and* have leaky brain syndrome.

A TRIP DOWN YOUR GI TRACT

Now let's look at the most common painful GI autoimmune conditions to which grain contributes, starting with your mouth and moving through your esophagus, stomach, and small intestine, ending with your large intestine.

It begins in the mouth. People with celiac disease produce antibodies against wheat gluten that interfere with tooth enamel production,[31] which can cause cavities and wear and tear on teeth. Other oral diseases and conditions linked to gluten sensitivity include canker sores[32] (which can also occur in the GI tract), cracked lips, inflamed gums, and angular stomatitis, or inflamed corners of the mouth. Dentists are beginning to actively look for signs of gluten sensitivity.

The esophagus and stomach. One of the most common esophageal issues with grain is *acid reflux*, often referred to as heartburn. Symptoms include tightness in the chest, hoarseness, burning in the stomach or throat area, and indigestion. As discussed above, medications such as Nexium or Aciphex only mask the symptoms of acid reflux and can contribute to leaky gut, poor digestion of protein, other vitamin and mineral deficiencies, and increased risk of infections. *Gastroesophageal reflux disease* (GERD) refers to when the sphincter between the esophagus (the tube that leads to the stomach) and the stomach relaxes, allowing its contents, including stomach acid, to back up into the esophagus. Research suggests that people who suffer from GERD benefit greatly from a gluten-free diet. Chronic GERD can lead to a serious condition called *Barrett's esophagus*, in which the tissue of the esophagus comes to resemble that of the intestine.[33]

The small intestine. For years gastroenterologists used the term *irritable bowel syndrome (IBS)* as a catchall diagnosis for bowel dysfunction of unknown origin. Startlingly, from 11 to 24 percent of Americans have received such a diagnosis.[34] IBS typically involves diarrhea, although it can also cause constipation (or the two can alternate), and is also accompanied by mucus in the stool, tummy pain, cramping, and bloating, In most cases, an IBS patient's condition doesn't improve by adding fiber to her diet. Nor does medication relieve the pain and gut symptoms. All too often, such patients are told they are stressed and should seek psychological help.

However, there is proof that removing grains from the diet of IBS patients results in improvement in symptoms. For four weeks study subjects with IBS diarrhea followed either a diet free of BROW grains as well as corn, or one that contained all five.[35] The former reduced the incidence and severity of diarrhea, but the latter did not. There was also a noticeable and measurable increase (in terms of production of inflammatory markers) in leaky gut in the group that ate gluten. However, the subjects who had genes for gluten sensitivity had a worse response than those who did not.[36] These findings make it clear that there is a way to reverse IBS. By now, you know exactly what that way is: good-bye, grains.

It's hard to discuss gluten without talking about *celiac disease*, which is why I've mentioned it in earlier chapters, primarily to distinguish it from non-celiac gluten sensitivity. If you have the genetic predisposition, consuming wheat, barley, rye, or oats causes the body to attack itself. The damage to the small intestine makes it impossible to properly digest food. People with celiac disease often have diarrhea, develop anemia, feel weak, lose weight and, of course, experience pain. It can also lead to osteoporosis[37] and other serious diseases, including type 1 diabetes and lymphoma.[38] Celiac disease produces villous atrophy, interfering with the absorption of nutrients. By the time a person has *complete* villous atrophy, he has had the problem for a long time.

The disease can usually be diagnosed with blood lab tests that look for antibodies that have formed in response to the inflammation caused by gluten, but results from such tests (and also with a biopsy) are often misleading. They look for damage only in the intestinal tract, but many people with gluten issues don't experience gut issues, and gluten can also damage tissues in the brain, muscle, and elsewhere in the body. So just because a biopsy or a blood test (or both) comes back negative doesn't mean you don't have a problem. These tests typically give a negative result unless the gluten has severely affected the intestine.[39] More accurate tests for celiac disease are now available, as discussed in chapter 11.

GRAINS AND DAMAGE TO THE LARGE INTESTINE

In my clinical experience, grains play a major role in inflammatory diseases of the large intestine. Hundreds of people have come to see me with inflammatory bowel diseases (IBDs) and responded extremely well to a grain-free diet. Interestingly enough, both major forms of IBD are classified as autoimmune diseases. Let's take a look at them.

Ulcerative colitis attacks the left side of the large intestine (the colon) and the rectum, causing inflammation and ulcers (sores) on the lining. Again, there is often a genetic component. If a parent or another family member has the disease, you may be predisposed to it as well. Typical symptoms include stomach pain or cramps, diarrhea, and rectal bleeding. Some people lose their appetite and may lose weight; others may run a fever. The vast majority of people with colitis have periods of remission, but a few have unremitting symptoms. Colitis can also lead to other conditions, including joint pain, eye problems, or even liver disease.[40] To distinguish ulcerative colitis from other gut diseases, which display similar symptoms, doctors order a colonoscopy to view the colon lining and take a sample for a biopsy. Blood tests and stool tests are also performed to look for infection or inflammation (in the form of white blood cells). Corn antibodies have been found in the blood of patients with ulcerative colitis (as well as those with celiac disease or Crohn's disease), despite following a traditionally gluten-free diet.[41] This means that they had an autoimmune reaction to the corn. In my experience, removing corn from the diet of such patients always results in improvement.

Crohn's disease attacks the right side of the large intestine. Like colitis, Crohn's may lie dormant for months or years between flare-ups. Symptoms overlap with those of other gut diseases and include abdominal pain, diarrhea, rectal bleeding, and weight loss. Crohn's may also lead to fistulas (abnormal connections) between organs, and to intestinal obstructions. Patients with Crohn's often have other autoimmune inflammatory diseases attacking the eyes, joints, or skin. *Diverticulitis* is a painful condition that occurs when weakness in the colon wall enables small pockets (diverticulae) to form. Trapped fecal material and bacteria can lead to inflammation. Whether you've been diagnosed with ulcerative colitis, Crohn's, or diverticulitis, research shows that ditching the grain can be helpful.[42]

EXCRUCIATING HEADACHES AND INTESTINAL PROBLEMS

Mary is a perfect example of the link between the brain and the gut brain. A 32-year-old mother of two, she had enjoyed good health until she began experiencing heart palpitations, muscle twitching in her eyelids and shoulders, and difficulty waking in the morning. Her symptoms worsened over several months, and she found it an increasing challenge to cope with day-to-day activities. Her anxiety progressed into severe irritability, along with zero libido and depression so severe that she was unable to get out of bed.

Her doctor attributed her symptoms to stress and prescribed Zoloft, an antidepressant. After using it for several months, Mary's depression lifted somewhat, but her energy level did not. She was also experiencing brain fog, severe constipation, gas, and intestinal bloating. Her doctor then ran some standard blood tests, which revealed normal results. He shrugged his shoulders and referred her to a psychiatrist, who prescribed both an antidepressant and an antianxiety medication. They diminished her anxiety and irritability, but the lack of energy and brain fog never improved, and her battle with constipation continued.

About three months later, Mary fell to the floor writhing in agony with a sharp, stabbing headache. Her husband rushed her to the ER, where she was given IV pain medications, diagnosed with migraine headaches, and sent home with two new prescriptions for pain and migraine prevention. Nonetheless, over the next few months, Mary had two or three headaches a week, each time experiencing debilitating pain for twelve to twenty-four hours. Her only relief was to rest in a dark, quiet room.

Mary went to a neurologist, who ran many tests, including extensive blood tests and an MRI of her brain and neck. All results were normal, and the neurologist told her that her headaches were caused by stress and depression and referred her back to her psychiatrist. At this point, she had spent more than $40,000 without finding a solution. She then visited me. After reviewing her history and blood work, I found some abnormalities that her prior physicians had not discussed with Mary, including several vitamin deficiencies. Further tests revealed multiple vitamin and mineral deficiencies, gluten sensitivity, allergies to several foods, and inadequate production of an important digestive enzyme.

Two weeks after I put Mary on a nutritional regimen her headaches were gone, her brain fog and energy levels were dramatically improved, and she no longer needed to use laxatives. Within two months, her symptoms were virtually gone and she was medication free. She revisited her psychiatrist and neurologist to let them know what she was doing. Both promptly informed her that food had nothing to do with her condition, but if she felt better, she could continue with her new diet. Mary was happy to be healthy and functioning again, but sad that her doctors refused to acknowledge her path to wellness.

OTHER GRAIN PROTEIN TROUBLEMAKERS

Glutens are not the only proteins found in grains. In the past few years researchers have identified a whole new mechanism by which grains can damage the gut of people with gluten sensitivity. Certain proteins— amylase trypsin inhibitors (ATIs) are one of them—effectively switch off your pancreas right when it needs to be hard at work. ATIs, found in wheat, are similar to glutens, but they inhibit enzymes that the pancreas secretes to aid in digestion. This means that sitting undigested in your gut are not only grains, but also any other food you ate in the same meal. Essentially, your gut is acting like a distillery or sauerkraut factory! What are these powerful ATIs? They're natural pesticides that a plant uses to protect its seeds from being eaten by predators—and yes, that includes us. (Wheat is only one of numerous grains that produce such chemicals.) When your immune system identifies an ATI as an invader, it produces antibodies against it, which adds to gut inflammation.[43] Explosive or chronic diarrhea, chronic constipation, bloating, and flatulence are typical responses.

As we've discussed, celiac disease is diagnosed by measuring the antibody response to gluten in the gut. In addition, leaky gut enables bacteria, food, and viral proteins to leak beyond the intestine. Recent research has identified a different kind of damage through a completely different pathway.[44] ATIs don't create just gut inflammation but also non-intestinal inflammation, which could manifest as migraine head-aches, nerve damage, or muscle or joint problems. ATIs may well be a contributing factor to celiac disease and may also explain why people who test negative for celiac disease may nonetheless be sensitive to grain.

In 2015, another study identified still more families of non-gluten proteins found in wheat that produce inflammation in patients with celiac disease.[45] These serpins, purinins, globulins, and farinins, along with ATIs, add a giant clue to solving the mystery of why so many people who test negative for gluten antibodies respond favorably to a gluten-free diet. This discovery also confirms that ATIs are inflammatory. Glutenology, the study of grains and how we humans react to them, is clearly still in its infancy.

In the next chapter, we'll look at the link between a grain-heavy diet and our epidemic of obesity, and how to quit (or never join) the grain-besity gang.

WHAT YOU NEED TO KNOW

○ Your gut functions as a second brain, constantly relaying information to and from the brain in your head.

○ Grain inflicts pain and damage on the gut at least four ways: direct inflammation, intestinal permeability (leaky gut), inhibited digestion, and alteration of friendly bacteria.

○ Five barriers protect the rest of your body from the contents of your gut: GALT, tight junctions, the mucosal layer, good bacteria, and stomach acid.

○ When all five barriers are breached, it can lead to leaky gut, an extremely serious condition.

○ Stomach acid is essential to digest protein, neutralize bad bacteria, and ensure absorption of vitamins, minerals, and other nutrients. In fact, acid-blocking drugs can rob the body of vitamin B_{12}.

○ Gluten intolerance is a digestive issue, like lactose intolerance, and unlike a gluten allergy, which is an immune response; the gut cannot digest gluten.

O Gluten sensitivity encompasses both allergy and intolerance.

O The allergic reaction may be acute and immediate, or it can be less obvious and/or delayed for hours or days. The damage caused by the immune response contributes to a greater sensitivity, another vicious cycle.

O Painful GI autoimmune conditions caused by grain consumption range from canker sores and cavities in the mouth to ulcerative colitis, Crohn's disease, and diverticulitis in the large intestine.

O A newly discovered way the gut can be damaged involves ATIs, a protein similar to glutens, and other non-gluten proteins found in wheat.

BONUS FEATURES

"10 Steps to Heal Leaky Gut Syndrome Naturally" (glutenfree society.org/gluten-free-society-blog/10-steps-to-heal-leaky-gut -syndrome-naturally) and an interview with Alessio Fasano, PhD, of Harvard, an expert on leaky gut, which is a major contributor to autoimmune diseases: "Leaky Gut Syndrome: Is Gluten at the Root?" (glutenfreesociety.org/gluten-free-society-blog/leaky-gut -syndrome-is-gluten-at-the-root).

CHAPTER 5

PAIN CAUSED BY OBESITY

Blame It on "Grainbesity"

For the first fifty years of your life the food industry is trying to make you fat. Then, the second fifty years, the pharmaceutical industry is treating you for everything.

—Pierre Dukan, MD

What is *grainbesity*? It's my word for the condition of being overweight as a result of eating a grain-laden diet. If you are still assuming that grain is a healthy food and that your health problems and perhaps your weight issues have nothing to do with your diet, this chapter will be your wake-up call.

So what is the connection between excess weight and grain? Consider this: feeding cows, pigs, and other livestock grain (and soy) is the primary way to fatten them for slaughter. Ditto for poultry. Of course, confining their movement helps as well. Why are we surprised that eating the same foods bulks us up, too?

In fact, our grain-based diet is an express train hurtling along the track to a station called obesity. No wonder two-thirds of American adults are overweight, including the 40 percent who are obese.[1] But you needn't be one of them. Once you let go of the myth that what you eat *doesn't* impact your health, you can eliminate your pain following my No-Grain, No-Pain program, all the while trimming your waistline. That change alone can reduce pain-producing stress on your joints and muscles.

THE PAIN OF DIABETES, OBESITY, ASTHMA, AND MORE

Linda was suffering with chronic back pain and metabolic syndrome, and diabetes had caused severe neuropathy that wracked her entire lower body and made her feet swell so badly she could barely walk. Severe asthma led to frequent hospitalizations for steroid treatments, and vocal cord inflammation required anti-inflammatory drugs and speech therapy to allow her to communicate. And if that wasn't enough discomfort for one person, Linda also had stomach pain and bloating, elevated blood pressure, and severe fatigue. Her gallbladder had been removed, her fingernails were splitting, and although she is only 5 feet, 4 inches tall, she weighed about 225 pounds.

Linda described her history, saying "My body started falling apart when I turned thirty." Twenty years later, she was under the care of three doctors and taking eight different medications to "treat" her pain and other symptoms. Nonetheless, she was getting progressively worse, and feared she was out of options. A thorough investigation revealed that Linda had a gluten-sensitive gene pattern, was allergic to both sugar and dairy products, and had a whopping twenty different vitamin and mineral deficiencies.

I put her on the No-Grain, No-Pain program immediately, along with supplements to address her vitamin and mineral deficiencies. Selenium, vitamin B_1, chromium, and vitamin D were absolutely necessary because such deficiencies interfere with the body's ability to regulate inflammation and blood sugar, and to produce thyroid hormone.

Linda's results were dramatic, shocking her doctors. When I followed up with her six weeks later, she had lost 45 pounds, her blood pressure was normal, and the nerve pain in her legs was gone, as were the stomach problems, episodic asthma attacks, swollen feet, and split nails. She was able to move around easily, and her energy had returned. Her vocal cord inflammation was also almost completely healed. Four months later, Linda was down to 164 pounds and virtually symptom free. She reported that she had attempted a "cheat meal" between appointments, which occasioned a four-day flare-up in asthma, leg, and back pain. She has learned her lesson. Today she is off of all eight medications and is living an active life, feeling better in her fifties than ever. Again, no grain, no pain.

MORE VICIOUS CYCLES

In previous chapters I've introduced a number of vicious cycles. We've discussed how poaching muscle to feed the immune system and combat the inflammatory effects of certain foods only creates more inflammation and pain as muscle shrinks and increases stress on joints. You now know that many of the drugs used to mask pain or reduce inflammation interfere with long-term healing and can over time actually damage the gut, causing more pain and inflammation. Moreover, such drugs deplete stores of vitamin B_{12} and other vital nutrients essential to healing. Another catch-22: increased pain leads to decreased activity, which makes you more likely to gain weight, making it harder and more painful to be active. Not unlike the use of NSAIDs and other painkillers and anti-inflammatory drugs, continuing to eat grains sets up a vicious cycle that impedes the body's natural healing capacity. It does so in part by stimulating weight gain, which deters activity (just as being in pain does), which leads to further weight gain.

That said, it bears repeating that people suffering from celiac disease can't keep weight on. Nonetheless, the vast majority of people with non-celiac gluten sensitivity (NCGS) struggle to keep their weight *down*.[2] Do you remember the old nursery rhyme about Jack Sprat and his wife? ("Jack Sprat could eat no fat. His wife could eat no lean. And so between them both, you see, they licked the platter clean.") The good news is that my No-Grain, No-Pain program helps both the Jack

Sprats with celiac disease and the Mrs. Jack Sprats (both male and female) with NCGS.

FLAWED ASSUMPTIONS YIELD FLAWED CONCLUSIONS

It's time to puncture another myth.

Myth 14: **If you eat the standard American diet, as exemplified by "My Plate," you're eating a balanced and varied diet.**
Not true! The overwhelming quantity of grain and grain-based processed junk that passes for variety actually delivers singularity. If it's any comfort, you're not alone in thinking you were eating a healthy diet. Nor are you foolish to have been duped. Remember that the Food Guide Pyramid, which most of us grew up with (replaced recently by My Plate), recommended 6 to 11 servings of grains every day. This despite the fact that there is little scientific evidence that confirms that eating grains (whole or otherwise) promotes good health, other than being a good source of fiber, which is also in good supply in vegetables and fruits. In fact, much of the "research" upon which these guidelines are based has been funded by the cereal industry.

By the way, unlike grain and other quickly metabolized carbohydrates, dietary fat actually helps us maintain our weight. The low-fat and no-fat craze of the 1990s led to more obesity than ever before. If you've been cutting back on fat, thinking that's all you need to do to slim down, think again. It does appear that the most recent food guidelines, which are in the process of being revised, are likely to no longer instruct us to restrict fat intake, and instead to acknowledge that fat is not inherently bad, although certain fats (as well as added sugars) are detrimental to health.[3] But these anticipated changes are unlikely to be reflected in My Plate any time soon.

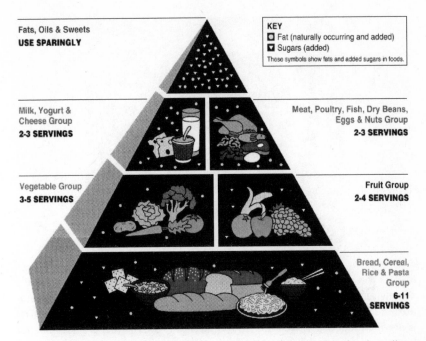

The 1992 Food Guide Pyramid emphasized grains over all other foods, calling for up to eleven servings a day.

GRAIN SURPLUS

In previous chapters, I have explained the problems many people experience when they eat grain, whether they are gluten sensitive or gluten intolerant. Now it's time to look at the other impacts of eating grain, which can affect anyone—and everyone.

Impact 1: Eating grain elevates blood sugar levels, which makes your body store sugar as fat. There is a large body of research on nutrition that strongly links the intake of refined grains to metabolic syndrome, as well as diabetes.[4]

Impact 2: Grains are super-high in calories. Taking in too many calories and expending too few in activity make you fat.

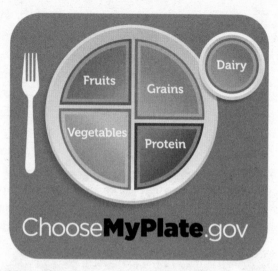

In 2011 the USDA replaced the Food Guide Pyramid with My Plate, which only slightly reduces the amount of grains relative to other foods but still perpetuates the flawed recommendations it has provided for 30 years. Note that fat is not mentioned despite the fact that the right kinds of fats are essential for health and weight management.

Impact 3: Grains are simply not a good source of nutrition because they are hard to digest, contain anti-nutrients and mycotoxins, and contribute to vitamin and mineral deficiencies.[5]

REFINED GRAIN AND UNINTENDED CONSEQUENCES

Whole wheat contains vitamins B_1 (thiamine), B_2 (riboflavin), B_6 (pyridoxine), and niacin, as well as vitamin E, iron, and zinc. However, these nutrients are mostly found in the fibrous outer layers, meaning the wheat bran. When it became easy to refine grain using a mechanical process that removed both the fibrous hull and the germ, which contains fat and protein, most people eschewed whole grains. White bread was considered more refined (in terms of social class) and therefore desirable. The flour produced light, white bread and other wheat products, but its overuse resulted in a serious case of unintended consequences. The processing procedure, which involves extrusion and high heat, destroys the vitamins, minerals, and other nutrients, leaving only empty calories. Thousands of people died of malnutrition (from a deficit of thiamine called beriberi) in the United States in the early 1900s because this vital nutrient was missing from refined grain.[6] (It remained a huge problem in undeveloped parts of the world for decades.) In 1943 the U.S. government banned the sale of unfortified grain. Flour manufacturers then replaced many of the nutrients removed by the refining process, including vitamins B_1 and B_2, niacin, and iron. Sometimes vitamins A and D are also added. The fact that grains are fortified with vitamins and minerals has added to the myth that they are healthy foods, when in actuality what was removed has simply been replaced with synthetic versions.

COLLATERAL DAMAGE: METABOLIC SYNDROME

All you have to do is walk through a shopping mall or airport terminal to see that we have an epidemic of grainbesity. Two-thirds of American adults are overweight and almost 40 percent are obese, based on body mass index (BMI), the ratio of weight to height, which roughly ascertains how much fat is on your body. A BMI of 25 to 29.9 is considered overweight, while a BMI of 30 and above makes you technically obese. (That said, the BMI is an enormously inexact measurement because total weight alone does not determine being overweight. A heavily muscled man would appear obese on paper, thanks to the weight of his muscle mass, despite having very little body fat.) To make this a bit more understandable, a man or woman who is 5 feet, 6 inches tall who weighs between 115 and 154 pounds is considered of normal weight.

The top three causes of death in this country are cancer, heart disease, and stroke, in that order. And absolutely, hands down, obesity contributes to all of these diseases. Heavy people are at greater risk for developing all types of chronic diseases. That's a fact, but the $64,000 (adjusted for inflation) question is why. What is in our food supply that triggers these causes of death? And why have these diseases become such major killers only in the past fifty years?[7]

Metabolic syndrome refers to being overweight in combination with at least two of the following factors: high blood sugar, high blood pressure (hypertension), and high triglycerides or high cholesterol. All of them can prove deadly. Metabolic syndrome is not a disease in and of itself; rather, it is the confluence of at least three disease states. As a result, your metabolic ability to process calories, keep weight off, and maintain muscle mass is impaired. Metabolic syndrome can be a precursor to type 2 diabetes, which is why it is also referred to as prediabetes.

Metabolic syndrome shows up as a certain pattern of weight gain: concentrated around the waist. On a man it presents as a potbelly, aka a beer belly, whether or not he is a teetotaler. On a woman it may look like a spare tire around her waist or a "muffin top" above her waistband. Arms and legs may remain relatively slim. Instead the fat is clustered around the vital organs, which is more of a health risk than more evenly distributed fat. If you receive a diagnosis of metabolic syndrome, it means that you have at least three of these four markers. In that case, your doctor will probably try to put you on a cardiovascular drug such as a statin. The theory is that taking such a drug will reduce your risk for a stroke or heart disease. But once again, instead of taking a drug with a host of side effects, some of them life threatening, you can beat metabolic syndrome by changing your diet, losing weight, becoming more active, and building muscle to raise your metabolism. That's exactly what the No-Grain, No-Pain program is all about.

In addition to the serious metabolic health risks, being overweight increases wear and tear on joints, leading to various forms of arthritis, with attendant pain, as we've already discussed. And you needn't be reminded that pain reduces both your inclination and your capacity for exercise as well as general activity. There we are again with another vicious cycle of pain, inactivity, increased weight gain, more pain, and so forth.

COLLATERAL DAMAGE:
AN IMBALANCE OF OMEGA FATS

Most people eat too much grain, which means they overconsume calories, but there is also the matter of omega-6 fats. Grains contain far more omega-6s than omega-3s, so eating lots of grain disrupts the balance of the two in your body.[8] Omega-3s are considered anti-inflammatory and omega-6s just the opposite. (An ideal ratio is 1 to 1 of omega-3s to omega-6s, although a ratio of 2 to 1 may be more achievable.) Most people eating the standard American diet actually have a ratio of 1 to 16![9] Such an imbalance increases inflammation, which in turn increases the amounts of insulin and cortisol, both hormones associated with fat storage. Even if you reduce your calorie intake, you're more prone to weight gain if your body remains inflamed. That's why so many people fail with Weight Watchers. They count their calories but don't counter the inflammation. As long as you continue to eat grain you'll continue to be inflamed, which perpetuates the grainbesity scenario.

BAD NEWS FOR OUR KIDS

Tragic as obesity and its health results are for adults, it's even worse for children. Rates of juvenile obesity have skyrocketed, doubling over the past thirty years.[10] In the 1970s, 5 percent of 2-to-5-year-olds were obese. By 2006, it was up to 10 percent. The number of obese 6-to-11-year-olds quadrupled in that same period, from 4 to 20 percent. Adolescent obesity rates (12 to 19 years of age) tripled from 6 to 18 percent.[11]

Researchers reporting in *The New England Journal of Medicine* believe that children of this generation will the first to have a shorter life span—as little as two years or as much as five years less—than their parents.[12] Today's average life expectancy is about 77 years. The authors of this 2005 study note that were obesity suddenly to vanish, we would live,

on average, at least four to nine months longer. And get this: as a cur-
tailer of average life span, obesity outranks accidents, murders, and
suicides combined.

People struggling with obesity are more likely to develop type 2
diabetes, heart disease, hypertension, joint deterioration, and cancer, among other ailments. The younger the age at which a person becomes obese, the earlier he or she is likely to develop such
conditions and therefore the more likely to die at a younger age.[13]
Once considered "adult" diseases, these catastrophic diseases now
increasingly appear in obese youngsters. Moreover, the child of an
obese parent has a 50 percent likelihood of being obese,[14] jumping
to 80 percent if both parents are obese.[15] Both genetics and lifestyle
(diet and activity) influence the "passing down" of obesity, but at
least the latter can be modified. Although youth obesity takes a personal toll, there is also a societal one. A staggering 27 percent of
young men and women are too heavy to serve in the military, with
about fifteen thousand potential soldiers failing recruitment physi-
cals annually.[16]

Not all obese children grow up to be obese adults. Nor is obesity
is not the only factor determining life span. Its partner in crime is lack
of fitness. In 2012 about one-third of Americans aged 12 to 19 did
not meet established cardiovascular physical fitness standards.[17] Obviously, the heavier you are and the greater pain you are in, the less active
you are apt to be.[18]

Nutritious School Lunches, Not!

With childhood obesity such a huge problem, it is instructive to take
a look at what schoolkids are eating. So I dropped in on a school
near my home to see for myself. The typical lunchroom menu is
dominated by pizza, pasta salads, bread and rolls, bagels, wraps,
spaghetti, grilled cheese sandwiches, fried chicken nuggets, potatoes in various forms, and processed meats and cheese. Yes, there
were some vegetables and fruit. Most kids who brought lunch to
school were eating processed junk food: sodas; fruit drinks made

with dyes, sugars, and artificial flavors; a vast array of chips cooked in GMO oils; sandwiches made with processed meat and cheese-like substances surrounded by a layer of hydrogenated mayo; fruit roll-ups; and cookies. This is no way to feed a growing body and developing brain.

Why are school lunches generally so bad? Many parents know nothing about nutrition—which is why so many are overweight—so they are in no position to teach their kids how to eat. Instead they leave it in the hands of the school dieticians. Not a good move. The schools are using My Plate, which is as flawed as the Food Guide Pyramid. Parents may also not realize that to keep costs down, school lunch menus are largely ruled by surpluses of grain sitting in warehouses. The National School Lunch Program started in 1946, and it's highly likely that the increase in obesity among children in the past seven decades is tied to the program's overemphasis on grains.[19]

Parents with gluten-sensitive children face a double dilemma. Instead of packing supposedly gluten-free food full of preservatives, artificial ingredients, and grains, send your kid to school with real food in his or her backpack, meaning fresh fruit, meat, nuts, and vegetables. My wife cooks extra dinner so that our son can take leftovers to school in a stainless steel thermos (to keep them warm) the next day. If you're worried about your child being "picked on" for bringing "different" food, let it go. Kids are going to be teased, regardless. Teach your child why food is important, and model the behavior that the proper care of his body starts with proper food.

BLAME IT ON HORMONES, NOT METABOLISM

I'm sure you've met people who complain about their weight and then in the next breath say, "But I eat like a bird, so it must be my metabolism." As we've already discussed, the more physically active you are, the higher your metabolism. What is really going on is hormonal. When you eat bread or pasta or pizza, you're effectively telling your pancreas to release the hormone insulin, which ferries blood glucose (blood sugar) into your cells. When there is an overabundance of glucose, the blood becomes thick and sticky, just as though you added syrup to water, coating the proteins in the bloodstream. That makes one protein, hemoglobin, which carries oxygen to the cells, work harder. The longer you repeatedly elevate your blood sugar by eating grains and other high-carb foods, the less efficiently the hemoglobin produces energy. As a result, the excess sugars and carbs convert into fat, which is stored in your liver, around other organs, and in fat cells, resulting in the truncal obesity associated with metabolic syndrome.

Some hormones, including insulin, are proteins. Hormones are always floating around in our blood, and they, too, can get bogged down with sugar, which interferes with their ability to travel to different tissues and the cells, where they signal appropriate actions to DNA. The breakdown of mega-calories into sugar produces excessive glucose and high blood sugar, which creates inflammatory stress on the body. Over time, this chronic process may also lead to diabetes.

AGEs AND AGING

When blood sugar binds with proteins, the process is referred to as glycation. Cells get rigid, less flexible, more subject to damage, and more likely to age prematurely. This produces what are called advanced glycation end products (AGEs), which make you age prematurely. When you burn meat on your grill, you create AGEs. Likewise, when you get a bad sunburn, AGEs form in your skin tissue. Not good. You don't want this going on inside your body either! AGEs appear to cause type 2 diabetes and may play a role in the development of Alzheimer's.[20]

A hemoglobin A1c (HbA1c) test measures how much sugar is coating your hemoglobin, the protein in your red blood cells that carries oxygen and produces energy. (If your fasting blood sugars are higher than 90, it merits concern.) Diabetics have trouble healing because their sticky blood can't transport oxygen to their cells efficiently. Nor can vitamins and minerals, which are carried by proteins in the blood, reach the cells. The outcome is often the development of what is called small blood vessel disease. It sounds benign but is anything but. The smaller blood vessels in certain parts of the body can't get the nourishment they need, which is why diabetics have a higher risk for eye and kidney disease. The blood vessels in these organs are very small. It's also why diabetics are apt to develop neuropathy in their toes and hands. When nutrients aren't available to the nerves in these parts of the body, they deteriorate. Neuropathy leads to an inability to feel your feet, so if you stub your toe or step on something sharp, you may not feel it. If it becomes infected, it could lead to gangrene and eventually amputation.

THE CORTISOL CONNECTION

As a natural defense mechanism when confronted with chronic inflammation, the adrenal glands make more of the hormone cortisol (a corticosteroid), in an effort to downregulate inflammation. This is an example of a normal response to an abnormal diet, but it is a short-term solution because corticosteroids are also catabolic. Catabolism refers to the body poaching its own muscle for energy. And since muscle sets the metabolic rate for the body, inflammation leads to a less favorable fat-to-muscle ratio, which produces a slower resting metabolism. Even cutting calories won't allow you to lose weight if your cortisol levels are out of whack. This is the sequence of events: bad food increases cortisol levels, which causes persistent inflammation, leading to weight gain, which leads to a permanent hormonal imbalance. So the very hormone that should reduce inflammation actually aggravates it.

What most people don't understand is that obesity *is* inflammation. Perhaps it really should be called "obeseitis," conjoining obesity and inflammation. Anyone who is lugging around excess pounds is actually over-inflamed, meaning that his or her body is the battlefield for an internal war waged by the enemy combatants of diet load, stress load, and lack of muscle. And every time he or she eats lots of sugar or grain, it perpetuates the "obeseitis" scenario.

MORE HORMONAL ISSUES

Grain consumption also impacts other hormones that help regulate weight. Overeating grain can contribute to a dysfunctional thyroid gland. The thyroid is the master organ that regulates the body's metabolism, and a deficiency of certain thyroid hormones can lead to excessive weight gain, as well as fatigue, bloating, dry skin and hair, joint pain, elevated cholesterol, sleep disruption, infertility, depression, and cold feet and hands. Several mechanisms of gluten sensitivity contribute to hypothyroidism, including gluten-induced GI damage. This can lead to a domino-like effect of leaky gut, followed by a cascade of inflammation and an exaggerated autoimmune response, over time leading to Hashimoto's disease. More than 10 percent of American women have this condition, and that figure rises to almost 25 percent for women over 65.[21]

We also know that eating grain can impact the hormones known as sex steroids. For a man, this can influence how well he makes testosterone, which is important for maintaining muscle and therefore a high metabolism that will keep weight off. (You've probably seen low-T centers popping up, as well as commercials hawking low-T remedies.) Well, vitamin and mineral deficiencies caused by eating gluten directly impact the ability to produce testosterone. The incidence of low T in men has almost doubled in recent years.[22] In 2002, 3.2 percent of the men tested had low T; by 2011, it was 5.8 percent.

When it comes to estrogen, there is substantial evidence that pesticides used on grains and other crops mimic estrogen.[23] Consuming such grains can create estrogen dominance.[24] For women, that can result in premenstrual syndrome (PMS), polycystic ovary syndrome, painful fibroids, and other conditions. I'm not saying that grain is the only culprit in such cases, but it is definitely a potential factor. I've had patients whose fibroids have gone away once they went totally gluten free, and I've had others whose fibroids remained. It's my belief that we never want to move on to medication or surgery unless we've entertained diet as a potential cause of a problem.

Estrogen dominance doesn't affect just women. When men are exposed to estrogen mimics, they can mute the effects of testosterone. That's why some guys have man boobs, commonly referred to as gynecomastia, the growth of breast tissue, along with cottage-cheese cellulite forming underneath the breasts. Estrogen dominance likely also plays a role in erectile dysfunction.[25]

THE THYROID CONNECTION

At age 23, Kristin had already been diagnosed with gluten sensitivity by her primary doctor and was following a traditional gluten-free diet. When she came to see me, she was 30 pounds overweight and suffered from severe stomachaches, a mysterious skin rash, and autoimmune hypothyroid disease. Despite her change to a supposedly gluten-free diet, her symptoms persisted. She was taking a variety of medications, including creams for her rash and thyroid pills.

Kristin's case is a classic example of how avoiding only wheat, barley, rye, and oats can be completely ineffective. In their place, she was consuming large amounts of corn and rice, and continued to have inflammatory issues, a perfect example of gluten-free whiplash. We eliminated all grains for a *true* gluten-free diet. After several months, despite moving and traveling, both of which can challenge diet compliance, Kristin's symptoms were completely gone. She lost 30 pounds, her skin was clear, and her thyroid levels had normalized, meaning she no longer requires medication. Again, no grain, no pain.

THE PAIN OF JOINT COMPRESSION

You may be thinking this is all very interesting and scary, but how does it relate to pain? I'm glad you asked. You already know that the vicious cycle of muscle loss and weight gain compresses the joints. Muscles connect your joints. When muscles deteriorate, they get shorter. If the muscle is shorter, that compresses the joint. Every extra pound you're carrying around puts greater gravitational compression on the joint. Having less muscle mass aggravates the situation. The double whammy of muscle atrophy combined with excessive weight creates another vicious cycle of pain and inflammation. Because the joints are overworked, overstrained, and grinding together, any exercise is painful. So the very thing that could help save you from being overweight and in pain becomes a contributing factor to more inflammation, pain, and extra pounds.

So what's the solution? First of all, everyone needs to have a minimum quantity of motion, mobility, and movement in the course of the day. The average American works and sits for eight hours a day. You can't work out for twenty minutes (or even an hour) and then sit for eight hours and expect that the former will offset the latter. It simply doesn't compute. You need to find ways to move regularly, whether or not you have a sedentary job. This is where the activities of daily living come into play. We need to consistently and constantly be conscious of ways to be in motion. I'm talking about deliberately parking farther away from the entrance to a store, climbing up and down stairs instead of taking the elevator, walking instead of driving whenever possible, walking in a zigzag pattern instead of in a straight line, getting off the bus or subway a stop before your destination, and the like. By themselves, these are all small things, but they can add up big in terms of mobility and motion.

Let's do some math. If a 160-pound man walks five miles a day, he burns about 350 extra calories a day more than if he just sat around on the sofa. That's the equivalent of a pound every ten days, which is three pounds a month, which is 36 pounds a year. The average person usually takes only about two thousand steps a day, which is what I see with many of my patients. Using a digital tracking device such as a Fitbit or even an old-fashioned pedometer can help you be conscious of how active you are. If you try to guesstimate, you're almost certainly going to overestimate your activity level (and underestimate your calorie intake). Once you have tracked yourself for several weeks, you should have a good idea of your normal day-to-day activity level.

Then you can add what is necessary to achieve a level of activity that helps prevent obesity.

IT HURTS TO BE FAT

Obesity creates pain because being overweight and being inflamed are two sides of the same coin. Obesity is an inflammatory disease. As long as the body is systemically inflamed, it's more prone to chronic pain in the muscles, joints, tendons, and ligaments. This is why weekend warriors get injured. They don't realize that they can't do what they did when they were eighteen, because they have ten (or twenty or thirty) more years of accumulated inflammatory damage. Trying to turn back the clock to what they did once upon a time is like the proverbial needle that breaks the camel's back.

When you combine grainbesity with the resultant wear and tear on the muscles and other tissues, in combination with "obeseitis," you have a perfect prescription for pain. If you're not overweight yet but are grain intolerant, your body is in a favored state to become fat. And as long you continue to eat grain, you will stay chronically inflamed and you will be in chronic pain. Now add to this the medication you have probably been using. If you're overweight, your joints hurt, so you're taking ibuprofen, which little by little destroys your gut, which leads to more leaky gut and leaches out the very vitamin C you need to help heal your muscles and joints. So now you're just stuck. How do you dig yourself out of that hole?

The vicious cycles comprise not just obesity, joint compression, and joint wear and tear, but also neuropathy. If your spine's joints are being broken down, they press against and pinch the nerves exiting the spine, which gives the nerve less wiggle room to maneuver. This can result in neuropathies, so nerve pain joins the pain pity party. Meanwhile, because you're overeating or eating foods that are inflammatory, your gut is going to be inflamed and painful as well.

EMOTIONAL PAIN

Being overweight is a pain in the neck, back, and everywhere else, but it also produces psychological pain in the form of depression and low self-image, which, all too often lead to overeating. Gluteomorphin, also known as gliadorphin, is a peptide found in wheat gluten (gliadin). Another peptide called casomorphin is found in casein, a milk protein. Elevated levels of these peptides (short chains of proteins) have been found in the urine of individuals with celiac disease, schizophrenia, and autism. The researchers who made this discovery suspect that elevated levels of both peptides may also be found in the urine of people with chronic fatigue syndrome. If gluteomorphin and casomorphin sound like opiates, you're right on. Both react with opiate receptors in the brain, so they mimic the effects of drugs like heroin and morphine, as Dr. William Davis explains in *Wheat Belly*. Dr. David Perlmutter also explores the gut-brain connection in his pivotal book *Grain Brain*. Eating grains and dairy products presumably soothes individuals with depression and other emotional or mental disorders. It is suspected that when such foods are not properly digested, they aggravate such conditions, leading to more weight gain—and more pain and inflammation. Yet another vicious cycle.

An Ancient Culture Meets the Standard American Diet

A longitudinal study on the Pima Indians of the Southwest, a culture that traditionally did not eat grains, has demonstrated the disastrous results when its people switched to the standard American diet (SAD) and lifestyle. Over roughly three decades, a population that had not experienced diabetes or obesity while following its traditional diet based on farming, hunting, and fishing gradually switched to the SAD. The result was an astronomical incidence of obesity and diabetes. Geneticist James Neel proposed that the Pimas had what he called a "thrifty" gene.[26] By this he meant that their bodies were accustomed to a cycle of feast or famine and were able to store energy as fat during lean times and then use it when needed, much as hibernating animals do. A pair of epidemiologists who followed the Pimas during this transition period as they began to consume more grain, more processed fats, more sugar, and more soda—and adopt a more sedentary lifestyle—concluded that the Pimas' old friend, the thrifty geneotype, had became its enemy.[27] With no period of famine, they packed on fat that they never needed to tap for energy in lean times. By 1990, more than 75 percent of Pimas were obese and more than 45 percent of them had type 2 diabetes. The initial study of the change in eating habits of Aleuts (Eskimos) reached similar conclusions.[28] Both cultures continue to be the subject of extensive research on diet and disease.

WHAT YOU NEED TO KNOW

O Our grain-centric diet is intimately related to the current epidemic of obesity.

O Eating grain elevates blood sugar levels, encouraging fat storage, which is linked to metabolic syndrome and type 2 diabetes.

O Too much sugar in the blood makes it syrupy, which can lead to glycation, which ages you prematurely, as well as impaired ability to deliver oxygen to the cells to make energy and disperse nutrients to nerves.

O Glutens can induce joint pain in susceptible individuals, which makes exercise difficult, discouraging the very thing that could help relieve inflammation and pare pounds.

O The combination of reduced muscle mass, as a result of inflammation, and excess body fat is a double whammy in terms of achieving a healthy metabolism.

O Grains also deliver an imbalance of inflammatory omega-6 fats.

O The hormonal impacts of eating grains are far reaching, including insulin resistance that can lead to type 2 diabetes, hypothyroidism, excess cortisol production, low testosterone, and estrogen dominance, all of which can pile on pounds.

○ Obesity is an inflammatory disease that can be cured with a change of diet and regular exercise.

In part 2 you'll learn about all the wonderful foods you *can* eat on the No-Grain, No-Pain program.

BONUS FEATURE

Video on nutrition and the thyroid: glutenfreesociety.org/no-grain -no-pain-thyroid-function-and-nutrition.

THE 30-DAY NO-GRAIN, NO-PAIN PROGRAM

Tell me what you eat, and I shall tell you what you are.

—Jean Anthelme Brillat-Savarin

I can almost hear you saying to yourself, "Okay, Dr. Osborne, I get it. I want to rid myself of pain, but what am I going to eat once I give up grain?" Not to fear. This section is not just about what you will *not* be eating; it also contains plenty of delicious and satisfying options to replace those problematic foods in the form of lists and meal plans. My dietary and supplement program is based on the Triangle of Health fundamentals. Going truly gluten free is essential to restore health, but critical as it is, changing your diet alone is not enough. Three factors interact with your own DNA to determine your health.

- Your physical side: exercise, overall activity, regular exposure to sunlight, etc.

- Your biochemistry: what you eat and drink, the air you breathe, toxins you're exposed to, etc.

- Your mental influences: Knowing that your condition can be reversed is essential to the healing process. Likewise, bad relationships and other unpleasant situations can negatively impact your health.

The two-phase, 30-day program, which includes dietary and other lifestyle changes including regular physical activity, presented in this section will allow you to begin the process of becoming what I call a *true* Gluten-Free Warrior: healthy in body, mind, and spirit. Follow this program for 30 days, and not only will you see dramatic pain reduction, but you will also experience across-the-board improvements in your health. In part 3, we'll delve into other important factors that may be necessary to completely relieve pain and inflammation.

THE THREE CARDINAL RULES OF NUTRITION

Regardless of whether or not a food contains gluten, there are some fundamental rules of nutrition to always keep in mind:

1. You can't get (and stay) healthy without eating healthy food, which does not include processed, genetically modified, packaged food, what I call "frood." Your body simply is not adapted to handle it.

2. Eat nothing to which you're allergic, sensitive, or intolerant.

3. If you feel pain or discomfort after eating a certain food, stop eating it!

Eating properly protects your gut and keeps it functioning well. In addition, we're equipped with senses that protect it—and us. Always:

- Smell food first and then taste. Both stimulate the release of saliva and gastric acids, which aid in digestion.
- Chew thoroughly. The more you break down the pieces of food, the less stress you put on your digestive organs.
- Eat mindfully and without distraction or stressful situations, which activate your autonomic nervous system, shunting blood away from the GI tract and making it harder to process and digest food.

•Just as you need to rest after exercising, you need to take a break from eating by allowing time between meals, as well as periodically and intermittently fasting.

If you break rules, there are consequences; in this case, consequences for your health. We're all human, so we do break them sometimes, but getting better requires an understanding that eating is a form of warfare: It's us versus the food we're eating!

Be forewarned: As you embark on the dietary and supplement protocol, there's a very real and likely possibility that your conventional medicines—whether painkillers, anti-inflammatories, or antibiotics—could become too strong, which could create a whole other set of symptoms. That's why it's important that you have a good relationship with a doctor who can walk you through and alert you to which signals could indicate that you need to change the dosage or stop certain medications. If your regular physician isn't willing to work with you on this, I suggest you go to MyFunctionalMedicineDoctor.org to find a functional medicine doctor who might be more willing to do so. At a certain point, you'll also want to ask whether you need to keep taking certain medications. Once you're feeling better, you're probably going to want to get off synthetic drugs (both over-the-counter and prescription) sooner rather than later.

CHAPTER 6

WHAT TO EAT—AND NOT TO EAT

Change Your Diet and Banish Your Pain

One man's meat is another man's poison.

—Lucretius, first-century
BCE Roman poet

Each person is biochemically unique. Never make the assumption that a food is safe or healthy for everyone. That is why the third rule of nutrition exists: If you feel bad after eating something, stop eating it. That will begin when you initiate the healing process in the 15-day Kickoff phase of the No-Grain, No-Pain program. In this phase, you'll remove a number of problematic foods and make several important lifestyle changes. Even in two weeks, the results can be transformational.

I can't promise that you'll see your world completely turn around, but you will almost certainly experience some of the following:

- Reduced pain and stiffness
- Reduced muscle aches
- Reduced fatigue

119

- Improved energy
- Enhanced mental clarity (less brain fog)
- Reduced gastrointestinal symptoms
- Improved bowel function
- Less frequent headaches (if you were plagued with them before)
- Loss of anywhere from 5 to 10 pounds, depending upon your former weight (much of that will be inflammatory water weight, not necessarily fat)

Again, not everyone will experience all these improvements in the first phase, nor may you need some of them.

After completing the second phase, the 15-day Challenge, in which you will eliminate additional foods and make other lifestyle changes we'll discuss in this chapter, including intermittent fasting, you will see profound changes in your overall health. That being said, 30 days is just the beginning. The road to complete health requires changing habits for a lifetime. If that seems hard to imagine, consider the alternative: years of pain, illness, and medications that do absolutely nothing to treat the origin of the pain, which all too often is the grain you eat at almost every meal. One of my patients was convinced that changing her diet couldn't help her and that she was just too old for any treatment to work. Her story follows.

A SKEPTIC NO MORE

A classic skeptic, Leona came to me originally only because her daughter dragged her into my office. Leona suffered from chronic arthritic pain in her neck, back, and hips. She had severe and uncontrolled type 2 diabetes and emphysema and, as a result, unrelenting fatigue. She needed help walking, sometimes using a cane and other times a wheelchair. She weighed more than 200 pounds and was unable to exercise because it made her emphysema flare up. Leona was on medication for high cholesterol, high blood pressure, and diabetes, and used a steroid to help her breathe.

But when I introduced her to functional medicine, this skeptic turned over a new leaf. Leona did everything I asked her to do. She was gluten sensitive and allergic to figs, MSG, and peanuts. She also had an intestinal yeast overgrowth and high levels of lead in her system. Her hemoglobin test for diabetes (HbA1c) was very high at 6.4. Plus she was deficient in zinc and magnesium, which was critical since both minerals are necessary to help regulate blood sugar, insulin, and inflammation.

Within a month of changing her diet and following her supplement protocol, Leona's joint pain was gone. Her energy improved dramatically, along with her breathing capacity. She no longer needed to use her steroid inhaler regularly. She also lost 15 pounds and her blood pressure dropped significantly.

Within three months, Leona was off of her medications. Her blood pressure level had normalized, as had her blood sugar levels, meaning her diabetes was finally under control, and she had dropped 50 pounds. She was able to move around without the need for her cane or wheelchair. She was exercising, getting outside, sleeping better, and still had no pain. Within eight months, Leona was down 80 pounds, her joint pain remained absent, and we spent an entire appointment learning new exercises to build muscle. Leona is a *true* Gluten-Free Warrior. She never complained about the diet change. Not once. For more of Leona's story, visit youtube.com/watch?v=LAM-Sc2zE-I.

RUNNING ON GRAIN

To get a handle on how deeply ingrained grain is in the American diet, let's take a quick look at how most of us currently eat. Then ask yourself how much of it lives up to the third cardinal rule of nutrition, and the logic for significantly changing your diet should be clear.

Your day might begin with a bowl of cold cereal or hot oatmeal and a glass of OJ. The cereal is made with GMO grains and is probably full of added sugar. The OJ might as well be liquid sugar, since the fruit's fiber has been removed. The milk you splash over your Wheaties or whatever is from cows that are almost certainly raised in a factory barn and fed only genetically modified (GMO) grain and soy. Or perhaps you grab a breakfast bar or a toasted bagel, both made with grains. A fast-food breakfast sandwich contains not just GMO grain but also eggs from chickens and bacon or sausage from pigs raised on grain. To keep the powdered sugar dusted on a doughnut from clumping, it's mixed with cornstarch. Pancakes are another gluten bomb, and the syrup is almost certainly made from corn syrup and an array of chemicals. Perhaps we should rename the first meal of the day "grainfest."

The reality is that most of the foods we consider traditional breakfast foods have been around for only half a century. And it's not just the foods that are different; the manufacturing processes and ingredients have also morphed over time. Our habits and palate have changed as well. Convenience is king, and sweet foods are no longer a treat but the norm. Our forefathers were definitely not having the equivalent of a breakfast tart to fuel their mornings.

A Brief History of Breakfast

Cold cereals appeared on the scene only about 125 years ago. Until then, breakfast was typically bacon or sausage and eggs, or perhaps pancakes. But in 1892 Henry Drushel Perky figured out how to boil and reconstitute wheat into a palatable form, and with his partner, machinist William Henry Ford, changed the course of culinary history. The machine they invented shreds whole wheat into crisp packets. Presto changeo: the first packaged breakfast cereal.

Two years later, Dr. John Kellogg, the superintendent of a sanitarium, and his brother, Will Keith Kellogg, invented cornflakes. Many of Dr. Kellogg's patients suffered from constipation, likely due in part to the heavy meat diet of the day. He believed the fiber in whole grains could alleviate the problem, although adding more vegetables to the diet would have been a much healthier decision. In accordance with the law of unintended consequences, Dr. Kellogg helped create a cascade of other health problems. The company he founded now fills stomachs around the world with Pop-Tarts, Eggo breakfast sandwiches, Froot Loops, and hundreds of other "froods." By 1897, when C. W. Post began manufacturing Grape-Nuts, the die was cast. Breakfast was now almost synonymous with grains—and sugar. Dr. Kellogg and C. W. Post both hawked grain's supposed health benefits as part of their innovative marketing methods, enabling this misconception to gain a solid foothold.

The past few decades have somewhat chipped away at the supremacy of grains. Dr. Robert C. Atkins's pioneering work linked high carb consumption to excess weight and an increased risk for type 2 diabetes. Likewise, Dr. Perlmutter's and Dr. Davis's books on the effects of a grain-heavy diet on the brain and the belly, respectively, have challenged the assumptions that whole grains are healthy foods. The gluten-free and paleo trends have cut into sales of breakfast cereals, but at the same time, the grab-and-go eating trend has prompted cereal companies to diversify their product offerings with breakfast bars and breakfast drinks. Most of these products also contain grains, corn syrup or corn sugar solids, and dehydrated milk, as well as soy, plus a long list of artificial flavorings, sweeteners, and preservatives.

THE LUNCH HOUR

While breakfast may be the most egregious grainwise, lunch is a close runner-up. If you opt for a ham or roast beef sandwich, the meat is probably marbleized with the fat of grainbesity cows. Bologna, salami, and other luncheon meats are typically injected with grain fillers, so you get a double grain whammy: meat from grain-fed cows plus more grain as a thickening agent. Actually, it is a triple whammy, because a lot of these "Frankenmeats" are glazed with corn sugar solids or syrup. Add a slice or two of cheese from those same grain-fed cows and it's a quadruple whammy. And don't forget about the mayonnaise, most of which is made from GMO corn or vegetable oil mixed with eggs from chickens fed GMO grains, and probably topped off with some corn syrup. The same goes for condiments such as mustard or ketchup. How about a PB&J sandwich? Well, the peanut butter is almost certainly full of hydrogenated vegetable oil and added sugar, usually in the form of corn sugar; the jelly is mostly sugar and/or corn syrup.

A cup of soup is a natural accompaniment to a sandwich, but even if you pass on chicken noodle, tomato rice, mushroom barley, or any other soup with obvious grains, you're still unlikely to avoid them altogether. Almost all packaged or canned soups are thickened with wheat flour or another grain, and the flavor is boosted with corn syrup. Beef or chicken broth is made from grain-fed animals.

Surely a salad isn't a problem, right? Think again. To enhance the taste and look of freshness, most fast-food restaurants soak the lettuce, other veggies, and even cheese in corn sugar water. Croutons are made with grain, of course, but so, too, is the fake bacon. Salad dressing combines corn or vegetable oil and corn-based vinegar, boosted with corn syrup. If you wash lunch down with regular soda or ice tea, it's sweetened with high-fructose corn syrup, which, by the way, is high in the toxic heavy metal mercury. Some manufacturers now proudly proclaim that their soda uses "real sugar." Never mind that sugar consumption is linked to obesity, cancer, heart disease, and diabetes. Nor are artificially sweetened beverages any better. (To learn why, see "Avoid All Artificial Sugar Substitutes" on page 199.)

FAMILY DINNERTIME

You might expect dinner to be the most nutritious meal of the day, but for all too many families, it comes from the frozen food aisle—perhaps spaghetti, lasagna, or macaroni and cheese to pop in the microwave—or it's takeout: pizza, burgers (with fries), fried chicken, or Chinese. All are packed with grains, although you may not be aware of them.[1] (See "Grain in Disguise" on page 148.)

Fast food is the worst. Whether you opt for a beef or a turkey burger, the animal was grain fed, and the bun is made from wheat. To keep them crispy, fries are rolled in finely sifted wheat flour and then cooked in corn or vegetable oil, the same oil in which other foods, including breaded and battered chicken, are often fried, creating gluten cross-contamination. The kids' menu at such fast-food restaurants leans heavily on chicken nuggets and other fried food. Douse such a meal with ketchup, and you get another dose of corn sugar plus white vinegar made from corn, for a plate full of pain-inducing grains.

Say good-bye to all that fake food as you embark on your soon-to-be-pain-free new life.

Snacks Are Food, Too

At least they should be. Before you start the program, remove all crackers, cookies, chips, puffs, rice cakes, popcorn, and other grain bombs from your pantry. Not only are they empty of nutrients and full of grains (and in the case of potato chips, a nightshade plant), they are almost always made with vegetable or corn oil. (You'll learn why nightshades are problematic in chapter 9.) There is really no need for snacks if you are eating the right foods, the right amounts, and the right ratio of protein, carbohydrates, and fat. But I am not anti-snack. If you're ravenous between meals and feel the need for a snack, make sure it is real food with some protein in it. Think of snacks on my Grain-Free, Pain-Free program as no different from meals—protein, veggies, and fruits—just in smaller portions. Here are some ideas:

- A small can or packet of tuna fish or salmon
- A chicken wing
- Grass-fed beef, turkey, or venison jerky
- A hard-boiled egg (try duck eggs if you're allergic to chicken eggs)
- A small handful of macadamias or hazelnuts (preferably) or other true tree nuts (no peanuts* or cashews,* which are legumes and seeds, respectively)
- A small piece of fruit or portion of berries; locally grown and seasonal are always preferable
- Raw veggies with hummus*
- Half a Hass avocado

*Suitable for Phase 1 only.

- Dried organic fruit (in moderation and always with some protein or fat, such as nuts or seeds). Dried cherries are handy
  when traveling and are packed with magnesium, potassium,
  and vitamin A. As with nuts, count out a small portion.

- Roasted garbanzo beans*

Another option is my gluten-free, all-organic Warrior Bar
(glutenfreesociety.org/shop/general-health/honey-almond-warrior
-bars-12-bars), made with almond butter, pea protein, clover honey,
chicory root fiber, and vanilla. It contains 14 grams of protein and
200 calories, and is evenly balanced among protein, carbs, and fat.

EATING IN IS IN AND EATING OUT IS OUT

I ask my patients to not to eat out for the first three months on my program. Say what? I know this is a radical change for most of you, even
for the 30 days in the subtitle of this book. Here is my logic: in order to
heal your body, whether as a result of gluten sensitivity, gluten intolerance, or simply difficulty digesting gluten, you cannot continually
re-inflame it with problematic foods. If you never give your gut a rest,
you cannot heal. To do so, you need to be in *complete control* of what
you put in your mouth. In order to avoid corn, vegetable, soy, and other
bad oils; as well as hidden glutens, GMO foods, conventionally grown
foods with pesticides, and other toxins, you (or a family member who
is on board with the program) need to be the one shopping for ingredients and preparing the food. I realize that this can be a lot to ask in this
day and age, but it is essential for speedy and permanent healing. Once
you are well and your pain is but a memory, you can probably have the
occasional meal out without fear of relapsing.

Here are two more reasons to avoid eating out. The more choices
you have, the more likely you are to unwittingly stumble into the grain
(and other problematic ingredients) zone. Finally, as you well know,

* Suitable for Phase 1 only.

unless you're eating Frankenfood at a fast-food joint, you're lucky to get away with a tab of less than $30 per person.

I do realize that not dining out may not always be possible because of work, family, or travel obligations, but I will ask you to do so only when absolutely necessary. Try to clear your schedule as much as possible before you begin the program, and then follow these tips if you must dine out:

- Always eat before you go, either a good-size snack or a meal, to moderate your appetite and boost your self-control.
- Go for the social interaction, not for the food.
- Grab a drink instead of a meal at big parties and buffet dinners
- Bring a tray of gluten-free alternatives to help the host and provide a safe fallback for you.
- If there is a vegetable tray, enjoy. But pass on the soy-based ranch dressing and the like.
- Avoid alcohol made with grain, which includes beer, ale, sake, rye, bourbon, whiskey, and most other spirits. Instead, have a glass of wine or a cocktail made with rum, grape vodka, or tequila. Alcohol also tends to relax your inhibitions, so beware of straying from your dietary regimen.
- At sit-down events, simply serve yourself acceptable foods and avoid the others. If your hostess forces something on you, take a small portion and leave it on the plate.
- Before eating at a restaurant, check out the menu online, decide what you will order, and stick to it. All chain restaurants and most other dining spots now post menus online.
- Avoid restaurants with cuisines that rely on breading and battering foods. Pizza and pasta places and pancake houses are also danger zones.

BONUS FEATURE

Coping with social issues with eating gluten-free: visit glutenfreeso ciety.org/no-grain-no-pain-social-challenges-gluten-free/.

When I'm not at home, my usual lunch solution is reheated leftovers from the previous night's dinner packed in a wide-mouth metal thermos, which is easy to eat from. This means meat (or poultry or fish) and vegetables, perhaps as a stew, stir-fry, or hearty soup. Avoid plastic containers, which usually contain hormone disruptors (see chapter 10). A main-dish salad is another option. Making enough food for more than one meal is a great time- and money-saver. To avoid monotony, simply freeze single-size portions of different dishes (with the exception of salads, of course) and defrost the night before you plan to eat them.

If you're thinking you just don't have time to make dinner every night, think again. In addition to cooking up a big batch of stew on the weekends, you can minimize nightly cooking by roasting a ham, beef, leg of lamb, or chicken on a weekend and using it as the basis for several other meals during the week.

Once people understand that a change in diet can solve their health problems, eliminate pain, and give them a healthier, happier life, I've found that transitioning from medications to dietary changes is an easy choice to make. And therein lies the genesis of this book. This program works. Do it, share it, and everyone will benefit.

When You Absolutely, Positively Must Eat Out

Say your boss invites you out for lunch to discuss a big project and you cannot decline. What to do? You can't control the source of the food, but at least you can make the best choices from the available options.

- Obviously, ignore the breadbasket.

- Order a tossed salad topped with chicken or salmon. Ask for cider vinegar or lemon juice and olive oil on the side to dress it, and for no croutons, cheese, and fake bacon bits. In the Challenge phase, also ask that tomatoes, peppers, and any other nightshade-family vegetables not be used.

- Or have grilled or roasted chicken, fish, or meat (minus any gravy or sauce).

- Avoid any food that has been breaded or deep-fried.

- Ask for an additional vegetable instead of rice or pasta.
- Pass on dessert or order fruit.

KICK THE SANDWICH HABIT—OR INNOVATE

I admit it. Sandwiches are easy to prepare, portable, and can be infinitely varied in their contents. But if you are giving up all grains, conventional sandwiches have to go. Here are some solutions to segue into your new bread-free existence:

- Simply serve whichever acceptable foods you were going to have between sliced bread on a plate instead.
- Wrap a burger, sliced meat, poultry, or fish in a lettuce or Chinese cabbage leaf. Yes, it's likely to drip, so tuck in a napkin beneath your collar.
- Check out my recipe on page 287 for Topp Paleo Flatbread made with almond flour.
- Wrap tuna, slices of grass-fed beef, or another filling in a sheet of nori (Japanese seaweed).
- Scoop out the pulp and seeds of half a tomato,* fill with leftover cooked ground beef, and run under the broiler for a couple of minutes.
- Fill endive leaves with hummus.*
- Peel and scoop out halved cucumber boats and fill with egg salad.
- Fill half an avocado with crabmeat moistened with lemon juice.
- Top a broiled portobello mushroom cap with a poached egg and guacamole.
- Some people swear by coconut wraps made from organic coconut pulp. Others find them expensive and messy.

*Acceptable in Phase 1 only.

The objective is to get away from the hamburger, breaded fish, and other fast-food-fare mentality. If you can find a "delivery system" for what you might have once placed between two slices of bread, while complying with the acceptable-foods list for the phase you're in, go for it.

OPT FOR ORGANIC AND THEREFORE NON-GMO

Whenever possible, organic foods are definitely a better choice, both for their superior nutritional content and because they are less apt to be contaminated with pesticides that can trigger an immune system attack. Monsanto and other Big Ag companies have successfully pressured the FDA *not* to require labeling on food that contains genetically modified organisms (GMO). A GMO plant (or animal) has had a gene or genes inserted into its DNA to produce desirable features such as the ability to withstand drought or ripen faster. While such efforts to do Mother Nature one better is a boon to industrial farming, its impact on the animals and humans who consume such products, to say nothing of the environment, is unknown. It is estimated that 93 percent of all corn and soy is now genetically modified. The best way to avoid GMOs is to buy organic food, which does not (or should not) contain any.

In Europe, the situation is very different. If a food contains more than 0.9 percent GMO ingredients, it must be labeled as such. Around the world, sixty-four countries require GMO foods to be labeled.[2] Fourteen states in this country have introduced legislation that would require GMO labeling, but other than in Vermont, pro-GMO lobbyists have stalled such efforts. Beginning in July 2016, foods sold in Vermont must carry a label if they contain GMO ingredients. Meanwhile, some manufacturers have started to label verified *non*-GMO products, and Whole Foods is working to identify foods that contain GMO and eliminate them from its offerings. Again, with this crazy quilt of information, your best bet is to buy organic and inform yourself about which foods are most likely to contain GMOs. (See "Organic or Not Quite" opposite.) So-called organic canola oil is an exception, because by default it is made from genetically modified rapeseeds. This is the only case I am aware of in which something is blatantly called organic but can't possibly be organic. If you steer clear of processed foods, you will immediately and dramatically reduce the amount of GMOs you consume.

Organic or Not Quite

How do you know if a packaged food is 100 percent organic? Well, it's complicated.

- Don't be fooled. The USDA seal below only means that 95 percent or more of the ingredients in a product are organic.
- If it is completely organic, meaning all ingredients are organic, it will also include the words *100 percent organic.*
- Produce, as well as eggs, which are all called single-item foods—and therefore 100 percent organic—must also be labeled with the official USDA organic label sticker.
- Although it is not mandatory, fruits and vegetables often have a numbered sticker affixed to them. Organic produce wears a five-digit number that starts with a 9. Any conventionally grown produce has a four-digit number. Any GMO produce has a five-digit number starting with an 8.
- Packaged foods that read "Made with organic ingredients" must contain 70 to 94 percent organic ingredients, of which up to three must be listed on the package front.

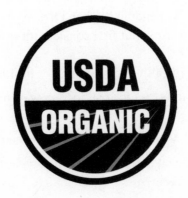

HIDDEN IN THE FINE PRINT

Become a label reader. Notice that on the label below five ingredients for "gluten-free" bread contain glutens that are or are derived from grains. They are called out in boldface type. No wonder eating such products is likely to produce gluten-free whiplash. The sugar and other highly processed ingredients are also unlikely to promote good health.

Ingredients: water, tapioca starch, **brown rice flour**, potato starch, canola oil, egg whites, sugar, **teff flour**, flaxseed meal, yeast, **xanthan gum**, apple cider vinegar, salt, baking powder (sodium bicarbonate, **cornstarch**, calcium sulfate, monocalcium phosphate), cultured dextrose, ascorbic acid (ascorbic acid, microcrystalline cellulose, **cornstarch**), enzymes

Contains: Eggs

A QUESTION OF PRIORITIES

Some of you may be rearing back, thinking, *I can't afford to buy organic vegetables, grass-fed beef, and free-range chickens and their eggs.* I'm not going to tell you how to spend your money, but I do want you to think about how you are currently spending it. Then I'll give you some suggestions about how to rein in costs. But first consider these questions:

- What are your health and your family's health worth?
- Would you rather pay for real food now or medical costs down the road?
- Is your cable TV subscription more important than good food?
- How much do you currently spend in a typical month eating out and getting takeout?

• Are you currently buying "frood" items such as breakfast cereal and chips with huge markups?

By changing your eating habits, you're making an investment. Instead of seeing your food budget as something left over after you've paid for your cable bill, your car loan, and all the other monthly costs that could be reduced if you really thought about them, consider what's really important. Your good health is priceless and is dependent upon what you eat. The number one reason for declaring bankruptcy in the United States is not because of defaulting on a mortgage. No, it's unanticipated and crushing medical expenses.[3] As a nation—and as families—we can't keep going that way. And can you justify the personal cost, as well, because you're going to bankrupt your health if you don't. If that sounds like tough love, it is. My message is "Wake up and reconsider your priorities."

Finally, once you stop spending $3 for 16 ounces of potato chips made of nightshade vegetables and GMO corn oil, $5 for a box of cereal that is full of sugar, and high markups on all those other processed foods to fund manufacturers' marketing campaigns and fancy packaging, you can instead purchase nutritious vegetables and fruit and quality sources of protein. You may actually find your weekly food bill is comparable to or only marginally higher than what it was before you embarked on your journey to health. And don't forget this: educating your family about nutrition is a priceless gift to share as you change your own eating and purchasing habits.

Nor must you sign over your paycheck to Whole Foods to eat the No-Grain, No-Pain way. There is a huge, booming grassroots market for "real" food no matter where you live. If there's nothing in your community, there are numerous online sources. Let's look at some ways to get the most bang for your organic and non-GMO food buck:

• Join a local food co-op or CSA (community-supported agriculture) group. For a state-by-state directory, visit organicaginfo.org/co-ops.

• Shop at farmers' markets. Some may be a little more expensive than the supermarket, but the food is fresh and locally grown, rather than trucked in from thousands of miles away, losing nutrients on the journey. To find one, besides checking your local news sources, check out Local Harvest (localharvest.org). This excellent organization maintains a database of farms, markets, and other sources of produce, meats, fish, poultry, and more.

• Join a buyers' club such as Thrive Market, Costco, Sam's Club, or BJ's. All have made a commitment to offering organic products.

• In addition to Whole Foods, other chains that sell grass-fed beef include HEB, Schnucks, and Dierbergs. Inquire at your store and/or contact the American Grassfed Association (american grassfed.org) for local sources of meat from grass-fed animals.

• Cut out the middleman by seeking out local farmers from whom you can purchase dairy and meat products.

• Support a hunter, perhaps by offering to barter groceries or a service, or asking if you can purchase venison or other game from him.

• Buy a share, with friends or neighbors, of a grass-fed cow or other meats from a local farmer. To learn about "cowpooling," visit marksdailyapple.com/where-to-buy-grass-fed-beef.

• Plant a vegetable garden (or some planters).

• Another great source is Slow Food USA, which has chapters in almost every state: slowfoodusa.org/local-chapters.

• Explore the resources offered by the Weston A. Price Foundation and/or join a local chapter: westonaprice.org.

MORE IS DEFINITELY NOT BETTER

A key part of the cost discussion is that when you eat better, you eat less. And when you eat less, you spend less. When food provides fewer calories but is more nourishing in terms of vitamins and minerals, your body becomes a more efficient fuel-burning machine and you're no longer just replacing calories burned with calories consumed. Your brain depresses your appetite when you feel more satisfied, often with the side effect of weight loss. So instead of having a great hunk of steak or roast or a three-quarters-of-a-pound burger from a grain-fed cow, why not have a quarter pound of sliced sirloin in a stir-fry from a grass-fed animal? The actual difference in cost may be minimal.

Satiety is interesting. All too often we think we're hungry and grab something to eat, but most of the time we're acting out of boredom, not real hunger. What appears to be hunger may also be a sign of thirst. It's also important to understand that it is okay to be hungry. Most of us have never been truly hungry, as in starving. How do you find satisfaction in your food if you've never really experienced hunger? Most people are so hell-bent on thinking they need to eat five or six small meals a day that they're never really hungry, with the result that they never have a calorie deficit. I realize I am up against another sacred cow here. In the past decade the powers that be have beamed out this message: never let yourself get too hungry because you'll lose control of your appetite and wind up overeating at your next meal.

Myth 15: **Having five or six small meals a day will keep your blood sugar on an even keel so you'll eat less in toto and be able to slim down.**
Not true! The reality is that the multi-meal-a-day fad is just that. More important, it hasn't worked or we wouldn't have today's 40 percent obesity rate.

Are You *Really* Hungry?

When you feel ravenous, ask yourself these questions:

- *Am I thirsty?* Try having a glass of water or cup of herbal tea.
- *Am I bored?* Take a break from whatever you're doing, to take a short walk, do some yoga, or check in with a friend.
- *Am I stressed?* Take your mind off your problems by meditating, doing some deep breathing, or stretching.

- *Am I feeling social pressure?* If your office buddies are having their midmorning coffee break (with doughnuts), there's no
  reason you have to eat what they are having. Enjoy their company but not the grain and coffee.

Once you free yourself from these triggers, you will begin to distinguish between true hunger and other prompts.

THE BASICS OF THE NO-GRAIN, NO-PAIN PROGRAM

Once more, to be healthy and free of pain, you must eat only healthy food, which includes healthy animals that have not been fed geneti-cally modified organisms (GMOs). Instead, you will be eating the fol-lowing foods:

- Grass-fed/free-range meat and poultry, plus eggs from organic and/or free-range poultry
- Wild-caught fish
- Vegetables, fruit, and nuts, preferably organic, which are free (or more likely to be) of pesticides and other chemical trash that can damage the GI tract

A TWO-PHASE STRATEGY

Starting on Day 1 of the 15-day Kickoff phase, you'll begin to reap the rewards of a pain-free future by eliminating grains, dairy products, processed foods, and soy foods. On Day 16, as you begin the Chal-lenge phase, you'll also banish other inflammatory agents by saying good-bye to the following foods: vegetables in the nightshade fam-ily, all legumes, added sugar, and certain seeds, Just to be clear, you won't just be forgoing Wheat Chex for breakfast, a sandwich for lunch, and brown rice at dinner; you also won't be consuming *any* processed foods, including but not limited to those that contain grain in its many guises. "Gluten-free" bread is only one example. (See "Hidden in the Fine Print" on page 132.)

Why does the program consist of two phases? Quite frankly, I don't want you to feel overwhelmed from the get-go. Before you run, you need to learn to walk. Plus if I asked you to eliminate at once *all* the foods that are likely contributing to your pain and discomfort, it might be harder for you to comply. Once you see your aches and pains significantly moderate after the first couple of weeks on the Kickoff phase, you'll be hooked and motivated to knuckle down and really go for it in the next phase. Make the commitment, and when you experience the empowering changes and the realization that you hold the key to changing your life, you'll be rewarded.

Nonetheless, like tobacco, foods can be addictive. And the process of removing foods you've been eating for years is not unlike the challenge of quitting smoking. Again, my advice is always to keep the outcome top of mind: improved health and vitality, and likely a longer life span. Without question, changing your way of eating can be daunting at first, but I'm going to make it easier by providing lots of resources and complete lists of both foods to avoid and foods that are fine to eat, along with meal plans and delicious, easy-to-prepare recipes. Chapter 8 will focus on the Kickoff phase and chapter 9 on the Challenge phase.

OTHER ELIMINATION PATHS

My personal and professional opinion is that it is best to remove all suspect foods at one time, but I realize that is not something everyone can do. That's why I came up with the two-phase approach. But if you prefer to eliminate all problematic foods at the same time, go for it. However, I get that not everybody can go cold turkey. I would rather see you move toward the goal more slowly than continue to stay where you are, which actually means you're going backward, as you only feel worse over time as you continue to eat the same inflammatory foods.

When I tell a new patient the foods she needs to eliminate, there is often a moment of disbelief. I immediately add, "You're going to feel really good after that." Sometimes the person says, "I don't know if I can do that." At that point, I say what I am going to tell you: Don't feel overwhelmed. Don't let the stress of these changes paralyze you. If you feel like this is impossible and too daunting, I would rather see you first take wheat, barley, rye, oats, and corn out of your diet over the next few days. You're still going to experience some benefit, although not as much as you would if you went whole hog. Then remove sorghum, rice, and millet. As you see more results and get more comfortable with significantly changing eating your eating habits, you could then eliminate the pseudo-grains buckwheat, amaranth, and quinoa. Once you've eaten no grains for a week, move to Phase 2 to implement 100 percent of the program.

It will be challenging, but anyone can change a habit for 30 days. Many people assume that restrictive diets are hard, but my patients often find it a mind-blowing experience and don't want to go back to their old way of eating once they see the life-changing results. Almost all of them experience an almost immediate reduction in pain and improvement in symptoms. I firmly believe that will be your experience as well.

Despite all I have just said, there may be a little voice in your head nattering away at you, *I can't do this*. I can tell you that thousands of other people have heard similar chattering. They're not here to cheer you on, but I think that as you read their stories, you'll be inspired to hang in for 30 days. And let me add my own voice. You can do this, and I'm going to help you! Now listen to Phil's story.

A LESSON LEARNED

Phil was obese, chronically tired, and battled with suicidal depression. He also suffered from back pain, constant involuntary twitching of his muscles, and severe nerve pain on the left side of his body. Before seeing me he had surgery for his nerve and back pain, but ensuing complications only exacerbated his symptoms. He was on the brink of giving up.

A close friend of Phil's literally dragged him into my office. At first, Phil was a huge skeptic, arguing with me that diet had nothing to do with his problems and quick to blame the botched surgery. As I didn't need convincing, I simply told him, "You have two options. Either follow my protocol or don't. With the first option, you at least have hope. The alternative will only keep you in pain." The protocol was very simple: stop eating grain and supplement with 10,000 mcg of methylcobalamin, a form of vitamin B_{12}, in which he was deficient, known to cause nerve pain and depression.

Thankfully Phil decided on option one. Within a month of going grain free, he was almost pain free. Three months into treatment, his nerve and back pain were completely gone. He was also 45 pounds lighter, and his depression and brain fog were history. He was reenergized and, needless to say, had a new lease on life. Nonetheless, before fully recovering, Phil went off on a weekend binge of grain and alcohol. This set him back a few weeks, but it also served as an important lesson. He no longer "cheats" because he saw that eating grain reactivated his symptoms almost immediately. It took him about three days back on the wagon to recover. For more on Phil, visit glutenfreesociety .org/no-grain-no-pain-phils-story.

Crucial as diet is to your escape from the prison of pain, it's not the only factor. In the next chapter, you'll learn the importance of supplementation to help correct vitamin and mineral deficiencies to reduce inflammation and pain, as well as play a vital role in the healing process. There are also three other key components to the program:

GET MOVING

Motion and (initially gentle) exercise is critical to boost your metabolism and to bring oxygen and nutrients to both muscles and joints. The disadvantage of being sedentary is that it creates pain and inflammation in joints and muscles.

- Take a minimum of six thousand steps per day, preferably ten thousand steps. That's the equivalent of about 3 to 5 miles depending upon your height and therefore your gait.

- A simple pedometer or, if you prefer, an electronic tracker such as a Fitbit or a Jawbone, can be an effective motivation tool. Wear it all day so you track not just your walks, but also all your other daily activity.

- Whenever possible, stand rather than sit, and use every opportunity to stay in motion.

- Several short walks are better than a single long walk and being otherwise being inactive.

GET YOUR RAYS

Sunshine is critical for the production of vitamin D, which in turn helps control immune function and inflammation.[4] Sunshine also increases your level of the hormone melatonin, essential for adequate sleep. Sleep, in turn, regulates levels of the stress hormone cortisol, helping fight inflammation. Vitamin D deficiency is linked to chronic muscle pain and weakness, as well as insulin resistance.[5] And here's another motivator: getting adequate sunlight is even linked to greater life expectancy.[6]

- Spend a half hour a day outside, preferably first thing in the morning, exposed to sunlight.

- Otherwise, spend time outdoors as early as possible.

DRINK UP

Did you know that up to 66 percent of your body is composed of water? Even low-grade chronic dehydration can contribute to a sluggish metabolism. Being dehydrated can contribute to pain in the form of chronic muscle spasms; it also makes your blood thicker. Both leave you more prone to inflammation and can interfere with healing. Water also helps deliver nutrients to help heal tissues and to produce the mucous surfaces in the gut and lungs essential to immune protection. As a rule of thumb, if you're not urinating at least three or four times a day, you aren't consuming enough H_2O.

• Consume a minimum of 64 ounces (eight 8-ounce glasses) of water a day to enhance your kidneys' ability to eliminate toxins.

• Staying well hydrated helps moderate appetite so you eat less often, taxing your gut less frequently.

• Eating more vegetables also increases your fluid intake.

FREQUENTLY ASKED QUESTIONS

Q. When is the best time to start the program?
A. The trick is to set yourself up for success. Check your calendar to figure out when you can map out a relatively stress-free 30-day period without many work or social obligations. For that reason it's a good idea to avoid holidays or vacations. On the other hand, don't keep coming up with excuses not to begin. You may find it easier to start on a Saturday morning to get comfortable with the program before returning to work.

Q. Can some of the recommended water intake be in the form of other beverages?
A. Yes, you can substitute herbal teas and any of the other acceptable beverages (except coffee or black tea) listed on page 171.

Q. Can I use paleo recipes on the program?
A. Many but not all paleo recipes are acceptable, and you can certainly adapt them if necessary to comply with the No-Grain, No-Pain program. But your best bet when starting out is to use the recipes that start on page 257 and those you'll find at glutenfreesociety.org /forum/true-gluten-free-recipes-no-grains-please.

Q. Can a vegetarian do the No-Grain, No-Pain program?
A. Yes, although it is more difficult for vegans, who don't eat eggs. Protein will come from primarily from vegetables. Pea protein is the least allergenic of the legume proteins. Pescatarians will have it easier.

Before we get to the specifics and meal plans of the Kickoff and Challenge phases in chapters 8 and 9, turn the page to learn about the supplements I often prescribe to my patients to bring their vitamin, mineral, and other micronutrient status up to par. They are as important to reducing pain and inflammation as dietary changes.

BONUS FEATURE

A video of seven highly effective healthy habits of Gluten-Free Warriors: glutenfreesociety.org/effective-habits-video-giveaway.

CHAPTER 7

WHICH SUPPLEMENTS HELP ELIMINATE PAIN?

Speed Healing by Replacing Meds with Vitamins, Minerals, and Other Nutrients

I believe that you can, by taking some simple and inexpensive measures, lead a longer life and extend your years of well-being. My most important recommendation is that you take vitamins every day in optimum amounts to supplement the vitamins that you receive in your food.

—Linus Pauling

Could nutritional deficiencies be contributing to your pain? It's extremely likely. All too often, I find that my patients suffering from chronic pain and autoimmune conditions have multiple deficiencies that aggravate their discomfort and prevent or delay their body's natural healing process. Nutritional supplements alone won't eliminate pain, of course, but they're an important component of the No-Grain, No-Pain program. They enhance your body's ability to detox and repair itself, which will make it easier to follow the rest of the program.

There are several reasons why you might have inadequate levels of certain vitamins, minerals, and other nutrients. You may simply not be consuming a nutrient-rich diet. Alternatively, you may not be absorbing the nutrients in your food and/or supplements. Or the very medications most doctors use to treat chronic pain and autoimmune disease may be causing the deficiencies.[1] Remember that both NSAIDs and steroids are linked to GI problems, soft-tissue damage, and depletion of vitamin and mineral stores. In this chapter, I'll spell out which supplements are needed as a foundation to help you heal, and which can be used for their own anti-inflammatory and pain-reducing properties so you can reduce your reliance on—and ultimately eliminate—prescribed pain-blocking medications.

REASON 1: CORRECT NUTRITIONAL DEFICIENCIES

Supplementation is not just, ahem, supplemental to the No-Grain, No-Pain program; it is integral. That's why I'm detailing it before we get into the specifics of the Kickoff and Challenge phases of the diet itself. If you are like most people with chronic pain, you've been hurting for years and may be on multiple medications. That means that by now, you've probably already developed several of the nutritional deficiencies linked to either grain consumption or medication use. You may feel as though you're trapped in a pit. Even though your arms aren't long enough to reach the top, you have to dig your way out. Think of vitamins and minerals as the ladder that will make it easier for you to escape the deep, dark hole of pain. Even if you never again touch another kernel of grain, it would take you far longer to heal yourself without the support of the right vitamin and mineral supplements.

Some people can get better with food alone, but if you have neuropathy caused by vitamin B_{12} deficiency, for example, a grain-free regimen is not going to be enough to correct it because your gut is already damaged. And that damage would interfere with the proper absorption of nutrients a healthy gut would allow. You might have 70 percent functionality, maybe less, and perhaps much less. And the resultant damage could have been accumulating over many years before you even realized there was a problem. Supplementation is extremely helpful to allow the body to both repair damage and accelerate the overall healing process. I've frequently seen patients unable to heal until we implement supplementation. That said, supplements are never a replacement for whole food.

REASON 2: REDUCE PAIN AND INFLAMMATION

Often I find myself working with a patient who is on perhaps five medications prescribed by one or more other doctors. "Where do I begin?" she asks. "How do I stop the medicine that's causing the zinc deficiency that's causing the collagen breakdown that's causing the pain for which I need medicine?" She has been trapped in this vicious cycle. Fortunately, we can use supplements as an adjuvant to minimize pain and inflammation while aiding in the healing process. Unlike drugs, vitamins and minerals are essential for your body to heal, repair, and function normally. Additionally, supplements don't come with the same risks and side effects that drugs do. In the right doses, supplements can be used to help reduce pain and inflammation, thus helping wean you off medications.

If you're trying to get off a NSAID but are in pain every time you stop taking it, what can you do to attenuate the pain during this process? One approach might be to use high-dose curcumin and omega-3 fatty acids, along with glucosamine and MSM. All block inflammation, but without the detrimental effects of a NSAID. Such a combination allows you to get the inflammation- and pain-blocking benefit while moving in the right direction by changing your diet.

THE PAINFUL PRICE OF MULTIPLE
NUTRITIONAL DEFICIENCIES

One of my patients is a perfect example of the importance of targeted supplementation as integral to a cure. From early childhood, Rachel suffered from gastrointestinal problems. In 1995 she developed lymphoma. She underwent treatment and thankfully recovered. Over the next decade she had several precancerous lesions removed, as well as her gallbladder, and continued to have GI problems.

Several years later Rachel started to develop nerve pain, numbness, tingling, and muscle weakness in her arms and legs. Ascending paralysis made it difficult to keep her balance and to walk. The symptoms progressed over several months until one day she passed out in a doctor's office and was hospitalized, kept alive on a ventilator. During her three-week stay, she was diagnosed with epilepsy and breast cancer. Over the next year she started to develop more muscle weakness as well as memory problems. Her treatment for breast cancer continued for the next year, but her other symptoms continued to worsen. She was in and out of the hospital several times, including a bout in the ICU.

Rachel came to see me after her other doctors told her they could do no more for her. Through the course of my investigation, we found that she could tolerate no grain. And although this was the most important change for her—gluten is a known factor in the development of epilepsy, neuropathy, and lymphoma—we also found that she was allergic to beans, dairy products, beef, carrageenan gum (a thickener found in many foods), garlic, watermelon, and peanuts, as well as pesticides. She had severe inflammation in her GI tract, and her pancreas was not producing enough digestive enzymes to properly digest her food. Without her gallbladder, she was at a serious nutritional disadvantage. She was also deficient in vitamins B_{12}, C, D, and K, as well as biotin, glutamine, carnitine, cysteine, choline, and many other nutrients, likely due to her chemotherapy treatments. Her nutritional status was so severe that without supplementation, she would not have made a proper recovery.

Rachel literally went from a ventilator and a wheelchair to dancing, driving, and living life again. Her muscle pain and gastrointestinal problems were gone in a matter of weeks. After several months of supplementation and dietary change, instead of multiple seizures a day, she experienced only mild episodes months apart. In Rachel's case, high doses of vitamin B_{12} were required to help her nervous system repair itself, and she stays on this critical vitamin even a year later to prevent nerve problems from creeping back. The moral of this story: supplementation plus no grain equals no pain. For more of Rachel's story, visit youtube.com/watch?v=3cI7vaCcZus.

YOU GET WHAT YOU PAY FOR

If you have ever stood paralyzed in front of the dozens of choices for a single supplement in your pharmacy or natural products store, you know how confusing a purchasing decision it can be. And how can you be assured that the supplements you do select will deliver the promised results and that you are not just paying for expensive urine?[2]

When you select supplements, you want to avoid any that contain:

- Genetically modified organisms (GMO)
- Grain, in the form of corn- or other grain-based fillers* (see: glutenfreesociety.org/hidden-corn-based-ingredients)
- Yeast
- Artificial colors or flavors
- Added sugars or sugar substitutes
- Iron (unless you've been diagnosed as iron deficient)

Instead look for products that contain none of the offending ingredients above and:

- Are taken in multiple doses (not just once a day)
- In the case of B vitamins, contain only the most effective forms (see pages 152, 153 and 159)

Bottom line: Read labels. Then reread them!

---

*Products labeled "gluten-free" contain no wheat, barley, or rye, but may contain other grains.

Grain in Disguise

All supplements contain fillers in addition to nutrients. But many of the fillers commonly used are sourced from grain. To avoid consuming hidden grains, avoid any supplements unless the manufacturer confirms that they are grain free. The following ingredients are, may be made from, or may contain, one or more grains:

Citric acid (may be corn)
Corn
Dextrin
Dextrose
Food starch
High-fructose corn syrup
   (HFCS)
Hydroxypropylated starch
Maize
Malt
Maltodextrin (wheat or corn
   based)
Maltose
Pregelatinized starch
Propylene glycol
Rice flour

Saccharin
Splenda
Sucralose
Syrup (commonly from
   sorghum, rice, corn, and
   barley)
Talc
Vanillin
Vegetable gum
Vegetable oil (usually corn
   and soy)
Vegetable protein
Xanthan gum
Xylitol
Yeast
Zein

Let's explore some of the no-nos listed in "Grain in Disguise." Fillers are found not just in multivitamins, but also in targeted supplements. In addition to those derived from GMO corn, rice powder, wheat, and maltodextrin are also common. Not all starches are necessarily bad. Some non-GMO starches, including potato starch or root starches, are fine. But avoid GMO cornstarch at all costs: it makes it really hard to digest some of these pills, to say nothing of introducing the very grains that are causing your problems. One of the most frequent problems with supplement-related inflammation and pain is gluten contamination.[3] I see it regularly in my practice.

Then there is the lacquer, perhaps made of acrylic, which manufacturers sometimes use to contain the odor of B vitamins, making them more palatable and easier to swallow. If a person's gut is already damaged, a highly lacquered pill will be hard to break down in order to release the nutrients. If the coating remains, you're wasting your money and not helping yourself get better. Many of the heavily advertised multivitamins are sprayed with such a glaze. Artificial dyes and colors—especially blue and red—are also common, particularly in brands such as Centrum and Flintstones and gummy vitamins for kids, along with added sugars and artificial sweeteners.

You want the highest quality in any supplement you are taking, of course, but specificity is the real issue. Do you need it? Is it something that will help you in particular, or is it just a general recommendation? So while I will cite certain supplements in the following pages, along with therapeutic dosage ranges, I recommend you work with a functional medicine practitioner who will run appropriate tests to ascertain any nutritional deficiencies you may have and tailor the dosage ranges to address these particular shortfalls.

That said, there's little risk in taking most supplements. Of course, there are a few exceptions, such as remedies sold to promote weight loss that could contain ingredients not listed on the label, some with the same effects as amphetamines. Heavy media coverage of these products in early 2015 led to their removal from store shelves. The nutrients we are talking about are not at risk of such contamination. Rather, what you should be concerned about is that if you're taking a supplement but not using a therapeutic dose, you're very possibly wasting your time—and money. Like spitting on a forest fire, it's an exercise in futility. You may need a much higher dose. For example, with vitamin B_{12}, oftentimes a multivitamin will contain 100 mcg, but you may require 10,000 to 15,000 mcg to correct a deficiency that may be contributing to elevated homocysteine, which is linked to inflammation and tissue damage.

A GOOD MULTIVITAMIN IS A MUST

I recommend a multivitamin as a general agent of health, while I recommend specific vitamins for an individual's unique needs. Most multivitamins/minerals contain grain, so check carefully to ensure

yours is grain free. (Again, check out glutenfreesociety.org/hidden
-corn-based-ingredients.) Vitamins C, D, B_{12}, and B_1, as well as zinc,
CoQ_{10}, and omega-3 are likely to be in your multivitamin. All are critical to recovery and repair of pain and inflammation, but the quantities in a multi are insufficient for therapeutic purposes, in part because
many of the pain-relieving drugs you may have been taking block these
nutrients. Nonsteroidal anti-inflammatory drugs block vitamin C, steroids block vitamin D, and high blood pressure medications block
vitamins C, B_{12}, and B_1, as well as zinc and CoQ_{10}. Chronic damage
to the gut from grain inhibits the absorption of all nutrients. Most
multivitamins contain poor forms of nutrients the body barely recognizes. Most also provide meaningless doses, are synthetic, and contain
GMOs, grain fillers, and artificial sweeteners. Bottom line: they just
aren't good for you.

The science and art of making good vitamins is complicated and
beyond the scope of this book, but it is important to understand that
all forms of a vitamin aren't the same. For example, there are four different kinds of B_{12}. Which one are you getting? Most people are getting the cheapest one because manufacturers assume the consumer is
ignorant of the differences among them. In this case, you want methylcobalamin or hydroxycobalamin, rather than cyanocobalamin or ade-
nosylcobalamin.

NUTRITIONALLY BASED PAIN REMEDIES

Now let's discuss the therapeutic use of supplements. Many people
suffering from chronic pain are deficient in the following nutrients.

Vitamin C is an anti-inflammatory,[4] an antioxidant, and a major
player in the repair and recovery process of those with gluten sensitivity.[5] No multivitamin contains enough.

- *Preferred form:* Ascorbate
- *Signs of deficiency:* Bleeding gums, joint pain and swelling, tendency to bruise easily, fatigue, and rough skin

- *Key functions:* Helps reduce gluten-induced inflammation, detoxify the liver, protect against cell damage, promote adrenal health, prevent constriction of blood vessels, repair tissues, regulate neurotransmitter production, reduce heavy metal accumulation, and destroy cancer cells
- *Therapeutic daily dose:* 1–10 grams

Vitamin D₃ production by your body requires regular exposure to sunshine. Its deficiency can exacerbate and contribute to the development of autoimmune diseases in gluten-sensitive individuals. If you have celiac disease or are gluten sensitive, work indoors, avoid sunshine, live in a northern climate, or overuse sunscreen, you are likely deficient.

- *Preferred form:* Cholecalciferol
- *Signs of deficiency:* Muscle pain and/or weakness, poor immune function, sinus and other chronic infections, eczema, acne, cancer, and cardiovascular disease; poor growth or bowed legs in children
- *Key functions:* Helps regulate many vital body functions, including building strong bones and muscles, and prevents autoimmune disease by regulating immune cells
- *Therapeutic daily dose:* 6,000–10,000 IU (make sure you have your levels checked after three months to reduce the risk of toxicity)

Zinc is a mineral and an antioxidant. Its deficiency is rampant in gluten-sensitive individuals, and is often why many people who eliminate all grains without supplementation don't fully recover.

- *Preferred forms:* Picolinate and citrate
- *Signs of deficiency:* Reduced immunity, hair loss, fatigue, poor blood sugar control, malabsorption of nutrients, digestive disruption, and loose bowels
- *Key functions:* Helps make digestive enzymes that enable absorption of nutrients in food; helps protect against free radicals;

essential to metabolism of omega-3 fats and enables a vegetarian to convert plant sources of omega-3 to ones the body can use; helps offset insulin resistance

- *Therapeutic daily dose:* 50–150 mg

Vitamin B$_{12}$ deficiency is extremely common in those with gluten issues, even when they eat sufficient animal protein, because gluten can damage the stomach's acid-producing cells, which make the intrinsic factor that ferries B$_{12}$ to the intestines, where it is absorbed. Gluten can also damage the area of the small intestine where most B$_{12}$ is absorbed into the bloodstream. Vegetarians and older people are also at high risk of deficiency.

- *Preferred forms:* Methylcobalamin or hydroxycobalamin
- *Signs of deficiency:* Fatigue, headaches, weight gain, brain fog, lack of mental clarity, poor memory, sleep disorders, joint and muscle pain, depression, irritability, neuropathy, ringing in the ears, and dizziness
- *Key functions:* Repairs and replicates DNA and RNA; produces insulation surrounding nerves in the brain and spinal cord; protects against cardiovascular disease, dementia, and neuropathy; maintains energy production; helps produce melatonin to regulate sleep
- *Therapeutic daily dose:* 2,000 to 15,000 mcg

Vitamin B$_1$, an essential (meaning that your body can't produce it) nutrient, is found in most foods, especially meats, mushrooms, cruciferous vegetables, asparagus, and peas. Gluten damages the GI tract, causing malabsorption of nutrients, and the resulting inflammation increases the body's demand for all eight B vitamins in order to heal. Processed grains, especially "gluten-free" substitutes, contain very little vitamin B and must be fortified with synthetic thiamine. Medications that cause deficiency include digoxin (Lanoxin), furosemide (Lasix), and other loop diuretics (Bumex, Demadex, hydrochlorothiazide) that lower blood pressure. So can chronic alcohol use.

- *Preferred forms:* Thiamine or benfotiamine

- *Signs of deficiency:* Difficulty digesting carbs (sugars); may contribute to glucose intolerance, muscle pains, poor appetite and weight loss, fatigue and weakness, loss of mental alertness, depression, impaired breathing, peripheral neuropathy, uncontrolled eye movements, and cataracts

- *Key functions:* Helps generate energy from food and prevent many serious conditions including depression, cataracts (in combination with other vitamins), heart failure, cirrhosis, and anorexia

- *Therapeutic daily dose:* 100–300 mg

Coenzyme Q$_{10}$ is an antioxidant your body produces, and eating meat provides more, but supplementation may be needed to overcome damage. Nerve drugs and those for hypertension, high cholesterol, and depression, among others, also block CoQ$_{10}$. It is primarily concentrated in liver, brain, and muscle tissue because they use the most energy.

- *Preferred form:* Ubiquinone

- *Signs of deficiency:* Fatigue, muscle pain, brain fog, and neuropathy and nerve damage

- *Key functions:* Helps preserve the integrity of the nucleic materials within DNA and acts as a "spark plug" to convert energy to a usable form

- *Therapeutic daily dose:* 50–300 mg

Magnesium is an essential mineral, meaning that your body can't produce it. Chronic stress depletes stores, as do diuretics, including caffeine, alcohol, and blood pressure medications. A high intake of refined carbohydrates also causes deficiency.

- *Preferred forms:* Glycinate, citrate, malate, and threonate

- *Signs of deficiency:* Depression; hypertension; bone loss (osteopenia and osteoporosis); muscle spasms in the eyes or elsewhere, with resultant pain and inflammation; thickened blood; elevated cholesterol

• *Key functions:* Among more than three hundred functions, enables protein synthesis and proper muscle and nerve function, as well as regulation of blood sugar and blood pressure; also essential for energy production, normal heart rhythm, and bone development

• *Therapeutic daily dose:* 200–600 mg

MSM (methylsulfonylmethane) is a sulfur compound found in meat, seafood, and vegetables that helps keeps tendons, ligaments, and muscles healthy by decreasing the pressure within the cells of those connective tissues.

• *Preferred form:* Lignin from pine trees

• *Key functions:* Relief from chronic pain from various forms of arthritis, joint inflammation, and muscle pain

• *Therapeutic daily dose:* 1,000–3,000 mg

Glucosamine is one of the building blocks of joint cartilage.

• *Preferred form:* Sulfate

• *Key functions:* In addition to being necessary for cartilage repair and resilience, it also works another way. Wheat germ agglutinin (WGA) is actually a lectin, a protein that is a sort of second cousin to gluten, and can provoke a similar inflammatory response. WGA is what makes wheat difficult for many people to digest, regardless of whether they are gluten sensitive. WGA tends to go after cartilaginous tissue, where it can create inflammation—and therefore joint pain. (There is actually more WGA in whole-wheat products than in refined wheat, from which the fibrous coating has been removed.) Here's where glucosamine comes in. By binding to WGA, it blocks the inflammatory effect, helping relieve the joint pain. People who are extremely gluten sensitive or who otherwise have an issue with WGA are most likely to benefit from using this supplement.[6]

• *Therapeutic daily dose:* 500–2,000 mg

Deplete It and Then Charge to Replace It

If you, like 25 percent of American adults over the age of 45, are taking a statin drug such as Pravachol or Lipitor to lower your cholesterol, you'll see a warning on the information sheet stating that a possible side effect is depletion of CoQ_{10}. Here's why: the statin blocks an enzyme called HMG-CoA reductase, which makes cholesterol, but the statin also blocks production of CoQ_{10} and vitamin D. Insufficient CoQ_{10} can weaken your heart's pumping capacity and circulatory system, with potentially devastating results. For this reason, physicians often advise taking a CoQ_{10} supplement to replace what it blocks. Merck, which makes the statin drug Zocor, seeing a potential marketing opportunity, took out a patent on a statin fortified with CoQ_{10}. Although Merck hasn't yet released such a product, the patent ensures that for the time being no other drug company can sell such a product.[7]

Omega-3 fatty acids are essential, meaning the body cannot make them. The best sources are fatty cold-water fish such as salmon, mackerel, herring, sardines, and anchovies.

• *Preferred form:* A combination *of* eicosapentaenoic acid (EPA) and docosahexaenoic acid (DHA)

• *Signs of deficiency:* Pain without injury, dry skin, hypertension, high cholesterol, elevated triglycerides, brain fog, and poor memory

• *Key functions:* DHA is the predominant essential fatty acid in the brain and is necessary for the production of myelin, a kind of fat that covers and protects the nerve fibers in the brain's white matter. EPA regulates inflammation and enhances healthy immune function by helping block the conversion of omega-6 fatty acids to arachidonic acid. Optimal levels of omega-3 therefore block the inflammatory action of omega-6s; they also regulate the consistency of blood, thinning it to its natural viscosity.

- *Therapeutic daily dose:* 2–10 grams

MOTHER NATURE'S PAINKILLERS AND ANTI-INFLAMMATORIES

A number of herbal and other plant-based medicines can be used to help reduce pain and inflammation while healing. Unlike zinc, omega-3s, and other nutrients discussed above, the following remedies are not essential to life, but they can most certainly enhance it. Three of my favorites are also culinary ingredients: turmeric (from which comes curcumin), ginger, and garlic. Turmeric is commonly used in Indian and other East Asian cuisines, lending a yellow hue to curries. Feel free to use these ingredients in meals, but at that "dosage," they're unlikely to provide any medicinal value. Instead, for pain and inflammation relief, you will need medicinal grade, which is more concentrated.

- *Turmeric:* The active ingredient in turmeric is curcuminoid, so turmeric and curcumin are essentially one and the same. A very powerful anti-inflammatory compound, it can be of great benefit to those in chronic pain.[8] *Preferred form:* Standardized to 95 percent per curcuminoid. *Therapeutic daily dose:* 500–2,000 mg.

- *Ginger root* has traditionally been used to help relieve nausea, indigestion, and heart irregularities.[9] Another powerful anti-inflammatory, it works by blocking the enzyme cyclooxygenase (COX), the same mechanism of action used in commonly prescribed NSAIDs, but without the side effect of gastric bleeding and thinned blood. *Therapeutic daily dose:* 500–2,000 mg.

- *Garlic*, a member of the onion family (genus *Allium*), contains strong anti-inflammatory compounds.[10] It also helps the body detoxify, protects against NSAID-induced stomach damage, and has anti-yeast and -bacterial properties. In addition, garlic has the ability to lower blood pressure and cholesterol, reduce the risk of cancer, and improve lymphatic flow. *Preferred form:* Standardized to contain allicin. *Therapeutic daily dose:* 200–600 mg.

• *Skullcap* is an herb that inhibits the COX-2 enzymes that lead to inflammation. It is known to help against antibiotic-resistant yeast and bacterial infections.[11] *Therapeutic daily dose:* 1–2 grams standardized to contain 30 percent *S. baicalensis.*

• *Proteolytic enzymes* are derived from digestive enzymes. Taken on an empty stomach (four hours after a meal), they actually enter your bloodstream, enabling their potent anti-inflammatory and healing properties to boost the natural inflammation process to eliminate damaged tissue and speed the growth of new tissue.[12] A lot of grains inhibit the action of enzymes. Your pancreas is generally responsible for producing proteolytic enzymes, but when a grain-heavy diet overburdens it, enzymatic deficiency can occur. Digestive enzymes can be helpful to digest food in the gut, but proteolytic enzymes actually help it heal. They may be as effective at reducing pain as NSAIDs without their side effects.

• *Probiotics* are another tool in the intestinal healing repair kit. A live culture of *Lactobacillus* and *Bifidobacterium* strains, they help restore healthy bacteria damaged by long-term gluten consumption.[13] However, a study presented at the 2015 Digestive Disease Week conference stated that analysis revealed that many top-selling probiotic products labeled as gluten free were actually contaminated with gluten.[14] This followed a study that found that people with celiac disease who take probiotics experience more bloating, cramping, and other symptoms of the disease than those who do not.[15] The latter study likely explains why and, rather than obviating the value of taking probiotics, makes it clear that not all supplements are created equal.

• *Therapeutic daily dose:* 1–400 billion CFUs.

THE GRAIN-FREE, PAIN-FREE
SUPPLEMENT PROTOCOL

I am not suggesting that anyone take all the supplements discussed above. However, I do highly recommend that everyone take a quality multivitamin and omega-3 supplement, and that everyone who is gluten sensitive take probiotics and digestive enzymes. In my experience, those who use targeted supplementation heal faster. And some others don't heal at all without supplementation.

PAIN AND ILLNESS HAD BECOME HER NORMAL

One of my favorite patient success stories is Candra, whose lifetime of health issues started as a child and included ten surgeries. She was so used to being sick that she thought it was her normal. She suffered from back pain, hair loss, low energy, hormone imbalances, and the inability to sleep well.

When she came to see me, Candra had already changed her diet and worked with various supplements to try to improve her health. Both of these approaches were helpful, but she had plateaued and couldn't figure out why. Candra tested positive for a gluten sensitive gene pattern as well as for multiple allergies including dairy products, black tea, basil, grape-seed oil, cinnamon, blue dyes, and pesticides. Because of vitamin B_{12} and folate deficiencies, her body wasn't producing enough white blood cells. She was also deficient in several other B vitamins and in glutamine. In essence, her immune system was not capable of supporting her needs.

Within weeks of additional diet changes and supplementation, Candra's symptoms dramatically changed. Her pain disappeared, her energy rebounded, and her severe symptoms of hormone imbalance all improved. Her results were so rapid that she brought in her daughter to see me as well—and this is my favorite part. Her little girl is as cute as they come. Sadly, she was dealing with severe gut, allergy, and skin problems. Removing grains and adding supplemental treatment led to a rapid resolution. Kids always heal faster than adults when you make the right changes. I'm happy to say that she no longer has stomach pains, and her immune system is so strong that she no longer has to avoid dogs—and what little girl wouldn't want a puppy? For more of Candra's story, visit youtube.com/watch?v=buQOmj7D7nY.

BONUS FEATURES

Gluten sensitivities and vitamin deficiencies: visit glutenfreesociety .org/gluten-sensitivity-and-vitamin-deficiencies.

Vitamin supplements contaminated with gluten: visit glutenfreeso ciety.org/vitamin-supplements-contaminated-with-gluten.

PILL OVERLOAD?

Many people take handfuls of pills in an effort to improve their symptoms. This is not always necessary. Don't assume that you need to take *all* the supplements described above. Your needs depend upon your individual nutritional status. For a protocol designed for your particular needs, I recommend you see a functional medicine practitioner. (See chapter 11 for more information.)

Now turn the page to learn how to begin the Kickoff phase of the No-Grain, No-Pain program.

CHAPTER 8

DAYS 1 TO 15

Kick Off Your Plan by Eliminating All Grains

Chronic disease is a foodborne illness. We ate our way into this mess, and we must eat our way out.

—Mark Hyman, MD

Okay, it's time to zero in on the food portion of the Kickoff phase of the No-Grain, No-Pain program. But I must remind you that eating certain foods and eliminating others is only one part of this program. Four other interlocking components, including the supplement protocol in the previous chapter, are key to your journey to wellness and freedom from pain. Follow this phase of the program for 15 days, and you'll likely see reduced pain and joint stiffness, particularly in the morning, as well as improved energy. Are you ready? Let's get going.

Eat right by eliminating:

- All grains and pseudo-grains (buckwheat, amaranth, and quinoa) and all foods that contain them

- Meat from grain- and soy-fed beef and other animals, as well as caged poultry raised on grain and soy (instead, eat grass-fed/pastured meat and free-range/organic poultry and eggs)
- All farm-raised fish and shellfish
- All dairy products, including fermented dairy products such as yogurt and kefir, as well as dairy derivatives (whey or casein protein powder)
- All processed and GMO foods, including so-called gluten-free products, and any other artificial ingredients
- All soy products, including fermented soy products such as soy sauce and tofu
- All manufactured sugars
- All artificial sweeteners

Instead, eat whole, preferably organic foods, including most vegetables and fruit. After 15 days, you'll move on to the Challenge phase, in which you'll remove additional problematic foods and learn how to practice intermittent fasting.

AT RISK OF LOSING HER SIGHT

Nancy was diagnosed with a painful autoimmune disease called ankylosing spondylitis (AS). In addition to causing severe joint pain and swelling, the AS was deteriorating her vision. Nancy had a long history of gastrointestinal problems, as well. She was on multiple medications to help alleviate her pain and swelling, including steroids, water pills, and acid reflux medications. She had been to multiple doctors who had performed countless medical tests, but to no avail. A test for celiac disease came back negative (of course), and her GI doctor insisted that she continue eating gluten. Her pain persisted.

Nancy came to see me at her wits' end. She was frustrated with her lack of improvement and was petrified about the next level of treatments that her doctors wanted to try.

What happened next? You guessed it. Nancy had a gluten-sensitive gene pattern, along with multiple nutritional problems, including deficiencies of the amino acid serine and vitamin C. She was allergic to squash, oranges, and a commonly used pesticide. Her cortisol levels were in the tank, making it impossible to fight inflammation. That's what made the vitamin C deficiency so important to recognize. You see, vitamin C is like fuel for the adrenal glands. Without it, the adrenals have a hard time making the hormone cortisol, and the body's ability to combat inflammation is greatly hindered.

I put Nancy on a grain-free, allergen-free diet, supplemented her nutritional deficiencies, and talked with her about stress management to aid in adrenal recovery. Within days, Nancy started to feel better. After suffering for more than a decade, a no-grain diet led to complete remission of Nancy's disease. For more of Nancy's story, visit youtube .com/watch?v=OXdJBcRPPes.

FIRST, THINK HEALTHY

Once more, the traditional gluten-free approach is to avoid wheat, rye, barley, and perhaps oats, but otherwise continue eating as usual, simply replacing wheat pasta with pasta made with corn or rice, wheat bread with "gluten-free" bread, and so forth. But to be a *true* Gluten-Free Warrior battling to restore your health requires a different approach. That means that you are looking first for healthy food and only second for gluten-free choices.

What do I mean by that? Well, the first requirement automatically eliminates almost all "gluten-free" foods, which are typically as processed as the "frood" that comprises 95 percent of what you'll find on supermarket shelves. Processed "gluten-free" food is rarely made with organic ingredients and typically contains GMO soy flour, soy and other manufactured "vegetable" oils, added sugar, and other grains, which will likely only fan the flames of your inflammation and pain. (By the way, organic processed foods are also often full of empty calories.) In order to make your food pass the healthy test, follow these guidelines:

- Make it organic whenever possible.
- The less processing and packaging, the better.
- Read ingredient lists and avoid anything full of chemicals. If you can't pronounce it, don't buy it.

Remember, you can't get healthy eating unhealthy food.

TOUGH LOVE ON FOOD SUBSTITUTIONS

Unlike most diet books, this will not offer a long list of "eat this instead of that" foods. The conventional reasoning is that providing substitutes makes it easier to follow a diet plan. I beg to disagree. It may be easier, but if it doesn't deliver the results you are after, what's the point? You already know about the gluten-free whiplash phenomenon, attributed to substituting one kind of grain for another, but that's only part of my rationale. If food has been chemically bleached, genetically modified, and packed with pesticides, it's still processed food. You're sick because you're doing what you're doing, so if you don't change what you're doing, you're going to continue to be ill. That's why we're not going to substitute this processed food for that processed food merely because it contains a different grain or grains. Instead, let's change the behavior. My program offers a whole different mind-set from the grain-centric way we've come to believe is the only way to eat. Once your diet consists of wild-caught fish, grass-fed meat and free-range organic poultry, and lots of great vegetables and some fruit, you're going to feel better. Note that *my* short list of *"True* Gluten-Free Substitutes" includes only whole foods.

True Gluten-Free Substitutes

Instead of this	Have this
Milk and other dairy products	Organic coconut "milk" or almond "milk"*
Oatmeal	Ground organic flaxseed with coconut milk
Cold cereal	Ground organic nuts, shredded organic coconut, fruit
Rice	Wild rice (a grass, not a grain)
Pasta	Spaghetti squash, shredded zucchini
White vinegar and rice vinegar	Organic cider vinegar, balsamic vinegar†
Bread, crackers, chips	Nuts and seeds, paleo trail mix
Soy sauce	Organic Coconut Aminos‡

Now let's look at the other delicious foods you *will* be eating in the first 15 days, as well as more gluten-filled foods you will eliminate from your meals.

KICKOFF PHASE ACCEPTABLE FOODS

ACCEPTABLE MEAT

Any variety and cut is okay, but you must consider the source. If the cow or pig or lamb has been grain fed, steer clear. You want to eat only meat from grass-fed or free-range animals, including bison.

*Use only unflavored, unsweetened products without carrageenan gum.
†Phase 1 only.
‡Made from fermented coconut and available at Amazon.com. One brand is Coconut Secret.

ACCEPTABLE POULTRY

It is hard to find totally free-range chickens in most regions, but if they eat organic feed, at least they aren't full of GMO grain and soybeans spiked with fertilizers and pesticides. Likewise, consume only eggs from free-range and organic hens and ducks. (Some people who are unable to tolerate hen eggs have no problem with duck eggs.)

ACCEPTABLE WILD GAME

In addition to bison, venison, elk, boar, pheasant, grouse, and other fowl are great protein sources. However, be sure they are truly wild and not from a ranch where they were simply pumped full of GMO corn and soy.

ACCEPTABLE FISH

Eat only wild-caught fish and shellfish. Farm-raised fish are restrained in nets and fed fish meal, a slurry of ground-up fish mixed with GMO corn and soy. Corn and soy are not the foods Mother Nature intended finned creatures to eat. I've never seen a fish jump out of the water and levitate into a soybean or wheat field! Avoid all farm-raised seafood, if only for their enormous imbalance of omega-6 to omega-3 fats.

Sounds Fishy to Me

The pink or red flesh of wild salmon comes from the shells of the minute shellfish called krill upon which they feed. In contrast, farm-raised salmon have white flesh, which is dyed pink. Those tiny krill, which eat plankton, are what make salmon such a good source of inflammation-soothing omega-3 fatty acids. Needless to say, red dye doesn't do the trick. Setting a disturbing precedent, the FDA has approved the first GMO animal protein, called AquAdvantage salmon. This "Frankenfish" is derived from Atlantic salmon, with an added growth-hormone gene from the Chinook salmon inserted. The GMO salmon grows in half the time to twice the size of a natural Atlantic salmon. Some major food chains, including Kroger and Safeway, have announced they will refuse to sell AquAdvantage salmon. If it is of any comfort, it must carry a GMO label.

ACCEPTABLE VEGETABLES

Organic is key, because conventionally grown produce has been treated with fungicides, pesticides, herbicides, fertilizers, and other chemicals. Opt for in-season vegetables for their superior taste and nutrient content. Finally, buy local produce whenever possible, not just because it is fresher, but also to keep independent farmers in business. They're the ones doing things right. When fresh organic is not available or is out of season, frozen organic veggies are an acceptable substitute, assuming they aren't in a sauce. Note that you will eliminate some of the vegetables listed below in the Challenge phase. In this phase, enjoy any vegetable (except corn, which is really a grain) to which you are not allergic or reactive, including:

Artichoke	Celery
Arugula	Chard
Asparagus	Collard greens
Bamboo shoots	Cucumber
Bean sprouts	Dandelion greens
Beets	Eggplant
Bell peppers	Garlic
Bok choy	Kale
Broccoli	Kohlrabi
Brussels sprouts	Lettuce (green or red leaf,
Cabbage (white, green, red, Chinese, savoy)	romaine, iceberg, Bibb, butterhead, Boston, etc.)
Carrots	Mushrooms
Cauliflower	Okra

Onion (and leeks, shallots, and green onions)

Parsnips

Peas

Potatoes

Radishes

Rutabaga

Tomatoes (technically a fruit)

Turnips

Spinach

Squash (yellow, butternut, spaghetti, acorn, pumpkin, etc.)

String beans

Sweet potatoes

Turnips

Water chestnuts

Watercress

Yams

Zucchini (and other summer squash)

ACCEPTABLE FRUITS

The same advice applies to fruits as to veggies: eat organic, seasonal, and local, whenever possible. Dried fruits without sulfates or added sugar are acceptable in extreme moderation. Frozen organic fruit without added sugar is also acceptable. (Check out my recipe for No-Pain Ice "Cream" made with frozen organic fruit and coconut milk on page 288.) Enjoy any organic fruit to which you are not allergic or reactive, including:

Apples

Apricots (and nectarines)

Avocado (botanically a fruit)

Bananas (including plantains)

Berries (acai berries, blueberries, blackberries, boysenberries, cranberries, goji berries, raspberries, and strawberries)

Cherries

Dates

Figs

Grapefruit

Guava

Kiwifruit

Kumquats

Lemons

Limes

Mango

Melons (cantaloupe, honeydew, watermelon)

Oranges, tangerines, clementines

Papaya

Passion fruit   Plantains

Peaches   Plums

Pears   Pomegranate

Pineapple

ACCEPTABLE BEANS AND LEGUMES

In this phase you can have any of the many varieties of beans, with the exception of soybeans, which are almost always GMO. Rinse, then soak in fresh water for several hours or overnight, then drain the water and cook in fresh water. Sprouting or fermenting legumes also improves their overall digestability and removes toxins. (See *Nourishing Traditions* by Sally Fallon [Washington, DC: New Trends, 2001] for more ways to prepare beans to make them easier to digest.) You may be surprised to learn that coffee beans are actually legumes. Other common varieties include:

Black beans   Mung beans

Black-eyed peas   Navy beans

Chickpeas (garbanzos)   Peas

Kidney beans   Pinto beans

Lentils (multiple varieties)   Red beans

Lima beans   White beans

ACCEPTABLE NUTS AND NON-GRAIN SEEDS

Any organic variety to which you are not allergic or reactive, including:

Almonds   Chia seeds

Brazil nuts   Coconuts

Cacao seeds (cocoa nibs)   Flaxseed

Cashews (a seed, not a true nut)   Hazelnuts

Chestnuts   Macadamias

Peanuts (a legume, not a true nut)*

Pecans

Pine nuts (pinyons)

Pistachios

Pumpkin seeds (pepitas)

Sunflower seeds

Walnuts

ACCEPTABLE OILS

Purchase only cold-pressed, organic oils, and only extra-virgin cold-pressed organic olive oil.

Avocado oil

Coconut oil

Grape-seed oil

Macadamia nut oil

Olive oil

Palm oil

Sesame oil

ACCEPTABLE CONDIMENTS

Most sauces and marinades are packed with sugar or corn syrup, and many also contain cornstarch and other forms of grain. Herbs and spices, however are free of sugars and grains, but do avoid spice or herb mixtures, which are often enhanced with sugar. Rely primarily on sea salt, pepper, parsley, basil, thyme, and other herbs such as garlic, cumin, and turmeric to flavor your foods. Also acceptable are:

Apple cider vinegar

Coconut Aminos (see *"True Gluten-Free Substitutes"* on page 165)

Homemade mayonnaise made with olive oil and cider vinegar or lemon juice

Horseradish

Mustard made with apple cider vinegar such as Eden Foods organic yellow mustard

Organic tomato paste* in lieu of ketchup such as Bionaturae

Pesto (minus the cheese, of course)

Red wine vinegar and balsamic vinegar*

*Acceptable in Phase 1 only.

ACCEPTABLE BEVERAGES

Most teas are contaminated with pesticides, so use only organic brands and do not add dairy or soy milk, or grain-based milk substitutes.

Fresh-squeezed or unpasteurized fruit juice with no added sugars

Organic black,* green, or herbal tea (unsweetened)

Organic coffee*

Water (filtered, mineral, sparkling) and unflavored seltzer (avoid brands with sodium benzoate as a preservative)

Prepare for Caffeine Withdrawal

If you must, you may drink coffee in moderation in this phase. The coffee bean is actually a legume, so that cuppa joe is really bean juice! If you've been eating gluten-free and are still experiencing certain symptoms, the culprit may be coffee, so you may want to eliminate it now. Otherwise, start cutting back, as you'll be eliminating it altogether in a couple of weeks. Here's why:

- Coffee is one of several foods that cause what's called gluten cross-reactivity. Basically, your body perceives them as mimicking gluten.[1] Instant coffee and some ground coffees appear to be the most cross-reactive, but organic, whole-bean coffees do not produce this problem. If you must have coffee, buy organic beans and grind them yourself.

- Coffee beans may be contaminated with mycotoxins, a mold toxin also found in corn.[2] Roasting the beans could reduce the quantity of these toxins. Nor is everyone is sensitive to them.

- Coffee is one of the crops most heavily treated with pesticides, which can cause intestinal damage and leaky gut, and disrupt estrogen[3] and other hormone levels.

*Acceptable in Phase 1 only.

• Caffeine can affect the GI tract in a number of ways, including increased gastroesophageal reflux disease (GERD) and reduction of blood flow to the intestines.[4]

• Caffeine can overstimulate the adrenal glands, allowing certain symptoms to persist and inhibit the recovery process.

• Coffee acts as a diuretic, which can lead to dehydration.[5] It can also wash out water-soluble vitamins and minerals that are important in the healing process.[6]

Finally, the caffeine in coffee can cause stress and anxiety. My advice is to give it a pass.

ACCEPTABLE SWEETENERS

Once you eliminate all processed foods, as you do in this phase, you automatically eliminate most manufactured sugar and artificial or chemically enhanced sugars from your diet, including both corn syrup and high-fructose corn syrup. In the Challenge phase, which follows, you'll remove all sugars. Following are the acceptable sweeteners for now:

Agave syrup or crystals

Honey

Maple syrup

Monk fruit (luo han)

Stevia (pure stevia only with no hidden grains such as maltodextrin); SweetLeaf offers an organic product with no fillers

Sugar alcohols (xylitol and others)

KICKOFF PHASE UNACCEPTABLE FOODS

Following are comprehensive (but not complete) lists of foods that contain (or may contain) gluten or added sugar and sugar substitutes. Avoid them all.

ALL TRUE GRAINS

To follow a *true* gluten-free diet, avoid the following grains, several of which are varieties of wheat. Regardless of the name, wheat is wheat. Wild rice is acceptable.

Barley (malt)

Corn (maize; traditionally considered gluten free, but contains gluten)

Durum wheat (semolina)

Einkorn (an ancient wheat that has recently been revived)

Emmer (another ancient wheat)

Ezekiel breads

Graham flour (whole-wheat flour)

Groats (any hulled grain, broken into pieces)

Millet (traditionally considered gluten free, but contains gluten)

Oats

Rice (white, brown, red, black, etc.; traditionally considered gluten free, but contains gluten)

Rye

Soaked or sprouted grains

Sorghum (traditionally considered gluten free, but contains gluten)

Spelt (another ancient form of wheat)

Teff (traditionally considered gluten free, but contains gluten)

Triticale (a blend of rye and wheat)

Wheat

ALL PSEUDO-GRAINS

These look like grain but are technically vegetables. Nonetheless, they contain gluten-like proteins and may be cross-contaminated with gluten from true grains.

Amaranth

Buckwheat

Quinoa

ALL DAIRY PRODUCTS

Your immune system "reads" milk and other dairy products from grain-fed cows (and sheep and goats) as gluten. In their natural habitat, these animals graze on grass. Feeding them grain and soy inflames their gut. And if you're gluten sensitive, you may react to conventional dairy products just as you do to gluten in grains because the proteins are so similar. Lactose is hard for anyone over the age of 3 to digest, and it becomes increasingly difficult with passing years. One of the main proteins in dairy products, casein has been shown to contribute to autoimmune diseases of the skin, including eczema and psoriasis.[7] Many people are also allergic to casein. The majority of dairy products sold in this country are from cows that have been fed GMO feed and pumped full of hormones.

Moreover, most dairy products contain thickening agents made with grains. Pasteurizing milk denatures the proteins and damages the other immune-boosting properties of milk. The fat is removed from most milk, making it devoid of nutrients. Fat is not the problem, but fat derived from grain the animal ate is highly inflammatory, thus promoting and perpetuating chronic disease. Many dairy products contain added sugar or artificial sweeteners and flavors, which aren't conducive to good health. Finally, dairy products are processed with an enzyme (microbial transglutaminase) that makes the casein "look" like gluten.[8] Clinically speaking, people who go dairy free at the same time they go gluten free typically recover faster from their illnesses than those who eliminate only gluten. Avoid all dairy foods from cows, goats, and sheep, including but not limited to:

Butter	Milk
Cheese of all kinds	Sherbet
Cream	Sour cream
Ice cream, gelato, and ice milk	Whey or casein protein powders
Kefir	Yogurt

Also eliminate margarine, which is not a dairy product but contains unhealthy fats.

Why No Soy?

You already know that eating grain can cause villous atrophy, which occurs when the minute tendrils (villi) that line your gut wear down, hindering the ability to absorb nutrients. A diagnosis of villous atrophy is a marker for celiac disease. It turns out that soy (as well as corn) can also produce this condition.[9] Soy flour, soy milk, soy creamers, and other by-products are major ingredients in countless processed foods, including many so-called gluten-free products. Anyone who knows (or suspects) that she is gluten sensitive should avoid soy at any cost. On top of its specific impact on your gut, more than 90 percent of soy is GMO and has been heavily treated with chemical herbicides and pesticides. Soybeans in any form are not a healthy food. As a vegetable source of protein, soy turns up in thousands of processed foods. The following short list is just the tip of the iceberg. Be sure to read any list of ingredients to avoid hidden soy. Following is a short list of the major soy foods to avoid:

Edamame (green soy beans)	Soy protein powder
Miso	Tempeh
Nondairy creamer	Tofu (bean curd)
Soy milk	

For more on soy, see video youtube.com/watch?v=EiLT4y-CjTM.

UNACCEPTABLE BEVERAGES

Canned or bottled iced tea

Cocktail mixers

Cocoa and chocolate drinks

Flavored seltzers

Juice drinks

Lattes and other coffee drinks with milk

Pasteurized apple, orange, and other juices

Soda in any form

Vitaminwater and similar drinks

DETECTING GLUTEN IN PROCESSED FOODS

One of the many reasons to remove "frood" from your diet is that it's full of chemical additives. Here are the most common chemicals in processed foods, but the names are not always very helpful. In some cases, the same name may or may not refer to an ingredient that contains gluten or may include more than one ingredient. The only way to be sure is to contact the manufacturer for more detail. Alternatively, just avoid any foods that list these items:

Artificial colors

Artificial flavors (including artificial sugars/sugar substitutes)

Caramel color and flavoring

Dextrin

Extenders and binders

Hydrogenated starch

Hydrolysate

Hydrolyzed plant (or vegetable) protein

Hydroxypropylated starch

Maltodextrin (wheat or corn based)

Maltose

Modified food starch

Monosodium glutamate (MSG)

Natural colors

Natural flavors

Pregelatinized starch

Seasonings (check labels)

Smoke flavors

Textured vegetable protein

Vegetable gum

Vegetable protein

PROCESSED FOODS THAT CONTAIN GLUTEN

You can find flour and grain-based ingredients in the most unlikely places. Here are some of the most common foods you'll want to remove from your pantry before you embark on the No-Grain, No Pain program.

Alcoholic beverages derived from grain, including beer and ale, malted beverages, and grain-derived hard liquor (whiskey, bourbon, rye, some vodka)

Baking powder (usually contains wheat or corn)

Bouillon or stock cubes

Candy (may be dusted with wheat flour)

Canned soups

Cheese spreads and other processed cheese foods

Chocolate (may contain malt flavoring)

Cold cuts, wieners, sausages (may have cereal fillers)

Dip mixes

Dry-roasted and honey-roasted nuts

Dry sauce mixes

French fries (restaurants may use the same oil used for wheat-containing items)

Gravy (check thickening agent and liquid base)

Honey hams (may have wheat starch in coating, as well as added sugar)

Ice cream and frozen yogurt (grass-fed dairy recommended, or avoid altogether)

Instant teas and coffees (may include cereal products or added sugar)

Margarine (typically made with corn and soy oil)

Mayonnaise (may have thickener and grain-based vinegar ingredients)

Meat (check flavorings and basting and inquire about transglutaminase, aka "meat glue")

Milk, yogurt, cheese, ice cream, and frozen yogurt from cows, sheep, and goats

Miso paste

Mustard (mustard powder may contain gluten)

Nondairy creamer

Most oil for frying (corn, soy, cottonseed, safflower, or vegetable, all of which may be grain-based or cross-contaminated; see "Acceptable Oils" on page 170 for acceptable oils)

Poultry (check flavorings and basting liquid)

Sour cream (may contain modified food starch)

Soy sauce (most brands contain wheat)

Spice and herb mixtures and other seasonings

Vitamin supplements (some brands contain grain-based ingredients)

This list is obviously incomplete. When in doubt, leave it out!

PORTION CONTROL

Now that you have a good idea of *what* you will and won't be eating, let's talk about the *hows*. You'll be pleased to hear that there's no need to count calories on the No-Grain, No-Pain program. Our society's obsession with calories has resulted in an epidemic of overweight and obesity, accompanied by a companion epidemic of type 2 diabetes and other metabolic conditions. Counting calories is ineffective for most people; we all also tend to underestimate how much we eat and how many calories those portions represent.

Counting calories just confuses matters and bogs you down; it could also become an excuse to not follow the program. Instead, initially be guided by your hunger mechanism. If you are really and truly hungry, eat something. And let's face it, one of the reasons you have a problem may be that you're eating too much. In the second phase you'll likely reduce the volume of the food you consume, especially with the intermittent fasting. But not to worry; as I explained earlier, the more nutrient-rich food and the relative amounts of protein and fat you will be eating are more satiating than the way you have probably been eating, so you'll actually want less. Read on.

HOW MUCH OF THIS? HOW MUCH OF THAT?

How should you apportion the components of your meals? You'll generally follow what I call the rule of thirds, meaning your plate will hold a roughly equal distribution of proteins, fats, and carbohydrates. Meat, of course, combines fat and protein, and vegetables combine carbs and protein. Regard fruit as just carbs. Nuts have some protein but are higher in fat. (Only oils and fats are 100 percent fat.) Of course there are exceptions to those rules. For example, avocado is a fruit but contains more fat than carbs. It is harder to visualize fat than protein and carbs, as it's in nuts, salad dressings, and meat and fish, but you'll soon get the hang of it. Start with the rule of thirds, but remember I referred to "roughly equal distribution." Don't worry about exact proportions; rather, this is a way to start paying attention to the way food makes you feel. If you find you're dragging by midafternoon or early evening, you may need to up your carb intake to closer to 40 percent. Or if you're working out a lot and building muscle, you might need more protein and more calories in general to support your immune system. Listen to your body.

Nor need you hew hard and fast to the proportions of protein, carbs, and fat at every meal. If your protein intake is a bit low at lunch, make it up at dinner, and so forth. Over the course of the day, as long as you're getting a roughly equal distribution of the three energy sources, you should be in good shape. But if you find that you're not healing quite fast enough, you can tweak your volume and the ratio of the three. I suggest increasing protein slightly if healing is slow.

How does the rule of thirds compare to what you have been eating? The National Academy of Sciences (NAS) provides broad guidelines for what it regards as desirable: 10 to 35 percent protein, 45 to 65 percent carbohydrate, and 20 to 35 percent fat. That means that the rule of thirds is in accordance with what you may have already been eating with respect to protein and fat. However, the carb guideline is far too high. Also, some dietary programs continue to glorify grains and demonize fat, ignoring the NAS guidelines and instead recommending a 60-30-10 ratio of carbs, protein, and fats. With such a ratio, the carbs and fat are way out of whack, and we all know where that has led: grainbesity. But what is less well known is that it has also led to an epidemic of autoimmune diseases. Think of your body as a highly specialized machine requiring a high-test fuel. People with gluten sensitivity tend to respond best to the 33-33-33 fuel ratio.

Even the (misguided) goal of eating only 20 percent fat is notoriously hard to maintain—to say nothing about what it does to your health. You are most likely already eating about a third of your calories as fat, but the real question is, Which fats are you eating? Most people are eating the wrong kinds. So-called vegetable oils are actually made from corn, soy, and other non-vegetables, and tend to have a high concentration of inflammatory omega-6 fats. Eating foods rich in omega-3s such as fatty fish like salmon and sardines, as well as macadamia nuts, hazelnuts, walnuts and other tree nuts, can help redress the balance between the two omegas so as not to suppress the natural healing process of inflammation. Oils made from grains contribute to an omega-6-to-omega-3 ratio that can be as high as 16 to 1. The ideal is a ratio of 1 to 1, which is impossible for anyone eating a grain-based diet. One of the many benefits of eliminating grains is that it redresses the balance. So rather than obsessing about fat, instead pay attention to eating the right fats (see "Acceptable Oils" on page 170).

FAMILY MEALS

Whether or not you're the primary cook, I recommend that if at all possible, your partner follow the same dietary program. There's no question that it's always easier to follow a dietary regimen if the family joins in. Certainly, your significant other and any other adults in the family are free to have their own opinions and actions, but having their support unquestionably will help you stick with the program and achieve the desired results more quickly. And, by the way, if your mate eats the way you will be eating for the next 30 days (and hopefully beyond), he or she will likely also feel better and perhaps change old habits for good. I encourage this because everybody, regardless of whether they are gluten sensitive, is going to benefit from the No-Grain, No-Pain program. When Candra's daughter began eating the way her mother did, she began to feel better. The same occurred with Shanna and her daughter Jessica, whose success stories have appeared in previous chapters. I've repeatedly seen such shared improvements with spouses as well as youngsters.

Things get a bit more complicated in social situations. Let's assume that your in-laws have invited you for dinner. How do you stay with the program without ruffling any feathers? Just as with any holiday or other social event, you're never completely in control of the situation when you aren't the chief cook and bottle-washer. Whether or not you get into an explanation depends upon your relationship with your host or hostess and how much you want to reveal about your health. Fortunately, the idea of avoiding gluten is no longer considered weird, although most people are misinformed about what it means. You might just explain that you are following such a program to deal with some health issues (or not). Tell your in-laws (or any host or hostess) that there's no need to modify the menu, but you will not be eating anything with grains and/or dairy products. Don't let someone pressure you with the "just one bite" argument. Instead, politely but firmly say that such and such a food simply doesn't agree with you. (For more on eating out, see "When You Absolutely, Positively Must Eat Out" and "Eating In Is In and Eating Out Is Out," on pages 128 and 126, respectively.)

BONUS FEATURE
Being gluten free and social: visit glutenfreesociety.org/video-tuto rial/being-gluten-free-and-social-at-the-same-time.

WHY NO GRAINS AT ALL?

Wheat, rye, and barley are only three of many grains that contain glutens. To understand why you need to remove all grains on the Grain-Free, Pain-Free program, let's take a closer look at some of the other grains (and one pseudo-grain) that play dominant roles in the standard American diet (aptly abbreviated to SAD). When you're in pain, you feel sad. When you eat the SAD, you will become even sadder because it's almost certain to include foods that stimulate an autoimmune response and, over time, lead to inflammation and pain.

DEMYTHOLOGIZING OATS

You have probably seen oats or oat bran labeled as "gluten free." Is that possible? Well, if you believe that the only reason that gluten has crept into oats is because they were cross-contaminated with wheat—meaning the oats came in contact with wheat, perhaps in the field or while being processed—the answer is yes. (It can just as easily occur in your kitchen or a restaurant via a cutting board, a countertop, or a utensil.) But the truth is that oats contain a gluten called avenin. Even oats that are not cross-contaminated cause an inflammatory reaction in patients diagnosed with gluten sensitivity.[10]

Nonetheless, both doctors and the "gluten-free" food industry completely ignore this research, and continue to claim that oats are a safe substitute food for wheat, barley, and rye. Some forms of oat protein have also been shown to trigger an antibody reaction.[11] One study found that two types of oat proteins were responsible for increased production markers for inflammation, which can cause mineral deficiencies and numerous other health problems.[12] In one small study, researchers purchased and tested products labeled as gluten-free, only to discover that 41 percent of them had enough gluten cross-contamination to create a health problem for those with gluten sensitivity.[13]

BONUS FEATURE

Video on oats: visit glutenfreesociety.org/no-grain-no-pain-hidden -danger-oats.

THE TRUTH ABOUT CORN

It's real simple. Corn is a grain. Corn contains gluten. And guess which grain is among the most commonly found in most so-called gluten-free products? Corn also hides in countless other processed foods, often where you would least expect it. (See "Corn Is Everywhere" on page 183.) Corn is a severe problem for the majority of people who cannot handle "traditional" gluten. Corn gluten is similar enough to wheat gluten that it stimulates an inflammatory response in gluten-sensitive individuals,[14] including those with celiac disease,[15] ulcerative colitis, and Crohn's disease. Gluten-free bread, specifically, has been found to cause problems.[16] Corn oil can cause gastrointestinal inflammation[17] and villous atrophy.[18] Again, villi are those minuscule tentacles that line the small intestine and help move its contents along. Corn also tends to be high in a toxin called fumonisin,[19] which can be particularly dangerous for people with type 2 diabetes and heart disease. Gluten-free products may contain high levels of this toxin.[20] Finally, corn is one of the most commonly genetically modified plants on the planet.

BONUS FEATURE

Video on corn: visit glutenfreesociety.org/no-grain-no-pain-dangers -corn.

Corn Is Everywhere

Corn is truly ubiquitous in our diet. In addition to the obvious foods like popcorn; corn on the cob; corn tortillas, tamales, and taco shells; corn fritters; polenta, grits, hominy, corn flour, and cornmeal; canned and frozen corn niblets; corn chips; cornflakes and many other breakfast cereals; and corn oil and margarine made with it, corn (maize) is a common ingredient in countless processed foods. You'll find it under the following names:

Corn alcohol

Corn extract

Corn gluten

Cornstarch and modified cornstarch

Corn sugar (dextrose, Dyno, Cerelose, Puretose, Sweetose, glucose)

Corn sweetener

Corn syrup, corn syrup solids, and high-fructose corn syrup (HFCS)

Hydrolyzed corn and hydrolyzed corn protein

Maize

Vegetable oil

Zea mays

Zein

THE SCOOP ON RICE

The United States has a much higher incidence of overweight and obesity than Japan, but in our country about 8 percent of the population has type 2 diabetes, compared to 11 percent in Japan.[21] South Korea and China also beat the United States.[22] How come? It's simple:

White rice is a staple of Asian cuisine and Asians eat far more, on average, than do Westerners. A review of four studies comprising more than 352,000 individuals found the more white rice people consumed, the more likely they were to develop diabetes.[23] Only a baked potato has a higher glycemic index (GI), which refers to how quickly a carb food converts to glucose, aka sugar, in your body, than does an equal portion of white rice. (Brown rice, which includes the fiber, which is where the gluten resides, has a lower GI.) White rice consumption also appears to increase the risk of breast cancer, according to research on South Korean women.[24] Rice is also highly likely to be contaminated with heavy metals, in part because it is grown in water, which may contain industrial runoff. Arsenic contamination is common in rice grown in many parts of the world,[25] as is cadmium contamination.[26] (Chapter 10 discusses the connection of heavy metals with pain and inflammation.) Rice milk contains gluten and additional proteins, which can create an allergic response that results in severe gastrointestinal inflammation and pain similar to that caused by dairy products or soy milk.[27]

BONUS FEATURE

Video on rice: visit glutenfreesociety.org/no-grain-no-pain-dangers -rice.

THE REAL DEAL ON QUINOA

Quinoa is often marketed as a gluten-free grain. Not true on two counts. First, it is the seed of a pseudo-cereal, not a grain. Second, although quinoa doesn't contain gluten, it is often processed in a facility that also processes wheat and other grains and may be cross-contaminated with gluten. Moreover, quinoa has its own gluten-like storage proteins that can mimic those in wheat, barley, and rye, and have been found to cause an immune reaction in people with celiac disease or gluten sensitivity.[28] In one test, two of fifteen types of quinoa stimulated an immune response as potent as that observed with wheat gluten. These results disprove the traditional assumption that only proteins in wheat, barley, and rye are problematic for people with gluten sensitivity.

WHY NO PSEUDO-GRAINS?

The other two pseudo-grains, amaranth and buckwheat, are equally grain-like in their appearance, consistency, and texture, and they, too, are actually seeds of vegetables. Both are now being marketed in "gluten-free" breakfast cereal, pasta, and bread alternatives. I don't recommend pseudo-grains because of the risk for cross-contamination, and also because some studies show that people who eat these foods continue to have persistent inflammatory responses.[29] Finally, I want you to think really hard about the fact that seeds are designed to survive even a treacherous trip down your GI tract. In general, seeds are hard to digest and often contain gluten-like proteins and chemical compounds called lectins. These have been shown to create digestive and inflammatory problems, including leaky gut, and are known contributors to autoimmune disease. If you consume seeds en masse, there will always be a price to pay, and that price is typically going to be paid first in the gut. Pseudo or the real McCoy, grains spell pain and destruction. In fact, a recent study found that 41 percent of inherently gluten-free products randomly pulled from grocery shelves contain enough gluten to cause damage to those with gluten sensitivity.[30]

Grain-Free Breakfasts

If you love eggs, the obvious way to start the day is with one or two, whether boiled, poached, scrambled, or fried; or in an omelet, perhaps with mushrooms, spinach, sautéed onions, or last night's leftover veggies. Or make your own version of egg foo yong with sautéed green onions and mung beans. Add a couple of slices of free-range pork (uncured, no sugar added) or perhaps a venison sausage; serve with a slice of cantaloupe, berries, or another fruit, and you're in business. You can also make pancakes, using organic protein powder that doesn't contain gluten, soy, or added sugars. If you make almond or coconut flour pancakes, be sure to boost your protein intake with bacon or sausage from appropriately raised animals. You can whip up a smoothie, again using suitable protein powder, coconut milk beverage, fruit, and some veggies. Or how about zucchini stuffed with either sausage from a free-range animal, or leftover chopped-up organic chicken or turkey; veggie hashbrowns made with leftovers and topped with a poached egg, or grilled stuffed mushrooms. The recipe section on page 257 includes more breakfast options, including Garden Frittata and Super Simple Banana Pancakes.

KICKOFF PHASE MEAL PLANS

After seven days, repeat these meal plans for another week. On Day 15, repeat Day 1 again. Feel free to swap days and individual meals around or make logical replacements, such as broccoli for cauliflower or a seasonal vegetable, ground beef for ground bison, a burger for a chop, a pear instead of an apple, and the like. You can also simply comply with the following guidelines, referring to the acceptable food lists provided in this chapter.

Ideally, all vegetables and fruits should be organic. Likewise, beef and other meat should be from grass-fed or pastured animals. Chicken and eggs should be from free-range birds fed organic feed. Fish should be wild caught.

Make vinaigrette salad dressings using extra-virgin olive oil (EVOO) or avocado oil and either lemon or lime juice or apple cider vinegar or balsamic vinegar, preferably all organic. Don't use bottled or otherwise prepared salad dressings.

Dress cooked vegetables with EVOO.

Cook foods in organic coconut oil (or coconut butter) or EVOO.

Use sea salt and gluten-free seasonings (see "Acceptable Condiments" on page 170) as desired.

A morning snack is listed for each day, but that is optional. You can have it in the afternoon instead, or as dessert after lunch or dinner. Or have no snacks or two snacks. Let your appetite be your guide.

Recipes with an asterisk (*) start on page 257.

DAY 1

Breakfast

1 or 2 boiled eggs

1 cup blueberries

¼ cup almonds

Snack

Gluten-Free Warrior Approved Whole Food Honey Almond Bar

Lunch

tuna salad (6 ounces canned or vacuum-packed tuna) on mixed greens, with sliced onion and tomato

½ Hass avocado

lemon juice vinaigrette

green apple

Dinner

*Baked Italian Chicken Breast

baked Japanese sweet potato

steamed broccoli

DAY 2

Breakfast

*Kane's Ultra Pure Protein Smoothie

Snack

½ cup pumpkin seeds

½ cup dried cherries (without sugar)

Lunch

grilled chicken on romaine lettuce and arugula topped with slivered almonds and clementine or orange segments

balsamic vinaigrette

Dinner

*Poached Cod with Mango Salsa

butternut squash purée

DAY 3

Breakfast

6 oz. sautéed ground lamb and spinach

½ cup strawberries

Snack

½ cup macadamia nuts

Lunch

*Chicken Fajitas

*South-of-the-Border Slaw

Dinner

*Pineapple-Chicken Kabobs

DAY 4

Breakfast

*Kane's Ultra Pure Protein Smoothie

Snack

2 celery stalks with almond butter

Lunch

*Taco Salad

Dinner

*Dijon Salmon Fillets

baked cauliflower florets and baby carrots

DAY 5

Breakfast

*Banana-Almond Muffins

*Homemade Breakfast Sausage

Snack

½ cup almond milk

1 apple

Lunch

*Speedy Salmon Cakes

*Cucumber and Tomato Salad

Dinner

*Baked Almond-Dusted Pork Chops

*Cauliflower Rice

DAY 6

Breakfast

*Super Simple Banana Pancake

Snack

*Topp Paleo Flatbread (1 to 2 slices) with almond butter

Lunch

*Strawberry-Bacon-Avocado Salad

grilled chicken

Dinner

*Lemony Brussels Sprouts

beef brisket

DAY 7

Breakfast

*Garden Frittata

Snack

*Apricot Cookies

Lunch

*Sausage with Cabbage "Noodles"

Dinner

*Herb-Seasoned Shepherd's Pie

steamed asparagus

FREQUENTLY ASKED QUESTIONS

Q. **What do I do if I realize I ate something with gluten in it by mistake—or intentionally?**
A. Move on. If you couldn't resist something, ate it, and knew you shouldn't have, don't beat yourself up. Tomorrow is a new day. On the other hand, if you get into the habit of eating foods full of gluten, your best bet is to simply start the 15-day Kickoff phase again.

Q. **Which cooking methods do you recommend?**
A. Baking, broiling, grilling, roasting, stir-frying, steaming, and poaching are fine. I do not recommend deep-frying.

Q. **Can I eat homemade French fries?**
A. Even if you don't use corn, soy, vegetable, or other unhealthy oils, deep-fried food is bad for you. Instead, I recommend roast-

ing "fingers" of sweet potatoes—the Japanese type is quite similar to white potatoes in texture—with olive oil and seasonings. In the Challenge phase, you'll eliminate white potatoes in any case.

Q. Are there any kinds of pasta I can eat?
A. I prefer you to quit thinking about non-grain substitutes for pasta, bread, and cereal, and start thinking grass-fed meats and organic vegetables. Substitute products are usually chemically bleached and perhaps genetically modified, so they're unlikely to pass the "is it healthy?" test. However, if you simply must have an occasional plate of pasta, shirataki noodles made from an Asian yam are the least problematic. They're widely available in the refrigerated section of the natural foods section of most supermarkets, but the fishy taste can be off-putting. (A tofu shirataki variation contains soy, making it a no-no.) Dried cellophane noodles made from the same yam or from mung bean, cassava, canna, or potato starch taste better, but are found mostly in Asian groceries. You can use these in Phase 1, but would need to eliminate anything with mung beans or potato in Phase 2. Nonetheless, all still are processed foods. At first glance, pasta made from a tuber called Jerusalem artichoke looks acceptable but the first ingredient is durum semolina, a form of wheat.

Before we move on to chapter 9, which introduces the Challenge phase of the No-Grain, No-Pain program, ask yourself whether you've been compliant with the dietary aspect and supplement components of the Kickoff phase. Likewise, have you been drinking enough water, regularly walking, and getting enough sleep and morning sun? If not, it would be a good idea to remain in this phase to lay the groundwork before moving on the more rigorous second phase. Finally, be sure to take the pain test on page 19 to retest the intensity and frequency of your pain after 15 gluten-free days. Don't go back and look at your original answers until you gauge your current levels. I strongly suspect you'll be pleased and surprised.

CHAPTER 9

DAYS 16 TO 30

Banish the Last of Your Pain in the Challenge Phase

Always bear in mind that your own resolution to succeed, is more important than any other one thing.

—Abraham Lincoln

In this second phase of the program, you will continue your good efforts and can expect even more significant cessation of pain and improvement in overall well-being. You'll keep eating the protein sources you've been consuming for the past 15 days, along with most vegetables and fruits. However, you will now eliminate certain plant foods from your diet. The act of eating itself can hinder the healing process. One of the most important components to this program is to give your gut a rest with periodic breaks, which is why you'll also begin intermittent fasting. Finally, you'll raise the bar in the activity department.

In the Challenge phase, you'll eliminate the following potentially problematic foods from your meals:

• Vegetables in the nightshade family: white potatoes, tomatoes, sweet bell peppers, chile peppers, eggplant, and goji berries

• All legumes (in addition to soy), including peanuts

• Some nuts and seeds (and moderate intake of all nuts and seeds)

• Processed sugar in any form

• Most sugar substitutes

• Tobacco is also a nightshade plant, so no smoking or chewing it

• Coffee and black tea

You'll also continue to:

• Get at least seven hours of sleep a night.

• Spend at least half an hour outside each day, preferably in the morning.

• Drink at least eight 8-ounce glasses of water daily.

• Walk each day, but increase your number of steps to at least ten thousand.

In addition, you'll add an exercise component (see "Raise the Activity Bar" on page 210).

THE LAST PIECE OF THE PUZZLE

Ruby came to see me originally because of severe joint pain. She had been diagnosed with rheumatoid arthritis, an autoimmune disease. The pain made it hard to exercise and keep up with her small children. It got so bad that her rheumatologist prescribed a potent medication called methotrexate, which helped reduce Ruby's pain enough to function but was damaging her liver. Over time, the medication lost its effectiveness, and her doctor wanted her to take a powerful anti-immune drug. The side effects of the medications scared Ruby, so she decided to seek my help instead.

After a functional medicine workup, I found that Ruby had a gluten-sensitive gene pattern. She was also allergic to sugar, dairy, eggs, blueberries, olives, aspartame (an artificial sweetener), and vinyl chloride, a chemical used to make plastics. Her liver enzymes were elevated, indicating the damage being done to her liver. She also was deficient in chromium and vitamins B_1, B_2, B_5, B_6, and B_8.

I started Ruby on a grain-free and allergen-free diet and a course of nutritional supplementation. Her joint pain and fatigue improved to the point where she could cut her dose of methotrexate in half. However, Ruby did not get complete relief from her pain until she stopped eating nightshades and legumes. Both these food groups contained enough inflammatory compounds to enable her pain to persist. But once she eliminated tomatoes, peppers, and other vegetables in the nightshade family, along with legumes, Ruby's rheumatoid arthritis was gone, and with it the pain.

MEET THE NIGHTSHADE FAMILY

Ruby's story is a perfect example of how improvements can be limited even when following a completely grain-free diet. Gluten is not the only food component that can contribute to pain and inflammation. You've probably heard of the deadly nightshade plant known as belladonna, which the Romans used as a poison, although it also has medicinal uses. Tobacco is in the same plant family, and its edible relatives include eggplant, tomato, potato, and peppers in all their variations. Edible or not, many people are sensitive to these plants, which is why we eliminate them in this phase.[1] The pain- and inflammation-inducing culprit found in our beloved nightshade vegetables is a compound called solanine. These plants have protective immune systems to prevent "us" predators from eradicating them. This chemical has been shown to cause leaky gut, joint inflammation, and muscle stiffness, and can also lead to excessive calcium deposits in your tissues.[2] Some people can reintroduce nightshade plants after several months, but if you have any form of autoimmune arthritis, you'll always react badly to them.

It's relatively easy to avoid potatoes, although do read labels to make sure that potato starch isn't lurking in a product. Just to be clear, yams and sweet potatoes are not members of the nightshade family and you can continue to eat them. Japanese sweet potatoes, which have white or yellow flesh, are less sweet than other sweet potatoes and yams and have a starchy texture more like white potatoes, making them a great substitute. Eggplant is easy to spot in dishes such as eggplant Parmesan, caponata, and baba ghanoush.

Tomatoes and peppers are far sneakier and ubiquitous. Most Italian and Mexican dishes and many curries and other Indian dishes contain one or the other, and often both. Both bell and chile peppers are off-limits, but the seasoning we call pepper is in another plant family. The following products typically contain peppers and/or tomatoes. Read labels carefully to spot others.

All canned or jarred tomato products

Barbecue sauce

Cocktail sauces (as in shrimp cocktail)

Enchilada sauce

Ketchup

Pizza sauce

Red spaghetti sauce

Salsa

Tabasco and other hot sauces

ANOTHER LOOK AT LEGUMES

Review the "Acceptable Beans and Legumes" list on page 169. Although you have already omitted soybeans, you may have been eating some of these other beans in the Kickoff phase. That was fine, but now it's time to say good-bye to them. Whether the tiny lentil or the mighty lima bean, this subset of the vegetable family contains multiple chemical compounds that inhibit digestion, prevent absorption of nutrients, trigger leaky gut, cause inflammation, and eventually lead to painful autoimmune problems. Proteins called lectins in legumes cause gut bacteria to ferment and produce gas.

Lectins are not the only problem with legumes. They contain phytic acid, which prevents the bean from sprouting before conditions are optimal. But in your GI tract phytic acid binds to minerals like calcium, iron, magnesium, and zinc, preventing them (and the other nutrients in the bean) from being absorbed.[3] And that's not all: legumes also contain galacto-oligosaccharides, a type of difficult-to-digest carbohydrate known to cause digestive problems, especially in individuals with IBS or other gut conditions. Remember that peanuts are not true nuts, but rather legumes, and should also be avoided for all these reasons, and more. (See "The Poisonous Peanut" below.)

These beans are available (in some cases) as fresh vegetables, but more commonly they're found dried, canned, and, in some cases, frozen. Say sayonara to all of them. (You can continue to eat fresh or frozen string beans, pole beans, snow peas, and Chinese peapods, as well as bean sprouts. It is the seeds of legumes, such as lima beans or fava beans, that are problematic, so avoid them and even shelled fresh peas.) Indian cuisine relies heavily on dal, made from dried peas and other legumes. Avoid refried beans in Mexican restaurants. In addition to the soy products already eliminated, avoid:

Baked beans	Hummus
Bean, lentil, and pea soups	Lentil and other bean dips
Bean sprouts	Peanut butter
Chili con carne	Peanut oil
Chocolate (yes, the cacao bean is a legume)	Refried beans
Coffee (ditto for coffee beans)	Succotash

The Poisonous Peanut

What is more American than a PB&J sandwich? Most of us were raised on them. But in addition to the gut issues common to all legumes, peanuts present an additional concern: aflatoxins. These toxins aren't actually in the so-called nut; rather, they are found in a mold like the one that is often found in corn. Even organic peanuts are subject to this mold. Aflatoxin consumption has been linked to a greater risk for cancer, hepatitis B, and other diseases.[4] Aside from being one of the most common food allergens, peanuts also contain lectin anti-nutrient compounds, which enter the bloodstream and can damage the lining of the arteries.[5] Peanuts don't belong in your diet, regardless of your tolerance for gluten.

DON'T GO OVERBOARD WITH NUTS AND SEEDS

Seeds and nuts are great snacks and have a place in your meals as well, but not all are created equal. In this phase, you'll narrow down your choices somewhat to those with a better nutritional profile and less likelihood of gut damage. Seeds (as well as some nuts) also contain lectins, so we have the same issues with incomplete digestion and gut lining irritation and resultant inflammation. Nuts also contain phytic acid (as do grains and legumes) in varying amounts, with macadamias and chestnuts having among the least, and pine nuts and Brazil nuts on the high end. Remember that phytic acid binds to zinc, iron, magnesium, calcium, and other minerals in the GI tract, causing mineral deficiencies.[6] Some nuts and seeds also have an unfavorable ratio of unhealthy polyunsaturated fats to healthy monounsaturated fats, especially omega-3 fats. For both reasons, eliminate the seeds and nuts listed below in the Challenge phase. Also take care not to overuse nut flours, which can be tempting once flours made from grains are eliminated, as overuse can lead to digestive trouble. With a few exceptions, continue to enjoy nuts and seeds in moderation.

UNACCEPTABLE PHASE 2 "NUTS"

Neither is a true nut:

Cashews

Peanuts

SUGAR NATION

The average American consumes a staggering 155 pounds of sugar annually. Much of it comes from the obvious places: desserts, pastries, chocolate, and candy. But a lot comes from what I call "hidden" sugar in foods you would not suspect contain it, usually in the form of high-fructose corn syrup, which is omnipresent in beverages and processed foods, including savory foods. You already know that corn gluten is detrimental to your health in numerous ways (see "The Truth about Corn" on page 182), but high-fructose corn syrup is another toxic and poisonous substance that has gained a foothold in our food system and is the most common sweetener used in soft drinks.

The rapid rise in medical problems such as type 2 diabetes is directly related to the increased consumption of high-fructose corn syrup.[7] Even though it comes from a natural source, it's essentially an unnatural product. Our bodies cannot tolerate too much fructose. Once upon a time, when we consumed perhaps 15 grams a day from fruits and vegetables, there was no problem, but now that we're up about 80 grams a day on average, it's a different story. Fructose is metabolized in the liver, and when the body is swamped with fructose, it increases triglycerides in the liver and veins, contributing to fatty liver disease and increasing the risk for heart disease, respectively.[8] It has also been linked to obesity, cancer, leaky gut, accelerated aging, and more,[9] to say nothing of cavities.

SCOPING OUT HIDDEN SUGARS

Even though high-fructose corn syrup is the main "fake" sugar to look out, it is hardly alone. There are dozens of other sugars in our food supply. Manufacturers of packaged foods don't make it easy to scope out the source of sugars. For example, added sugar can be from a natural source, such as honey or fruit juice, but if it's showing up in a package of frozen berries, it's still added sugar. That's one of the many reasons you removed processed foods from your pantry and your plate in the Kickoff phase. Here are some of the numerous names under which hidden sugars hide in plain sight. None is allowed in the Challenge phase.

Agave syrup or crystals

Barley malt or barley sugar

Beet sugar

Brown sugar

Cane sugar, cane syrup, or cane juice crystals

Caramel

Carob syrup

Corn syrup, corn syrup solids, or corn sweetener

Date sugar

Demerara sugar

Dextran or dextrose

Diastase, diastic malt

Evaporated cane juice

Fructose

Fruit juice, fruit juice concentrate

Galactose

Glucose, glucose solids

Golden syrup

Granulated sugar

Grape sugar, grape juice concentrate

High-fructose corn syrup (HFCS)

Honey

Lactose

Maltodextrin

Malt syrup, maltose, maltol

Maple sugar or syrup

Molasses

Muscovado sugar

Raw sugar

Refiner's syrup

Rice syrup   Treacle

Sorghum syrup   Turbinado sugar

Sucrose

AVOID ALL ARTIFICIAL SUGAR SUBSTITUTES

Most sugar substitutes, aka sweeteners, are primarily artificial chemical concoctions. Stevia is made from the leaf of a plant, but is still a highly processed product, and at least one brand, Truvia, contains corn. Aspartame and saccharin have been linked to various health problems. Then there are sugar alcohols, which are natural compounds that appear in many "sugar-free" and diet foods such as gum and ice cream. Sugar alcohols are FODMAPs (fermentable oligosaccharides, disaccharides, monosaccharides, and polyols), which are also found in the cabbage family, lactose, and other foods. Largely indigestible carbs, FODMAPs can contribute to gas, bloating, and diarrhea as a result of gut bacteria fermentation. If you have persistent IBS or GI problems, you would be well advised to stay away from them. Sugar alcohols made from birchwood, instead of corn or milk, are acceptable in this phase, in moderation (2 to 3 packets a day). If you cannot tolerate them, eliminate them along with all of the following:

Acesulfame-K (Sweet One)   Saccharin (Sweet'N Low)

Advantame (coming soon, a   Stevia (Truvia contains corn)
derivative of aspartame)
                                             Sucralose (Splenda)
Aspartame (NutraSweet)
                                             Sugar alcohols such as xylitol,
Lactitol (a sugar alcohol sugar   sorbitol, mannitol, and erythritol
derived from milk)   derived from corn

Neotame

ACCEPTABLE CHALLENGE PHASE
SUGAR SUBSTITUTES

Neotame

Organic stevia (SweetLeaf packets only)

Xylitol made from birchwood (Swanson Xylitol Granules is one non-GMO product)

GIVE YOUR GUT A REST

In addition to removing these additional foods (and "froods" in the case of sugar substitutes), the introduction of intermittent fasting is an integral component of the healing process. Fasting has been linked to longevity and a reduced incidence of many chronic diseases.[10] Fasting or intermittent fasting has been shown to benefit patients with arthritis, pain syndromes, inflammatory conditions, anxiety, metabolic syndrome, and elevated blood pressure.[11] Many of my patients profiled in these pages performed intermittent fasting as part of their protocol, which helped them heal more quickly.

If it hurts every time you eat or you experience other unpleasant symptoms, you may have already figured out the connection. Many of my patients tell me, "Until I started intermittent fasting, I didn't notice the connection between eating and pain." Intermittent fasting gives you an opportunity to focus on this connection. Just to be clear, the hurting could be gastric pain, but for many people it's joint pain, especially when they eat corn. The same goes for neuropathy. Once you're paying attention to such signals, I believe you'll be more successful in the long term adhering to the No-Grain, No-Pain program. The absence of suffering is a powerful motivator.

You may have also discovered that one way to feel better, if only temporarily, is to skip a meal. Until you started reading this book, you likely didn't know whether what you have been eating was creating the pain or whether it's the act of eating itself that produced the pain. If you are occasionally skipping meals, you're already doing what is called intermittent fasting, as opposed to fasting for a full day or more. With intermittent fasting you pick an eight-hour window during which you eat all your meals. You don't have to eat fewer calories; you just eat them in a shorter time frame. Unlike fasting for a day or several days, you still give the GI tract a rest—again, one of the most profound ways to reduce inflammation and relieve pain is to not eat—but it also satisfies the need for nourishment. Most people already eat too much and too often. However, doing so with a broken gut is even more dangerous. By alleviating the stress and pressure on the GI tract, the gut can heal and recover.

A SIXTEEN-HOUR FOOD-FREE ZONE

Remember that a leaky gut allows food and other chemicals to penetrate the bloodstream, causing inflammation and pain. Intermittent fasting reduces the quantity of toxins that can pass into your blood. Intermittent fasting may sound intimidating, but it is really very simple. Here's how it works:

- Pick eight hours in the day during which you will eat, and don't eat outside of that time frame. That means you go food free for sixteen hours. However, it is important to continue to drink eight cups of water and/or herbal tea while fasting to stay hydrated and wash out toxins.

- The easiest way to accomplish this is to eat an early dinner so that the majority of your fast occurs while you're asleep: perhaps brunch at ten a.m., lunch at two p.m., and dinner at six p.m.

- If you've normally finished dinner by six p.m. and have breakfast at eight a.m., you're already going thirteen hours without eating, so the sixteen-hour fast is not all that different.

- Some people prefer to have two meals instead of three. Again, you're not depriving yourself of food; rather, you're ensuring that your gut gets a rest.

• Nor does intermittent fasting mean eating less food than you would otherwise, although I do find that when you are eating a better-quality diet you are satisfied with less quantity.

There are two ways you can approach intermittent fasting:

• *Fast Track:* For speedier results, start fasting in Week 3 as you simultaneously eliminate the remaining foods that may be irritants.

• *Slow and Steady:* If that feels too overwhelming and you want to get comfortable with eliminating more foods first, wait until Week 4 to introduce intermittent fasting.

Ideally, fast on a daily basis if you can tolerate it, which will initiate improvement more quickly. However, this is not necessary and can be adapted to your schedule and personal needs.

You now know that most people experience what they perceive as hunger out of boredom, so the best way to change your mind-set about when to eat is do something else to occupy your mind and body. If your internal time clock is saying, "I just got up and it's breakfast time," how do you override that? My advice is to take a walk, practice yoga, meditate, write in your journal, work in your garden, or anything else that takes your mind off food. Again, you may actually be thirsty, not hungry, so have a glass of water or a cup of herbal tea until the sixteen hours have elapsed. Pretty soon you will have established a new morning pattern.

Understand that intermittent fasting is not mandatory. If you find that it makes you feel worse, stop and simply continue to remove the additional foods from your diet.

"Traditional" Fasting

Fasting for more than sixteen hours is not part of the No-Grain, No-Pain Program, although I sometimes prescribe it to my patients. I find that men are better able than women to fast for twenty-four to forty-eight hours, which is not to say that women cannot also tolerate a day or two of fasting (or more) if done properly. The reason men are better equipped to fast for longer periods is that they have more muscle mass. Because of their relative lack of muscle mass, women tend to have a more exaggerated excretion of cortisol and insulin during a fast than men do, which can lead to dramatic blood sugar fluctuations. Before attempting a longer fast, women need to address any hormonal imbalance of cortisol and insulin under a doctor's care.

BREAKING YOUR FAST, AKA BREAKFAST

After not eating for sixteen hours, it's important to have your first meal of the new day rely primarily on protein, which provides the necessary building blocks in the form of amino acids for healing, repair, and immune system balance. Amino acids are also essential for neurotransmitter formation, enabling your brain to think and work clearly. Breakfast does not have to be a huge meal. In fact, if you don't feel like eating in the morning, that's fine.

Myth 16: **Breakfast is the most important meal of the day.**

Not true! I would even go so far as to say that if you don't feel like eating, don't. This whole idea has been hyped to sell breakfast products, namely cereal, and now all sorts of breakfast pastries, sandwiches, and shakes.

A century ago, when most people's jobs involved physical labor, a big breakfast was more important, but many people don't operate well on a heavy breakfast. I can't tell you how many times I see patients who say, "I just don't feel like eating first thing in the morning," but they do so because they have been told it is healthy. Personally, I am far more interested in eating midmorning. Call it brunch if you wish.

The meal plans don't provide portions for protein or vegetables. So, for example, a petite woman might find an egg and a small piece of sausage are plenty, but a tall guy might do better with two eggs and two pieces of sausage. And clearly a steelworker is going to need to eat more protein than a deskbound clerical worker. The meal plans do specify quantities for foods such as nuts that are particularly high in calories.

Sufficient protein will compensate for the carbohydrate blast you may be used to having at breakfast and sustain your energy until lunch or midafternoon, depending on when you're having your next meal. The biggest habit to break with breakfast is that of having toast, cereal, bagels, doughnuts, and anything else made with grains. After all, breakfast food is just food. It doesn't have to be the "traditional" breakfast foods made by cereal companies. Just eat real food. If you want a (free-range) turkey burger or a bowl of (grass-fed) beef-vegetable soup, go for it.

SAVOR A SMOOTHIE

A liquid breakfast can be a great way to break your fast. If you like to make smoothies, you're probably familiar with most types of protein powder:

Beef

Dairy (whey and casein)

Egg white (albumin)

Pea

Peanut

Soy

Whey, casein, and soy are out from the get-go as they all contain ingredients you removed in the Kickoff phase. Pea and peanut protein hit the dust in the Challenge phase, which seems to leave us with only egg white protein, but there is actually a superior powdered protein you may not be aware of unless you're a body builder: beef protein. Before you turn up your nose and say the last thing you want in your smoothie is something made from meat, let me assure you that it is tasteless and has a creamy texture and consistency comparable to whey protein powder. It is also higher in protein than any other protein powder. Seek out a hydrolyzed beef protein powder made from grass-fed beef, such as the one I offer on my website. Try it in the recipe for my Kane's Ultra Pure Protein Smoothie on page 260 (glutenfreesociety .org/shop/general-health/ultra-pure-protein).

EXPAND YOUR HORIZONS

Boredom can be the enemy of a new dietary program. Your initial concern on the Grain-Free, Pain-Free program may have been that you would get tired of eating a more limited array of foods. After the first two weeks on the program, I want you to think again.

There are hundreds of varieties of fruits, vegetables, and herbs out there for the tasting and the savoring. If you haven't already expanded your horizons by trying new foods in the Kickoff phase, I encourage you to do so now that you are beginning the Challenge phase. As your taste buds change throughout the program, you'll find that certain foods start to taste different. Foods you may have avoided or just tolerated may now appeal to you once you remove the grains that may have dominated your diet. And just because you occasionally get a woody asparagus spear or a sour peach, don't write off that vegetable or fruit because of one bad experience. Give it another try or cook it another way. Maybe you find arugula too sharp in a salad, but love its zest in a stir-fry. Yes, you're not going to be eating certain foods, but look at the world of other opportunities that opens up once vegetables take up more space on your plate. Consider these options:

- Instead of always picking up the iceberg lettuce, try romaine, red or green leaf, butterhead, Bibb, or Boston. Try adding some bitter greens such as watercress, radicchio, or arugula for contrast in color and taste. Fennel and jicama add distinctive textures and flavors.

• Celery root and jicama may not be the prettiest veggies in the produce section, but grated and combined with grated apple, they make a great slaw.

• Instead of always steaming spinach, swap it out occasionally for Swiss chard, mustard greens, or beet greens.

• If you reflexively pick up a bag of yellow onions, why not also explore the taste treats of shallots, spring onions, leeks, or green onions?

• If you always buy green cabbage, how about using Brussels sprouts, red cabbage, or savoy or Chinese cabbage instead? They're close relatives and are interchangeable in pretty much any recipe.

• If you never cooked an artichoke or broccoli rabe, now may be the time.

• If you love the tangy crunch of red radishes, give daikon, a big carrot-like Chinese radish, a try. Or grate daikon and use it instead of rice as the base for a stir-fry.

You may also want to explore options in game meats and fowl. Be open to the fact that your taste buds are going to change once you go on a *true* gluten-free diet, and that foods you may not have previously savored may now be appealing.

TO SNACK OR NOT TO SNACK

The meal plans for the Challenge phase include no snacks. Since you'll be fasting intermittently during this phase, you'll be having all your meals within an eight-hour time frame; you're less likely to feel the need for them. Your objective is to take pressure off, rather than impose more pressure on, your gut. Ideally you initially should eat less often, not more often, to get the pain under control. However, if you do feel the need for a snack within that window, you can certainly have one. (See "Snacks Are Food, Too" on page 125 for some ideas.) Just don't pick a snack that's off the charts in terms of omega-6s—or make it a petite portion. For example, almonds, pecans, and walnuts are all relatively high in omega-6s compared to macadamias and hazelnuts. In addition to their dense calorie content, it's notoriously easy to just keep eating them, particularly if you are used to eating lots of bread or pasta. Peanuts, of course, are off the menu altogether.

CHALLENGE PHASE MEAL PLANS

After seven days, repeat these meal plans for another week. On Day 30, repeat Day 1 again. As in Phase 1, feel free to swap days and individual meals around or make logical replacements. Simply follow the same general guidelines as outlined for Phase 1 in chapter 8.

- All produce should be organic, beef and other meat should be from grass-fed or pastured animals, chicken and eggs should be from free-range birds fed organic feed, and fish should be wild caught.

- Guidelines for making salad dressings remain the same, as well, as does dressing cooked vegetables with extra-virgin olive oil (EVOO) and using organic coconut oil or coconut butter and EVOO for cooking.

- Dress vegetables and salads with sea salt and gluten-free seasonings (see "Acceptable Condiments" on page 170), as desired.

Unlike in the Kickoff phase, there are no snacks listed because I recommend you fast intermittently in this phase, which means eating all meals within an eight-hour time frame. However, if you are hungry you can certainly have a snack from the Phase 1 meal plans (beginning on page 187) or from ""Snacks Are Food, Too" on page 125, assuming they are appropriate for Phase 2.

Recipes with an asterisk (*) can be found starting on page 257. Note that some have modifications to make them appropriate for this phase.

DAY 1

Breakfast

2 scrambled eggs

sliced cantaloupe

Lunch

*Chicken-Apple-Avocado Salad

*Black Sesame Seed Slaw (omit seeds)

Dinner

*Speedy Salmon Cakes

steamed zucchini or other summer squash

DAY 2

Breakfast

*Homemade Breakfast Sausage (omit red pepper)

banana

Lunch

grilled chicken

spinach, ½ Hass avocado, and dried cherries (without added sugar)

apple cider vinaigrette

Dinner

*Pancit with Glass Noodles

DAY 3

Breakfast

protein shake with banana and ½ cup baby spinach

Lunch

bison steak

sautéed mushrooms

zucchini "noodles"

Dinner

*Baked Almond-Dusted Pork Chops

sautéed spinach

*Cauliflower Rice

DAY 4

Breakfast

smoked wild salmon

1 cup cubed fresh pineapple

Lunch

*Chicken "Unwich"

sliced cucumbers

1 cup seasonal fruit

Dinner

*Poached Cod with Mango Salsa
(omit jalapeño)

DAY 5

Breakfast

2-egg omelet with sautéed
spinach, mushrooms, shallots,
and garlic

sliced peaches

Lunch

steamed veggies

6 ounces canned or vacuum-
packed tuna with ½ cubed Hass
avocado

lemon juice vinaigrette

Dinner

*Chicken Noodle Soup with a
Surprise

*Topp Paleo Flatbread

DAY 6

Breakfast

*Kane's Ultra Pure Protein
Smoothie

Lunch

grilled mahi mahi with lemon
juice and garlic

steamed asparagus

Dinner

beef burger

baked sweet potato

mixed green salad

apple cider vinaigrette

DAY 7

Breakfast

ground lamb patties

sautéed mushrooms

honeydew melon

Lunch

cooked shredded chicken
wrapped in cabbage leaf with
chopped onion, cucumbers,
olives, and ½ Hass avocado

Dinner

*Chicken Fajitas (omit peppers)

sautéed red chard

RAISE THE ACTIVITY BAR

I mentioned at the beginning of this chapter that the Challenge phase includes exercise in addition to your walking regimen, so here goes:

- Increase your daily steps to ten thousand if you are not already there.

- Engage in high-intensity interval training with 6 to 10 minutes of strength training and cardio at least five days a week, using your body weight: jump rope, do sit-ups, lunges, squats, etc. Follow the instructions provided in the video "Bonus Feature" below, "Exercise for the Gluten-Free Warrior." These exercises require no outlay for equipment or a gym membership. Options will be provided for scaling exercises to your fitness level. For example, more advanced exercisers can add a vibration platform.

BONUS FEATURE

Two-hour video: "Exercise for the Gluten-Free Warrior": gluten freesociety.org/no-grain-no-pain-hiit.

If you have any doubt at this time that embarking on the No-Grain, No-Pain program won't change your life, read the story of one of my most challenging patients.

ACCUSED OF BEING A HYPOCHONDRIAC

Sheryl was in a bad way. Hip pain, chronic headaches, muscle twitching all over her body, vertigo, ringing in her ears, severe fatigue, digestive problems with constipation, severe and erratic spikes in her blood pressure, swelling of her face and feet, swollen lymph nodes, and severe allergy flare-ups had landed her in the ER eleven times, and she had been hospitalized twice. She had been to GPs, naturopaths, allergists, gastroenterologists, and a host of other specialists, many of whom accused her of being a hypochondriac. All her traditional lab tests were normal. Completely incapacitated by fatigue, she was housebound much of the time. She searched for answers for three years before coming to my clinic.

After a full functional medicine evaluation, we discovered that Sheryl had a gluten-sensitive gene pattern as well as being allergic to many foods she ate regularly. She had nutritional deficiencies in vitamins E, A, and K, as well as coenzyme Q_{10}, the mineral selenium, and the amino acid carnitine. GI lab markers revealed that her intestines were severely inflamed by gluten, and she had low levels of *Bifidobacteria* ("good" bacteria). Her adrenal hormones were almost nonexistent, and her blood sugar levels were very high, although she was not overweight and didn't have a "sweet tooth." But that's not all. Sheryl also had high levels of lead and mercury coursing through her body.

I put her on a grain-free, allergen-free diet and began supplementation to immediately correct her nutritional deficiencies. In addition, I started her on a natural heavy metal chelation protocol to remove mercury and lead. Within a few weeks, her constipation was gone, her digestion improved, and her energy levels improved well enough for her to function normally. Within two months, her hip pain and headaches were completely gone, as were the ringing in her ears, the vertigo, and the muscle twitching. The swelling in her face and feet had also dissipated. Within four months, her blood pressure normalized.

One of the challenges in Sheryl's case was her need to take blood pressure medications during the protocol. Her medication had a hidden source of wheat in it and was one of the factors that delayed her healing process. She took the medicine for two months before discovering the problem, which was resolved by having a compounding pharmacist prepare the prescription. Today, Sheryl feels great! She is energized and no longer under care of the allergists and gastroenterologists, nor does she have the huge stress of being sick all the time. She is pain free because she is grain free. For more of Sheryl's story, visit youtube.com/watch?v=Tw63_F1FT9s.

FREQUENTLY ASKED QUESTIONS

Q. Where do I go from here?
A. After two weeks on the Challenge phase, I know that your level of pain will be significantly less and you will feel enormously better. If so, just keep doing what you're doing. Once your gut is completely healed, which could take several months—and only if you're not gluten sensitive—you may be able to occasionally eat grains or other problematic foods in moderation. On the other hand, if you return to your old habits, I can almost guarantee you that your pain and other symptoms will return.

Q. Can I start eating out again after Day 30?
A. If your strategy is to get back to doing everything as you used to, you may find yourself right back to square one. Continue to eat out only when necessary so you can maintain control of your intake and keep pain and inflammation at bay.

Q. How do I know when to stop taking conventional medicines once I am following a dietary and supplement program to eliminate pain and inflammation?
A. If you're currently taking painkillers, anti-inflammatories, and/ or antibiotics, it's important to understand that the doses could become too strong as you reduce your pain and inflammation. That could create a whole other set of symptoms. Ask your doctor to alert you to which signals could indicate that you need to change the dose or stop certain medications. If your regular physician isn't will-

ing to work with you on this, I suggest you go to MyFunctionalMed icineDoctor.org to find a doctor who might be more willing to do so.

Q. When and how can I try reintroducing certain foods?
A. If you are gluten sensitive, never. If not, wait at least three months. Then try one food at a time and let several days elapse before making any other changes.

In part 3, "Beyond 30 Days," we'll look at how to continue to heal, and also explore matters such as environmental toxins that may be standing in the way of vibrant health. I'll also familiarize you with the principles of functional medicine if you decide to take that path in your journey to wellness. But before you do, and after you have been in this phase for 15 days, once again take the pain test introduced on page 19. Don't refer back to your earlier results as you gauge both the intensity and frequency of your pain.

PART 3

BEYOND 30 DAYS

It's not what we do once in a while that shapes our lives.
It's what we do consistently.

—Anthony Robbins

First let me congratulate you on the good work you have done in the past 30 days. At this point, almost everyone feels significantly better and almost always shows dramatic improvement in pain relief and other symptoms. Now that you've eliminated grains and certain other problematic foods and started repairing years of damage, you're well on your way to joining the ranks of *true* Gluten-Free Warriors. You're also now in a better position to understand how your food and lifestyle impact chronic pain and autoimmune disease. Of course, 30 days are just the beginning; now it's time to set your sights on going beyond the improvements you achieved in the Kickoff and Challenge phases to achieve permanent relief. If you have been chronically sick and plagued with pain for years, it's unrealistic to think you can be completely cured in 30 days.

The next two chapters introduce additional changes (and challenges) that will continue to improve your health and the quality of your life. One or more of these factors might well have been ganging up with grain in causing your pain. As I've said on several occasions, the same symptoms can result from different causes. But before we go there, it's critical that you understand how important it is to continue all the good work you've been doing.

DIET

Continue to eat as you have been for the past two weeks, but also listen to your body by remaining vigilant about your response to foods and making small dietary adjustments, as you see more and more improvement in your overall health.

Now that you've eliminated grain, you may be able to identify reactions to other foods. I've seen patients react to a variety of other foods, but your reactions will be unique to you.

If you want to reintroduce dairy products, you can try to do so after six months on the program, using only unpasteurized products from grass-fed cows, goats, and sheep.

SUPPLEMENTS

Continue the No-Grain, No-Pain supplement program, taking omega-3s, probiotics, and digestive enzymes, as well as a quality multivitamin, each day.

ACTIVITY

Remain a body in motion, both in your day-to-day activities and by walking at least ten thousand steps a day. Also continue the strength-training program introduced in the Challenge phase (see "Raise the Activity Bar" on page 210), increasing endurance and intensity as you get stronger.

SLEEP AND SUNSHINE

Continue to get a minimum of seven and preferably eight hours of quality shut-eye a night, and normalize your body clock (and ability to make vitamin D) by getting half an hour of morning sun each day.

• • •

To optimize your healing process, there are additional changes you'll want to make, as discussed in the following two chapters. These range from swapping out toxic cleaning supplies and cosmetics for safer alternatives to meeting with a doctor who practices functional medicine. Read on to maximize your health and remove the word *pain* from your vocabulary.

CHAPTER 10

BEYOND FOOD

How to Minimize Damage from Toxins That Can Compound the Effects of Grain

A dream doesn't become reality through magic; it takes sweat, determination and hard work.

—Colin Powell

You're probably thinking you're done, but you're really just beginning your campaign to make yourself and your family as healthy and inflammation free as possible. You're definitely on the right path by eliminating grain and other pain stimulators from your diet and taking the supplements I've recommended. And assuming you're also getting more exercise, sleep, and sunlight, kudos on those changes as well. If you've put off reading this section until you began the No-Grain, No-Pain program, I trust you're already feeling dramatically better. Now I hope you will feel motivated to up the ante with additional lifestyle changes that will continue to make a difference in your health and comfort.

You may initially wonder why such subjects as pesticides and air and water quality are relevant in a book about the pain inherent in grain. Good question. While the book *is primarily* about grain-related problems, it's to your advantage to understand that there can be other triggers for similar problems, and be on the alert for them. If you're saying to yourself, *I've now been grain free for a month but I'm still not pain free*, it's time to carefully consider whether one or more of these factors is linked to those symptoms. They often gang up with grain, although another possibility is that one or more of these toxic exposures is at the root of your pain. And even if your pain has completely vanished or is just a dull ache, you can improve your overall health and immune resistance by removing as many of these toxins as possible from your home (and body). I'll tell you how and/or point you in the right direction to achieve that goal in this chapter.

You see, chemical exposure, whether in the air in your home, the plastic containers in which you microwave your food, or the toothpaste you use daily, can all inflame your immune system, just as grain and certain other foods can. That means that you could remove every kernel of grain and every ounce of dairy from your diet and continue to experience pain—although likely reduced pain. If you have a little bit of inflammation coming from here (plastics), there (pesticides), and everywhere (other environmental toxins), how much will your full recovery be hindered as a result of those persistent exposures? Leaky gut has clearly been linked to exposure to pesticides, food additives, processed chemicals, and plastics.[1]

I'm well aware that some aspects of our contemporary lifestyle are almost impossible to change without retreating to a log cabin and forgoing electricity, heat, and running water. Don't worry. I don't expect you to catch every fish or grow every leaf of lettuce that makes its way into your kitchen. That said, there are many positive changes you can make to reduce your exposure to environmental chemicals and poisons in your home. But sometimes it is relatively small changes that can make a huge difference.

THE BASICS ARE ESSENTIAL FOR HEALING

When Burt originally came to see me, he suffered from depression, severe irritability, and social phobia. His mother brought him in because his medications weren't working, and she was worried about their long-term side effects. Testing revealed that Burt had a gluten-sensitive gene pattern, along with deficiencies of vitamins D and B_{12}, as well as of niacin (vitamin B_3) and omega-3 fats.

After making changes to his diet and following his supplementation program, Burt's symptoms improved dramatically, but he didn't make a full recovery. You see, he was somewhat of a skeptic about the value of sleep. A night owl, he liked to stay up late, a habit he had formed because he had a hard time falling asleep. He thought that staying up late was just how his body functioned. After I measured his cortisol levels, the picture became clear. Burt's levels of the hormone were high in the morning, low during the day, and high again at night. This pattern leads to sleep disturbances, as well as irritability.

After showing Burt his test results, I convinced him to start a rigorous exercise program each morning, while also implementing a nine p.m. lights-out policy. He was to get twenty minutes of morning sunshine daily, and I prescribed 10 mg of melatonin to take an hour before bedtime. After sticking with this approach for several weeks, Burt was able to fall asleep at a decent hour, and after several more weeks could nod off at bedtime without the need to take melatonin. No long afterward, he made a full recovery.

Burt's story is a perfect example of how you can do everything right with your diet, but still not fully improve. Proper exercise, sunshine, and sleep are essential to the healing process, and cannot be overlooked if you want to achieve and maintain good health. Now let's look at some other changes I recommend.

ALL OR NOTHING, NOT!

This book is all about making changes, but please don't be intimidated. The right mind-set is the most important component to beginning this process. If you become so paralyzed thinking about all of the environmental toxins assaulting you on a daily basis, you could shut down and ask yourself, *I can't possibly do all of this, so what's the point of changing anything?* A better approach is to control what you can and pray—or meditate, if you prefer—about the rest.

The issue of control factors into why I recommend that you don't dine out in the initial 30 days of the No-Grain, No-Pain program—and preferably longer. Whenever you can choose not to eat out and thereby stay in control of what you put in your mouth, do so; but when you must eat out and therefore aren't in complete control, simply accept it and make the best choices you can. As long as you're in control most of the time, when circumstances mean that you occasionally can't be, so be it. Let me remind you that you've already taken giant steps in reducing the toxins in your system. As long as you're following my recommendations to eat organic and non-GMO, you've done a great job of removing the vast majority of toxins, including prior water-based and food-based antibiotic exposure. You've already accomplished a lot in just 30 days. Now let's talk about how we can take this to the next level.

First of all, you needn't implement all these other safeguards simultaneously. Take them one by one or several at a time, if you wish. The better you feel, the more inclined you will be to keep making improvements in your environment. You may want to do the ones that are easiest first, for example, ditching plastic containers and replacing them with glass. Swapping your household cleaning products for safer ones is relatively easy, as well.

In each case, I'll give a brief explanation of the damage a certain factor can inflict, and offer some solutions or alternatives. Some relate directly to grain. Others can produce symptoms that mimic those of grain or simply stand in the way of achieving relief from pain and good health. But first I want to make a blanket statement: heavy metals, environmental poisons, mold, and other toxins are everywhere. Some people go through life and despite exposure to one or more agents never have a problem because their bodies are really good detoxifiers; others aren't so lucky. It's the poor detoxifiers who are more apt to have autoimmune diseases, and they're the ones for whom dietary changes are most impactful. I say this because I don't want you to become so fearful of your environment that you shut down and become bubble-gal or bubble-guy, afraid of everything and unable to relax and lead a normal life. Already in the past 30 days, you've made yourself a better detoxifier. And the longer you continue to eat this way, the better you will become.

GET THE LEAD (AND MORE) OUT

Let me introduce you to Cheryl, who was referred to me by another functional medicine doctor. She suffered from severe foot and leg pain, which kept her bedridden most of the time. She also had chronic fatigue syndrome. After a functional medicine workup, we discovered that Cheryl had a gluten-sensitive gene pattern. She also had allergies to blueberries and cabbage, both foods that most people would agree are quite healthy, as well as to sugar. (Yes, you can be allergic to sugar.) Additionally, she was reacting to phthalates (the compounds found in plastic water bottles, cosmetics, Tupperware, and other petrochemical-based products). She had nutritional deficiencies in vitamins D and A, and in the thyroid-boosting mineral selenium. But that's not all. Cheryl also had high levels of lead in her system.

Within two weeks of implementing her diet, supplementation, and lifestyle protocol, eliminating grain and other problematic foods, and reducing her exposure to hormone-disrupting phthalates by eliminating certain types of cosmetics and no longer drinking or eating from plastics, Cheryl's crippling pain was completely gone. Within a month, her energy levels returned, and within a few months, she lost 30 pounds and reduced her body fat by 10 percent. Once more, good-bye grain, good-bye pain. For more of Cheryl's story, visit glutenfree society.org/Cheryls-no-grain-no-pain-testimonial/.

• • •

I see many people who have toxic levels of lead and other heavy metals in their body. You've already read about several other success-story people who faced this challenge. We're all daily exposed to heavy metals, which can build up in your body for years—what is called bio-accumulation—before the damage is evident. Many processed foods, including corn sugar,[2] contain heavy metals. If you're eating only real food, you're going to be better at getting rid of these toxins. Let's look at the four most common heavy metals.

MERCURY

Mercury displaces sulfur compounds, which help your body detoxify,[3] so it actually gums up your ability to excrete the toxins via the liver or kidneys. It also displaces zinc, copper, and iron, highjacking the functions of these nutrients, making it appear that you have a zinc, copper, calcium, or magnesium deficiency.[4] If you have any of these deficiencies, it would be worth testing your mercury levels with an environmental doctor before deciding on a course of treatment. (See "What Is Environmental Medicine?" on page 226.) The longer and greater the exposure to mercury, the more difficult is to get rid of it. Mercury can mimic symptoms caused by grain, including severe neurological problems,[5] or they can occur simultaneously. If you have not eaten grain for at least 30 days and still have some of the symptoms below, you may also be accumulating mercury. Or, possibly, grains were never your problem, and instead the culprit is mercury.

Sources: Primarily amalgam fillings, but also vaccines and seafood. I say this not to discourage you from eating fish or getting vaccinated, but to avoid mercury whenever possible. Eating fish is a problem only if you're also accumulating excessive mercury from junk foods. Don't stop eating fish. It's part of a healthy diet. Mercury accumulation over time contributes to disease. It is expensive to get amalgam fillings removed correctly, but if done improperly, mercury can spill into your bloodstream and digestive tract.

Symptoms of toxicity: Depression, anxiety, brain fog, and fatigue; also body odor from literally sweating out mercury; a metallic taste in the mouth; hormone disruption, creating an abnormal menstrual cycle; ringing in the ears.

LEAD

Lead toxicity is also extremely common.[6] Some older municipal water lines were soldered with lead, which can leach out and into the water supply. Lead is also ubiquitous in the petrochemical and battery industries and was once an ingredient in paint and gas. Those coming of age in the 1950s and '60s are sometimes called the lead generation. Lead displaces calcium and iron, so it gets stored in the bones. By age 35, women begin to lose bone mass, but if someone had a lot of lead exposure as a child, lead is now trickling into her bloodstream. If she also has a sedentary lifestyle and poor diet, the lead overload could be the proverbial straw that breaks the camel's back. Lead also crosses the placenta, so a pregnant woman exposed to lead may pass on the toxicity to her unborn child.[7]

Sources: Airborne lead particulates and water; also toys, especially those produced in China; ceramics with low-fire lead glazes. There have been numerous recalls after finding lead in products as diverse as pet foods and lipsticks.[8]

Symptoms of toxicity: Because lead displaces zinc, selenium, chromium, calcium, and iron, it can create persistent anemia, which causes fatigue and can interfere with hemoglobin production; also learning disorders, brain damage, and kidney problems, as well as cardiovascular inflammation and hypertension.

CADMIUM

Cadmium has been found in dangerous levels in rice,[9] another reason to avoid this grain. Cadmium is used in electroplating, so the electronics industry is reliant on it. Cadmium also displaces calcium and can lead to softening of the bones, thyroid disease,[10] and kidney damage.[11] Cadmium found in costume jewelry and children's jewelry, as well as in drinking glasses with painted designs used as promotional items at McDonald's, have led to recalls. Cadmium can displace zinc, and many of the symptoms linked to overexposure to this metal are similar to those of zinc deficiency, including weakened immunity, digestive problems, proneness to injury, slow healing, and muscle and joint pain.

Sources: Electroplating and electronics factories, electroplated costume jewelry, plastics, fertilizers, secondhand cigarette smoke, and agricultural crops that are grown in soil or water.

Symptoms of toxicity: Kidney and liver damage, bone loss, fatigue, anemia, joint pain, shortness of breath, brain fog, headaches, and dizziness.

ARSENIC

Arsenic poisoning is something I often see in my practice. Arsenic is a naturally occurring element in the earth's crust, so organic arsenic is found in soil and water. Inorganic (manufactured) arsenic appears mainly in fertilizers and pesticides.[12] Contamination can come from one or both sources. Like cadmium, this metal has also been found in rice.

Sources: Water supply, groundwater, soil, and rice and other grain crops grown in contaminated water or soil, respectively.

Symptoms of toxicity: Vitamin B_1 deficiency; high blood pressure due to its effects on arterial walls, which regulates the dilation of blood vessels; muscle pain; heart irregularities; nerve and brain damage; and lung cancer. (For more on heavy metals and how to eliminate them, see "Help Get the Metal Out" on page 253.)

There are four primary organs your body uses to detoxify. Priming these systems will boost the chelation process.

What Is Environmental Medicine?

A relatively new field, environmental medicine is a part of functional medicine, and addresses the interaction between humans and our

environment, specifically how we experience exposure to an exci-
tant, a provoking agent found in air, food, water, drugs, or the home
or other buildings. All these agents may adversely affect one or
more organ systems. If you have heavy metal toxicity or suspect
you do, you should see a physician who has had specific training
in environmental medicine. Unfortunately, most doctors have not
been trained to recognize anything other than acute toxicity, so bioaccumulation is not usually on their radar. To learn more about environmental medicine, visit the American Academy of Environmental
Medicine at aaemonline.org/introduction.php.

PLASTIC EQUALS PETROCHEMICALS

Would you add petroleum to your food or beverages? Of course not;
it belongs in your fuel tank, not your body. But every time you store
and reheat leftovers in your microwave oven in a plastic container, you
might as well be doing just that. You're probably aware that plastics
that contain BPA (bisphenol A) have been linked to cancer, but they
are just the tip of the iceberg. BPA is a phthalate, a petrochemical
that mimics estrogen and creates estrogen dominance in both females
and males.[13] It has also been linked to intestinal permeability[14] and
increases the risk of cancer for both sexes, to say nothing of encouraging weight gain.[15] Excess estrogen in birth control pills has been linked
to cardiovascular disease.[16]

When bottled water became popular, it was considered a healthier alternative to sugary soda. But as the bottles of water sit in warehouses in summer heat, the chemicals leach out of the plastic and into
the water. Heavy use of bottled water can lead to bioaccumulation just
as with heavy metals, creating hormone disruption and dysfunction.

Time to bust another myth:

Myth 17: **BPA-free plastic is safe to use.**

Not true! All plastics are made from petroleum products. Just
because we haven't identified a certain type of plastic as carcino-

genic or studied it well enough yet doesn't mean that it doesn't contain hormone disruptors and other dangerous compounds.

Now that the word is out that their estrogenic effects make BPA containers unsafe, there's a big push to make all plastic bottles BPA-free. But all plastics are made with petrochemicals and other toxic chemicals. Removing the BPA is like removing the fat from dairy products but adding sugar. The fat-free version isn't any healthier. The BPA situation is actually akin to the gluten/grain issue at the core of this book. As a culture, we've labeled certain grains as containing gluten and declared the others fine and dandy. Likewise, we've declared one plastic the bad guy and implied the others are good guys. Both assumptions are equally flawed. My advice is to quit looking for BPA-free plastic containers and purchase glass or stainless steel containers, which are nonreactive. Don't wait for the research to tell you a few years from now that other plastics presently used for water bottles and storage containers are also dangerous. It's not only better for your health to eschew plastic; it's also better for the planet. Buy filtered water in glass jugs and use it to refill your stainless steel or glass water bottle.

If you're following the No-Grain, No-Pain program, you won't be purchasing many packaged foods, but when you occasionally do, avoid those sold in plastic containers whenever possible. Chemical leaching is of greater concern with liquids than solids, so I'm not as concerned about salad greens in plastic containers, for example, at least from a health perspective. The reality is unless you have your own garden you're going to have to buy some things in plastic. Again, control what you can and pray about the rest. If you have the option to buy fresh fruit and vegetables not packaged in plastics, do so. If not, accept it.

On the other hand, here are the absolute no-nos with plastic, all of which are well within your control. Never:

- Drink bottled water
- Heat up food up in plastic
- Eat off or out of plastic

• Use plastic utensils

• Heat up a plastic baby bottle or feed your baby from it

To minimize exposure to plastics of any kind:

• Avoid produce wrapped in plastic.

• Bring string bags to the supermarket to hold greens and other large items.

• Bring small paper lunch bags to corral items such as string beans and cherries.

• Opt for glass containers over plastic ones or aluminum cans in the supermarket.

• Use glass storage containers for leftovers and to reheat.

• Use a stainless steel thermos and a glass water bottle to transport food and liquids.

Biodegradable plastic bags and other products made from corn may be environmentally "friendlier" if indeed they do compost, and depending on how much energy is required to produce them, but if you have removed all grains from your diet and are still sick, you might be hypersensitive even to such products. Stop using them to see if you experience improvement.

BPA has long been used to line the interiors of cans of acidic foods such as tomatoes. Recently, a number of manufacturers have switched to non-BPA linings, but they are still using some type of plastic. (Some tomato products do come in glass.) As far as I'm concerned, the only reason to have canned vegetables and fruit on hand is as emergency rations during a hurricane, tornado, or blizzard when you may lose power. Otherwise, fresh locally grown organic produce is the best choice, followed by fresh organic and then frozen, with canned produce a distant fourth. Of course, if you have the time, buying produce in bulk in season and putting it up in mason jars is a great option. Vegetables or fruit with no sugars, sauces, or seasonings are acceptable, but premade frozen meals and the like don't qualify as food in my book.

PESTICIDES ARE POISONS— AND HORMONE DISRUPTORS

Pesticide residue in foods is an enormous problem, but if you've been buying organic produce and avoiding most processed foods, you're already heading in the right direction. (Tim, one of our success stories, had pesticides in his system.)

The two most commonly used pesticides are glyphosate (Roundup) and the herbicide atrazine, which is the first line of defense used by conventional growers of corn, sorghum, and sugarcane. It has been shown to cause sex organ changes in fish, frogs, salamanders, and turtles.[17] That's another powerful reason to avoid these foods. These pesticides are designed to kill plants, so the crops on which they are used have been genetically modified to survive the poison, unlike us!

There are several ways pesticides poison us:

- They can interfere with sulfur pathways in our body, effectively shutting down the detoxification process.
- They can cause GI damage, the very thing we're trying to heal.
- Just like plastics and grains, they mimic estrogens.
- They can contain heavy metals.

Avoidance of pesticides is the way to justify the higher cost of buying organic. Paying for medical services now or down the road is unquestionably more costly than spending a little bit more today to avoid such expenses in the future.

Symptoms of toxicity: General fatigue, malaise, rashes, hives, and gastroesophageal reflux disease (GERD) and other gut problems. Severe reactions and dysfunction are also possible.

As I've mentioned earlier, there's a significant body of research on gluten that is attempting to untangle how much of the ill effects people experience are from gluten itself versus the result of harvesting methods. For example, farmers can now time the harvest of wheat, corn, and other grains by spraying the crops with Roundup.[18] Efficiency, not healthier plants—or people—is the driver. As an industry, agribusiness is all about producing more with less, which is where pesticides and GMO crops come into play. Some large landowners simply lease their land to Dow or Monsanto and use the procedures their corporate masters specify. Call it modern-day sharecropping. At the other extreme, most independent farmers are trying to capitalize on the organic industry. Buying organic is not just better for you; it also helps independent farmers remain in business.

Plastics and pesticides are just two forms of petrochemicals, which pollute our air and water, many of them acting as "obesogens."[19] As hormone disruptors, they make it easier to gain weight and keep it on. And, of course, obesity aggravates pain. Many petrochemicals mimic estrogen, increasing the risk of cancers and heart disease and other diseases linked to estrogen dominance. In men that leads to reduced muscle mass and likely increased docility, meaning that if a man's doctor tells him to take drugs he is more apt to do so. I needn't remind you that grain is also a hormone disrupter.

MORE DRUGS THAT CONTRIBUTE TO PAIN

In chapter 2 we discussed the deleterious side effects of prescription and over-the-counter painkillers and anti-inflammatories. Now let's look at other drugs that can contribute to chronic pain.

Antibiotics destroy good gut bacteria, and when you knock out all the good guys and don't replace them with a probiotic, it creates an opportunity for yeast overgrowth.[20] And what does yeast do? It creates inflammatory chemicals and chronic infection, which inflame the GI tract. Yeast also converts any sugar you eat into alcohol, so now your gut behaves as a distillery hammering your liver with alcohol.[21] Your liver is one of the organs responsible for pain control and inflammation, so the last thing you want to do is damage it. I'm not advocating against antibiotic use, but if you do need one, you must also take a probiotic for at least a month and preferably two months after completing the course of antibiotics. (Be sure to take the two four hours apart.) Antibiotics also cause deficiencies of vitamin K[22] and biotin[23], both of which are produced by good bacteria.

Antacids such as Nexium, Prilosec, Zantac, Aciphex, and even Tums and Rolaids can also cause big problems. (Nexium tops the list as the most commonly prescribed—and expensive—brand-name medication paid for by Medicare.[24]) A major problem associated with aging is reduced production of stomach acid, but the symptom of this is the same as that of making too much: acid reflux. Most doctors assume acid reflux is the result of excess stomach acid and prescribe an antacid. However, if you're already making less acid, taking an antacid could destroy your ability to digest protein, which is essential to repair, heal, and build new tissue. Protein is one of the main ingredients necessary to relieve muscle or joint pain and inflammation. Blocking stomach acid leads to malabsorption of protein and poor digestion, but it also can compound drug-induced nutritional deficiencies. As we've discussed earlier, when you block stomach acid, you also block vitamin B_{12}, calcium, iron, magnesium, zinc, and vitamin A, causing deficiencies of these essential nutrients.

Aside from the human cost, what are the consequences for taxpayers of the use of such drugs long term? The biggest cause of early mortality is loss of muscle, yet the number one drug we give our elderly population is one that blocks their protein absorption so their body has to steal from existing muscle to create antibodies to fight all the other stuff in their environment. This results in millions of dollars for medical care that wouldn't be necessary if the elderly were well nourished and stronger.

Antidepressants also interfere with nutrient absorption. Doctors often tell people that their pain is "all in their head" and prescribe an antidepressant, without thinking of the unintended consequences. These drugs affect how quickly food breaks down and moves through your GI tract, what is called gastric motility,[25] often with the side effect of IBS. Whether gastric motility is speeded up or slowed down, it impacts digestion and assimilation of nutrients. Two of the more common selective serotonin reuptake inhibitor (SSRI) antidepressants are Paxil and Prozac.

Blood pressure drugs, such as hydrochlorothiazide, often cause a zinc deficiency or block it altogether. If you're experiencing difficulty smelling and/or tasting food, you may be zinc deficient.[26] This reduces the ability to taste flavors, so there is a tendency to oversalt food and indulge in sugary treats, both of which contribute to inflammation and high blood pressure.

ACE inhibitors also block zinc, and many of them also block CoQ$_{10}$. Zinc plays a role in the taste buds and scent receptors in your nose,[27] which directly affect the way you eat and therefore impact nutrition.

Statins block CoQ10 and vitamin D, as discussed earlier, causing muscle degradation, contributing to pain. By trying to reduce the risk of heart disease with a drug to block cholesterol, you degrade muscles, reducing exercise capacity. Being sedentary means you're going to hurt more. I call this particular vicious cycle the pain-prescription trap.

You'll also recall that many supplements contain gluten or grain fillers, which could be a "hidden" source of pain for people with gluten sensitivity. The same is true of drugs. Be sure to read both lists on the label or information sheet. The active ingredients list tells which chemicals are in the drug; the inactive ingredients list provides the names of the fillers, sweeteners, dyes, and other ingredients that make the form of the drug distinctive in appearance and/or easier to swallow.

THE MOLD FACTOR

Industrially farmed grains are generally stored in huge bins, increasing the likelihood of mold growth and contamination. Many people have mold allergies and reactions, so although you might not be grain sensitive per se, you might very well be mold sensitive.

Some types of mold produce severe types of mycotoxins. Mold is a plant, although it reproduces with spores instead of seeds, as most plants do, and a mycotoxin is a poison the mold produces. Two of the foods that are most laden with molds that contain mycotoxins are grain and coffee.[28]

Molds comprise a huge family that include *Alternaria*, which often grow in our sinuses, mouth, and nose; *Candida* (*Candida albicans*), which appears as oral thrush or even thickened toenails, and can be caused by taking antibiotics; and athlete's foot and jock itch caused by *Trichophyton*. Our subject is environmental molds, and in particular one that grows predominantly on grains: *Fusarium*, which produces the myco-toxin fumonisin. It is extremely dangerous, and some people are very reactive, even to small amounts. *Fusarium* can suppress immune function and create inflammation and pain, making it yet another reason to avoid grain. The black discoloration you often see inside a house is *Aspergillus*. *Cladosporium*, which is typically seen growing on the side of a house, can trigger respiratory problems. Regardless of the source, if you are chronically sick, in pain, and your immune system is already on fire, the last thing you want is to be attacked by a mold toxin. If despite eliminating grain and certain other foods for 30 days you still don't feel up to snuff, you should consider the possibility that you have a toxic mold condition.

HOW TO MINIMIZE TOXIC EXPOSURE

Okay, we've discussed a number of disturbing possibilities that may be contributing to your pain and discomfort, or perhaps even be the driving force. It's scary stuff, especially since with the exception of mold, you can't see most of these attackers coming. In addition to eliminating plastics from your kitchen and as many other toxic products as you can and minimizing your intake of drugs, what can you do to protect yourself and your family from toxic exposure?

STEP 1: FILTER YOUR WATER

Most major cities have serious contamination of their drinking water from unmetabolized drug residue excreted in urine or unused drugs flushed down the toilet. There is no perfect way to filter your water. Nor has there been research on how to remove specific contaminants. What we do know is that a granular activated carbon filter works well at removing chlorines, bromines, and certain other compounds, and can remove some toxins. For removing metals and other chemical compounds, KDF (kinetic degradation fluxion), a copper-zinc alloy, is the most effective. A whole-house water filter typically uses a salt to soften water, but a combination granular activated carbon and KDF purifi-cation medium improves its quality. The KDF will remove chemical compounds from the water along with fungi, bacteria, chlorine, certain pesticides, and some heavy metals.

I recommend that you filter all the water in your home at the point of entry, rather than simply at your kitchen faucet. When you take a shower, you breathe in roughly a quarter of a gallon of steam, not including the toxins you may absorb through your skin. Nor do you want to wash your clothes in chemical-laden water. That said, a carbon/KDF filter is not going to remove fluoride. If your water is fluoridated, you'll also need to use a reverse osmosis (RO) filter to get rid of it, typ-ically in the form of a five-gallon RO tank under the kitchen sink. The RO system usually has a carbon and KDF prefilter on it. Otherwise, the chlorine in the water would destroy the RO filter. On the other hand, if you have your own well, you might have hundreds of feet of earth fil-tering your water, and may not need certain filters. Nonetheless, your well could be contaminated, especially with slant drilling, aka fracking, by the petroleum industry, so I would still recommend filtering well water with a KDF/carbon filter. It's also a good idea to have your water tested by an independent company.

STEP 2: FILTER YOUR AIR

Better-insulated homes have reduced our energy consumption, which is a good thing, but when a building doesn't "breathe" and windows remain shut, toxins are trapped inside. If your air conditioner uses recycled air, you're just recirculating those toxins. The result is mas-sive exposure to chemicals leached from your furniture, wall-to-wall carpeting, polyurethane-finished flooring, fabrics impregnated with flame-retardant chemicals, and other volatile organic compounds. Emissions from gas cooktops, heaters, furnaces, and other devices add to the toxic stew. According to the Environmental Protection Agency, off-gassing of numerous products has made the air inside our homes two to five times more toxic than our outdoor environment.[29] In some cases, indoor air is a hundred times more polluted than outdoor air![30]

Obviously, you aren't going to do away with your furniture and accessories. So what *can* you do?

If you can afford furniture made with all-natural organic components, go for it, but it's extremely expensive and, frankly, may not hold up as well or be as comfortable. Instead, filter your interior air and regularly open the windows to air out the house. An AC system that pulls from the outdoors is a healthier alternative than a recirculating one. Your objective is to filter both the air coming into the home from outside and the air within.

And get yourself a good vacuum cleaner. Again, control what you can and pray about the rest.

Air conditioning creates condensation, which can lead to humidity formation. An air conditioner also acts as a dehumidifier. Try to keep the relative humidity under 55 percent to avoid mold growth. A digital reader available at any hardware store lets you keep it in check. Even in a dry climate, I would advise using a humidifier only if you experience severe dry skin and persistent rashes. (Certain types of mold grow in dry climates.) Any air filtration system should be HEPA (high-efficiency particulate air) based, meaning the screen is small enough to capture mold spores. If you then subject them to UV light, you kill a lot of those that create problems for humans. An electrician can install a UV light to reduce the likelihood of mold circulating in the vents. (It's also a good idea to have a HEPA filter on your vacuum cleaner.) The Swiss-based company IQAir (iqair.com) makes a good whole-house air purification system, which is worth considering if you are building a new house.

STEP 3: CLEAN UP YOUR ACT

Most household and personal cleaning products contain petrochemicals, which again have estrogen-mimicking effects, as do the dyes and artificial scents used to make them more appealing. My patients are more apt to have migraine headaches and other problems triggered by inhaling the chemical perfumes than by the cleaning agents themselves. My suggestions for natural alternatives:

- Instead of ammonia-based window cleaning products, use vinegar and water.
- Instead of hand or facial soaps loaded with chemicals, use a coconut-derived agent or glycerin or castile soap.
- Instead of shampoos made with sodium lauryl sulfate (SLS), a sudsing agent, look for organic products and natural ingredients.
- Instead of antibacterial wipes full of triclosan, which plays havoc with our hormones and creates free radicals, which have an oxidizing effect in the body, opt for unscented products without this toxin.
- Avoid household cleaners with chlorine, artificial scents, and any unpronounceable chemicals.
- Seek out brands of toothpaste that are free of SLS, the antibacterial triclosan, and fluoride; or use baking soda.

Rather than provide a list of the chemicals and products currently in your medicine cabinets and under your sink to avoid (new entries are regularly being added), I recommend you use the resources provided by the Environmental Working Group (see "Bonus Features," on page 239). You'll want to also minimize exposure to most fertilizers, as well as herbicides, pesticides, and other chemicals in your garage or garden shed. To find more natural alternatives, visit transition-to-organics.org /safe-alternatives.

Too Clean for Their Own Good?

In recent years, antibacterial soaps, gels, and wipes have been big sellers. Most of them contain triclosan, which is also in dishwashing detergent and liquid hand soap, as well as toothpaste. According to the FDA, the use of antibacterial products has not been shown to provide any benefits over plain soap and water.[31] Moreover, the American Medical Association cautions that triclosan should not be used in the home.[32] We actually need good bacteria on our skin, in our homes, and in our environment.[33] When we sterilize our environment, we actually contribute to autoimmunity. In fact, a new theory about disease, the hygiene hypothesis, posits that being *too* clean actually causes health problems. Obsessively protecting young children from exposure to dirt, infectious agents, parasites, and certain common allergens, while simultaneously exposing them to antibiotics, means their immune system response isn't properly stimulated, making them more susceptible over time to a wide array of diseases and conditions.

A RUNNER RUNS INTO TROUBLE

Susan was a runner. She loved to run, and that's how she stayed in shape, until she started to limp. She hadn't had a physical injury; rather, one foot simply started to drag when she walked or ran. She noticed that all of her shoes were wearing out as a result. Her legs felt heavy, and she also developed dizziness. These symptoms are a classic form of gluten-induced nerve damage, but unfortunately, very few doctors recognize this or investigate the cause.

That's not all that was wrong. She had a litany of symptoms, including severe arthritic pain in joints throughout her body, fatigue, and brain fog. Before coming to see me, she had had MRIs, X-rays, and physical therapy. She had also been placed in an orthotic boot, but to no avail.

My evaluation revealed that Susan had gluten-sensitive genes, as well as multiple food allergies including dairy, pomegranate, cherry, and the sweetener xylitol. She was also deficient in calcium, vitamin D, and the B vitamins 1, 2, 3, 5, 9, and 12. Of particular note was her 15-year history as a vegetarian, which can create a deficiency of both vitamin B_1 and B_{12}. These two nutrients are vital for proper nerve function and maintenance. When combined with gluten-induced nerve damage, the outcome can be even more profound.

After a month without grain, Susan's foot drop improved dramatically and she noticed that her arthritis was alleviating. As an added bonus, many of the symptoms she had blamed on aging started going away. Moral of the story? The now familiar: no grain, no pain. For more of Susan's story, visit glutenfreesociety.org/no-grain-no-pain-review -Susans-story/.

BONUS FEATURES

The Environmental Working Group (ewg.org) offers a database of more than seventy thousand toxin-free products, including detergents, air fresheners, hair spray, lotions, sunscreens, cosmetics, and numerous other categories, as well as a guide to pesticides in produce and other helpful content. Also check out Campaign for Safe Cosmetics (safecosmetics.org), which covers personal care products for both men and women and describes the chemicals commonly found in such products, as well as the Personal Care Products Council (personalcarecouncil.org). Finally, you'll find gluten-free and toxin-free cosmetics and other products at glutenfreesociety.org/shop.

In the next and last chapter, we'll look at how seeing a practitioner of functional medicine can help you address pain and other serious problems related to grain and more.

CHAPTER 11

BEYOND SELF-HELP

Functional Medicine Is the Future of Medicine

The good physician treats the disease; the great physician treats the patient who has the disease.

—William Osler

The days of generic medicine are coming to an end. Each person is biochemically unique. As I've explained earlier, the role of a functional medicine doctor is to identify the origin of a health problem and treat it, rather than mask symptoms with chemical drugs. I trust that this book has opened your eyes to possibilities you may not have been aware existed. Hopefully, I've helped you to understand why you've been sick and in pain and encouraged you to start the process of healing that will put an end to your suffering. However, if you have an autoimmune disease or a chronic pain-based condition, you may want to work with a doctor experienced in functional medicine so that the two of you can individualize your treatment approach, not just guess at what you *might* need. Another important facet of functional medicine is that patient and doctor work as a team.

In this chapter, I'll paint a larger picture of how I work and provide you with resources to find a practitioner in your region. Although working with such a doctor is highly personalized, technology is an important piece of the process, as you'll understand as we delve into the various tests we functional medicine doctors use to help identify what each patient needs to do to get better. Overall, technology has taken the guessing out of the game and eliminates years of doctor shopping, pain, grief, wasted money, and fruitless trips to the ER.

THE ROLE OF DRUGS IN ACUTE VS. CHRONIC CONDITIONS

Although I am generally no fan of conventional medicines, not all drugs are useless or dangerous. Some have their time and place, primarily when somebody's life is at risk. Looking at drugs actually provides a lens with which to take a closer look at functional medicine. If you have a traumatic injury, such as a fractured bone, clearly surgery is warranted. Although the injury involves inflammation, it won't be banished by eliminating grain. This is the kind of situation in which conventional medicine shines. But when it comes to chronic conditions, which are the subject of this book, pharmaceuticals have little relevance.

In an acute situation, such as surgery in which you would need to be knocked out, a chemical painkiller is mandatory. And it would be needed for some time afterward while the incision knits. Antibiotics have their place, too, for example, to eliminate a serious life-threatening infection. If you were completely debilitated by a migraine headache, you might also need a painkiller—but only in the short run. On the other hand, if the injury and inflammation are caused by diet and have gone on for a long time, dietary changes can solve the problem. In some cases an injury compounds a chronic problem that has been neglected and has become acute over time. To feel better immediately, you might need conventional medicine, but in order to restore your health and stay better, you need a functional medicine approach.

THE LIMITS OF MOST LAB TESTS

In addition to this difference in philosophy about drugs, another factor that distinguishes functional medicine from conventional medicine is the lab tests used. The vast majority of tests conventional medicine doctors order can be helpful, but they can also be inaccurate. That's why so many chronically ill people see their doctor with a complaint, but when their blood-work results come in, they're told, "Everything is normal." And if that happens to you and you continue to insist that something is wrong, you're likely to hear "It's in your head. Go see a shrink." Blood work can appear normal but the patient can still be sick, either because there's an inaccuracy or inherent flaw in the blood work or because it has not been accurately interpreted.

Let me explain how this can happen. All lab tests have a range that is considered normal, but you may not realize that those ranges change every several months. The lab regularly recalculates normal ranges based on a sampling of people who get tested. As these ranges change—and the population is obviously a lot sicker today than in the past—what is considered normal changes, becoming the new norm. It's rather like "fat is the new thin": a weight that would have been considered overweight a few decades ago has become the norm. With more people diagnosed with diabetes, heart disease, and cancer than ever before, normal becomes degraded and being within the "normal" range doesn't necessarily equate with health.

Second, some ranges have been changed in an effort to sell more drugs. For example, it used to be that as long as your total cholesterol was below 250 mg/dl (milligrams per deciliter of blood), a statin drug wasn't recommended. But that number was revised down to 220, and then to 200. This enormous change had nothing to do with the average cholesterol levels of people in the tested population. Rather, it was the result of doctors being influenced by drug companies to change lab values to allow them to sell more drugs.[1] This means that ranges based on the average "healthy" population aren't really all that relevant for somebody who is sick. A third issue with the idea of so-called normal ranges is that such serum blood tests don't necessarily take into consideration whether you're male or female, whether you weigh 115 pounds or 215 pounds, whether you're 5 feet or 6 feet tall, or whether you're 20 or 60.[2] Twentysomething Jane Doe is grouped with her 50-year-old dad.

Some doctors don't consider all the possibilities that can throw test results off, particularly if the patient appears to be healthy. If he or she *is* actually healthy, the results are probably accurate. But with a chronically sick patient who has immune diseases, a doctor's head is in the sand if he or she doesn't question "normal" results. A doctor should always consider how the lab results interplay with the status and condition of the patient. Functional medicine involves thinking about the things that doctors tend to not think about, either because they didn't learn about them in medical school or because they haven't spent enough time with the patient.

Which would you prefer? A doctor who comes into the room and says, "Your lab tests are normal, but here's a prescription to reduce your stress," and exits the examining room in three minutes, or a doctor who says, "Your lab tests are normal, but tell me how you're feeling. You describe yourself as hypothyroid, but your thyroid tests all came back normal. Let's talk about what else might be going on and maybe run additional tests that might give us an answer to why you feel this way."

This second approach clearly takes more time, which is why I see only four patients a day. If I don't have the ability to deliver good care, what's the point in having a practice? Before I meet with a new patient, I have her fill out an extensive questionnaire to get a thorough background and medical history, which helps me tailor my questions when we do sit down together. Most people who see a functional medicine doctor have already had all the standard lab tests done, along with all the traditional drugs prescribed. They've usually have had very little or no benefit to date and are at their wits' end, which usually makes them very open to alternatives.

AN INDIVIDUALIZED APPROACH TO TESTING

In my practice, we use narrower ranges based on older data. We also use other tests that don't rely on such ranges. In *Biochemical Individuality*, Nobel Prize–winning biochemist Roger Williams challenges the assumption of normal.[3] Are you an average person? Of course, there is no such thing. Each one of us is unique. For example, after measuring blood volume, organ size, and skin surface area, Dr. Williams reports huge variables in the volume of numerous vitamins, minerals, and other chemicals, even among people of the same weight, height, and age. These potential variables aren't accounted for in standard lab testing.

For example, when I test for vitamin and mineral deficiencies, I don't compare a patient's range to everyone else's range. Instead, I need a marker that is going to give me a long-term view of her nutritional status. A serum blood test can't do this. When I test Jane Doe's blood cells, I actually measure the growth rate of her cells. Then I give those cells all the vitamins and minerals they will need to grow and I measure the rate at which the cells are capable of growing.[4] That's Jane's baseline: her cells at their optimal level. Then I can tailor her regimen to her individual potential. In contrast, if Jane came to me with a standard vitamin B_{12} test from her conventional doctor, all it would measure is how much B_{12} was floating around in her blood when her blood was drawn. It wouldn't tell me anything about what the level was the day before or the day after. And compared to ten thousand other people who are called "normal" because they fit into the range, her blood level of B_{12} would be probably appear within normal parameters.

The test that I use, on the other hand, might show that Jane is deficient in vitamin B_{12}, not because of the level in her blood at that moment, but instead based on how much B_{12} is being stored in her cells, where it works. Additionally, because the cells being used have a six-month life span, the test measures a patient's average nutritional status over that period. Instead of basing test results on whether she seems normal compared to other people, such tests are based on individual patient outcome, which is why they are called functional outcome tests. This particular test exemplifies cutting-edge medicine; it took seventeen years to develop at the University of Texas.

BONUS FEATURE

A video explains how functional outcome tests work: spectracell .com/clinicians.

WHAT GENETIC TESTING DOES AND DOESN'T REVEAL

You've undoubtedly noticed that my patients' success stories often refer to genetic test results that indicate that they're gluten sensitive. But that's only one genetic test. Just to be clear, genetic testing doesn't tell you whether or not you'll develop a certain disease. Unless you're born with a genetic disorder, such as cystic fibrosis, your DNA doesn't dictate that you'll have a disease, only that you may have certain weak links. If a person has a genetic pattern for gluten sensitivity and she eats gluten, there's the potential to develop an inflammatory response every time it's consumed. Or if you have genes that don't detoxify certain chemical toxins efficiently and you put yourself in an environment full of them, that weak link is going to have a tendency to show up in your life as some form of disease. A doctor must be careful with genetic testing not to lock a patient into a state of mind where he or she feels powerless to do anything about it because of a "bad set of genes."

Myth 18: **Through the luck of the draw, some people have just inherited bad genes.**

Not true! The idea that disease is inherent to our family history is a foolish notion that even medical professionals perpetuate because they aren't looking for real answers.

Imagine genes as light switches that can be turned off or on. Their expression isn't good or bad; rather, it is one of adaptation, meaning that the gene is adapting to your choices to keep you alive. For example, if you're diabetic and you overeat sugar, your body is going to make more insulin. This is a bad thing because too much insulin causes more weight gain. The lab abnormality that most doctors label as disease is an adaptive response by the person's genes to protect their body from their own behavior. In this case, that's eating too many foods that quickly turn to blood sugar, stimulating the release of more insulin to help ferry the sugar to the cells to make energy, and prevent the sugar from damaging the bloodstream. If you want your genes to promote good health, change your diet and your genes will adapt to do so. Doctors are often so hellbent on naming the condition or disease that they can victimize the patient. Effectively, they say "Poor you, you have XYZ." Instead, I would hope they would say, "You've been making bad choices. Nobody has taught you how to do it right, but I'm here to do that. You need to make these changes because even though you haven't realized it until now, your genes are just doing what you're telling them to do."

Just to be clear: Genes are expressed by the choices you make. If those choices lead to inflammatory expression of your genes, then you're going to end up with inflammatory disease. The premise of all genetic testing has to come from the right place: not because knowing your genetic weakness makes you powerless to make a change, but instead to understand that if you have a particular weakness, you have the power to make a lifestyle change accordingly. So if your genes reveal that you're not great at detoxifying chlorine, for example, you have to filter your water more aggressively than someone without that weakness. It gives us doctors the ability to set the right stage for a patient, not make them a victim of their genes.

THE DIAGNOSIS VS. THE CAUSE

Instead of focusing on a diagnosis as conventional doctors do, what I'm really looking for and what I try to convey in the first appointment is that my patient's and my shared job is to identify the reasons *why* he or she is sick. So instead of "Let's decide what to call this so that we can prescribe the right drug?," the real question is "What's causing your pain, and how can we change your life so that you stop experiencing these symptoms?" I believe that the old precept of teaching a man to fish rather than giving him a fish applies in medicine. When we give people drugs to allow them to continue their bad behavior, we're enabling them, rather than helping them. When a new patient comes to me, she's usually already been diagnosed with six or seven different disorders (none of which has been resolved or she wouldn't be in my office), and I say, "I don't really care what we call it, let's just figure out why it's there. If we can figure that part out, then the disease itself will go away and we won't have to worry about what to call it."

As you know, insurance companies require that any doctor visit get one or more codes on the paperwork to indicate which procedures, medications, and tests the patient received. But you may not know that the American Medical Association (AMA) owns and has copyrighted this labeling system, which is considered "the standard of care." It's absurd that one organization can have a monopoly on treatment and diagnoses.[5] That's why any protocols other than those used in conventional medicine are mocked and looked down on. It's akin to Monsanto trademarking seeds. How can an entity trademark or patent what God created? Okay, time to get off my soapbox.

THE GROWTH OF FUNCTIONAL MEDICINE

You're not doing anyone a favor by dispensing a disease label and a prescription to "treat it." The whole premise of medicine is that a physician is—or should be—someone who cares and wants the patient to get better. But if that were true, why don't doctors display more tough love? Instead of just prescribing a drug, they would tell each patient like it is: "You must make these dietary changes or else you simply won't get better." Allowing doctors to practice under the guise that they are experts in nutrition when in fact they haven't adequately studied the subject is an intrinsic flaw in our health-care system.[6] This is why functional medicine is starting to boom on a grassroots level. People are sick of being told something that is wrong and doesn't work. And the Internet is playing a major role in this sea change now that anyone can educate herself. Instead of blindly following a doctor's orders, more and more people are questioning their doctors and asking themselves, "Does that really make sense? I don't think so, so why should I do that?" Many people are so frustrated with conventional medicine that they're looking for practitioners who will take time with them, and who won't just run them through a mill that sees thirty or forty patients a day.

Not every patient is right for every doctor. I have a litmus test that I make patients pass, although they don't know they're being tested. (At least until now.) One of the first questions I ask is "Are you willing to change your diet above and beyond what you think is reasonably necessary?" If they answer, "No," I'll politely say, "If you're not willing to do that, I don't think I can help you. Instead, let me give you a referral." Yes, I practice tough love!

START WITH THE BASICS

There are some basic tests that I recommend for every patient with chronic illness and pain. One of them is a gluten sensitivity genetic test. We have to know whether or not gluten (grain) is going to be an ongoing problem. If so, the patient must understand the necessity of making a permanent change. Even though this book is about a 30-day program, if you're genetically sensitive to gluten, you'll have to eat this way for the rest of your life to avoid pain and inflammation. Thirty days lay the foundation, but you'll continue to build on that. Today there seems to be a greater realization that there's no such thing as a quick fix when it comes to diet, particularly when you're looking not just at weight loss, but rather at overall health. Obviously weight and health are connected, but this isn't a quick weight-loss program to take off ten pounds before your college reunion; this is something entirely different: your life.

TESTING FOR GLUTEN SENSITIVITY

Genetic testing for gluten sensitivity testing is ground zero as far as I'm concerned, but first let's look at the conventional test. Most labs measure only one kind of immunoglobulin (or antibody) response to just one type of gluten. You'll remember that there are hundreds of types of gluten. Traditional tests basically measure whether or not your immune system is producing antibodies against gluten—which, as you know, I like to refer to as shooting off missiles, bullets, and guns—at the moment of the blood draw. But your immune system might not be firing its arsenal at that moment, making it all too easy to get a false negative. Additionally, many people have a depleted immune system, so their body is too weak to even produce the antibody reaction to gluten, thus yielding a false-negative result. Or you could have a nutritional deficiency that is causing the immune system to malfunction, leading to an inadequate ability to respond. In any of these three situations what looks like a normal response is actually misleading.

In contrast, genetic testing (which involves a cheek swab you can do at home and send to a lab) identifies the genes that are responsible for looking at gluten as either friend or foe. If a person tests positive for a gluten-sensitive gene pattern, then his or her *normal* reaction to gluten (as a foe) is to produce an inflammatory response. To date scientists have identified numerous different types of inflammatory responses to gluten, as we discussed in part 1. No wonder so many tests come back negative even though a person may experience dramatic health improvements by cutting out gluten. The proof is in the results—not just your mind!

OTHER IMPORTANT TESTS

In addition to the fundamental tests most doctors run—a complete blood count and chemistry, and vitamin D as well as iron (ferritin) status—and a genetic gluten sensitivity test, I run a number of other tests to establish a blueprint for each patient's personal needs. These include tests to:

- Measure the immune system response to gluten as well as more than three hundred different things, including foods other than grains, dairy, and sugar, plus food additives and preservatives, pesticides and other environmental toxins, and various molds

• Detect the presence of heavy metals, including lead, mercury, and others

• Identify vitamin, mineral, and other nutrient deficiencies

• Determine the status of the gut to know its capacity for digestion and absorption

• Look for infections

Moreover, if a patient has already been diagnosed with a thyroid condition, I'll run some additional tests to find out what's going on. Sometimes patients bring me the results of traditional blood work, such as C-reactive protein or homocysteine, which both indicate inflammation levels. In that case, I might follow up and do another test after the patient has been on the diet for ten weeks so she can see a tangible improvement in the lab results and understand that the diet change actually stopped the inflammation. Seeing those tangible results will help her maintain greater compliance.

TESTING FOR ALLERGIES

The tests for food and other allergies are highly advanced, unlike the standard skin prick technique, which isn't a very accurate measure of a person's allergic response. There are actually seven different pathways in which the immune system can respond, which include IgE, IgA, IgD, IgM, IgG, immune complex, and T-cell response. The first test is to measure IgE antibody responses to foods, but instead of pricking the skin, we use blood. I can't tell you how many times skin prick tests come back negative when a blood test comes back positive. It's not that a skin prick allergy test is always inaccurate, but blood tests for IgE are more comprehensive. A single test is never the be-all and end-all, which is why a battery of tests is more accurate and nuanced. Figuring out how to improve a person's health is a puzzle, and a doctor must be a sleuth to get results. With functional medicine allergy tests

NO GRAIN, NO PAIN

we're actually directly measuring a patient's immune cells' response to a particular food, and not their response as compared to someone else's response.

TESTING FOR HEAVY METAL TOXICITY

This test involves a pre- and post-provocation. First we collect a urine sample to determine whether or not the patient has had any ongoing exposure. If he or she has, we start looking at the potential source. If we can't find the source and exposure to it is ongoing, the person will become more and more toxic. The second test allows us to identify whether or not there is bioaccumulation: the presence of heavy metals in bones and other tissues, which can cause a multitude of health problems. Doing both tests allows us to distinguish between recent exposure and long-term accumulation, or possibly both. Either way, we have to look for where it's coming from and/or advise how to avoid it. Then we have to design a protocol to get rid of it. When heavy metals build up, they displace important minerals like magnesium, zinc, and calcium. (For more detail, review the section on heavy metal toxicity in chapter 10.)

It can take some detective work, but I've always been able to find the source of the heavy metal(s). That may require testing the patient's water supply or looking at whether he works in a metal shop or machine shop or another situation where he is exposed. The conventional test for lead and other heavy metals is not a provocation test. It simply measures what's floating in the blood at a certain moment in time. But your body doesn't want metals in your bloodstream, where they do damage, so it punches them into your fat cells and tries to push them into your bones. That's why we do the test again after chelation. Chelation (pronounced "key-lation") is a natural process that uses pills—I use a proprietary product called Chelemax—containing certain nutrients and plant-based molecules to "grab" heavy metals and pull them out of the tissues and blood and into the urine, where we can measure what's coming out. These natural chelators are concentrated doses of garlic, cilantro, chlorella, calcium EDTA, alpha lipoic acid, and other natural agents. Both the provocation and the bioaccumulation tests I use involve urine, not blood.

Help Get the Metal Out

To support the chelation process, there are three ways to help your organs naturally eliminate heavy metals.

- *Kidneys:* Be sure to drink adequate water during chelation. Asparagus is a natural diuretic that helps increase urinary output of toxic metals.

- *Lungs:* Exercise increases respiration and helps the lungs expel chemical toxin buildup. Sweating also releases toxins through the skin. It's also a good idea to perform an intentional deep breathing exercise before each meal.

- *Skin:* Exercise pumps muscles and lymphatic fluids, helping drain toxic compounds. An infrared sauna helps induce sweating, especially if you can't exercise easily.

THE IMPORTANCE OF POOP

Don't giggle. Being able to measure bacteria in the gut is critical. I test stool samples taken on three different days because a single sample—which is standard procedure—might reflect a single bad meal. I tell new patients not to change anything about their diet until the tests are done, to get the best read on what's happening. Technology enables us to measure the kind of bacteria that live in a patient's intestine, the ratio of good guys to bad guys, and whether there are overgrowths of the wrong kind. Knowing the status of your bacteria is crucial for overall health: sealing leaky gut, regulating immune function, helping with digestion, and aiding in vitamin and mineral assimilation. Stool testing goes beyond problems with grains to the larger issue of gut health. It's a chicken-and-egg situation: Did the grain cause damage to the gut, or did the damage to the gut make the patient more susceptible to damage from eating the grain? Once we have the results of the test, we have to address both. Think of it as having a nail in your car's tire. You can pull out the nail, but the tire is still punctured. And unless you sweep the nails off the driveway and pull out the nail, there's no point in fixing the puncture. In essence, whether you have a broken gut or you are eating things that damage the gut, both have to change.

In addition to analyzing bacteria, I want to know if there's any kind of gut infection, how well the patient is digesting and processing food, and how well nutrients are being absorbed. Many people with gluten issues are deficient in digestive enzymes, which may be why their gut is broken. One of the most common reasons why dietary changes alone don't always result in recovery from pain and inflammation is that compromised enzyme production makes it impossible to process food properly. Instead, it sits in the gut and rots. In that case, we can supplement with enzymes for as long as necessary. We also can measure the pH, or the acid level, in the gut, which also impacts the ability to digest food.

That's why we do a battery of tests. Once I have all the results in hand, I have an overview of what's happening in the patient's GI tract and whether or not we need to make lifestyle adjustments and supplementation changes, and/or use therapeutic agents to overcome bad bacteria so as to get the gut working again. When called for, I also test for different kinds of bacterial and viral infections, as well as yeast and other mold infections. These tests cover 95 percent of the problems I find in my patients. With the remaining 5 percent who aren't getting better, I have to dig a layer deeper, which could involve other tests such as assessing adrenal, thyroid, and sex steroid hormone levels.

THE IMPORTANCE OF GENETIC TESTING

Dana was suffering with severe asthma, allergies, headaches, and chronic fatigue. She was also battling recurring respiratory infections and "living on antibiotics and steroids," as she put it, to keep her head above water. Despite taking a multitude of allergy, asthma, and anti-inflammatory medications, she wasn't seeing any positive results.

She came to see me as her "last hope" of getting better. Genetic tests showed she was gluten sensitive. Additionally, Dana had vitamin D, B_2, B_{12}, and A deficiencies. After putting her on a *true* gluten-free, meaning a completely grain-free, diet, her symptoms began to resolve in a matter of weeks. Dana was able to discontinue all of her medications, no longer having to use antibiotics and steroids to battle chronic infections. After correcting her vitamin B_{12} deficiency, her energy skyrocketed, and her headaches completely stopped. I should point out that vitamin B_{12} deficiency is the second most common deficiency caused by gluten sensitivity. Once again: no grain, no pain. For more of Dana's story, visit glutenfreesociety.org/danas-no-grain-no-pain-testimonial/.

EXPERIENCE COUNTS

As functional medicine increasingly becomes a hot field, some doctors jump on the bandwagon, not because they understand the specialty, love the detective work, or are passionate about getting people better, but because they're looking for a revenue source to make ends meet. For that reason, it's very important that you find somebody who is experienced in the field. The medical school curriculum gives doctors starting out a baseline of knowledge, but it doesn't qualify them to practice functional medicine. Some of the smartest doctors I know are chiropractors, naturopaths, or PhDs. They don't have a medical career education, but when it comes to functional medicine they've trained in it and have been immersed in it from the get-go.

At the other end of the spectrum, anyone can call himself a health or nutrition coach: there is no regulatory agency for certification. This might be someone who has worked as a fitness trainer, struggled with his own illnesses, or has a nutrition degree from an online coaching site, but that doesn't qualify such a person to practice functional medicine. That's not to say that all nutritional coaches are unqualified, but keep in mind that human nutrition is a complex and challenging field, and requires not just intelligence but also education and staying abreast of the ever-emerging research, plus the application of this knowledge to patients on a consistent basis. Beware of people who are not credentialed or don't come highly recommended.

I've had many patients tell me that they've been to other functional medicine practitioners, but they're still sick, and the advice they were given was just flat-out awful—and wasn't functional medicine at all. To be sure you are in the hands of a competent and experienced practitioner, ask him or her the following questions:

• *Where did you receive additional postgraduate training in nutrition?* Remember that medical doctors don't train in nutrition, and if they don't have additional postgraduate training, then the odds that they have any training at all is nil.

• *Did you do additional postgraduate training specifically in functional medicine?* There's nutrition, and then there's functional medicine. To me, they are almost one and the same because functional medicine is actually applied biochemistry, which is what nutrition is.

• *How long have you had a functional medicine practice?* There's no point in asking how long they've been in practice because he or she could have practiced for two decades and just started practicing functional medicine six months ago. I don't want to be too hard on new doctors because they need to get experience, too, but we're talking about chronic pain, we're talking about very sick people, so I would say that you're looking for somebody who has five years minimum of actual real-time functional medicine experience, and absolutely not less than two years.

BONUS FEATURE

Visit MyFunctionalMedicineDoctor.org to get a more intensive look at functional medicine and find a practitioner near you.

Turn to part 4, which offers an array of recipes, along with tips on gluten-free cooking, suitable for both the Kickoff and Challenge phases of the No-Grain, No-Pain program.

PART 4

GRAIN-FREE, PAIN-FREE RECIPES

Pineapple-Chicken Kabobs

Speedy Salmon Cakes

Dijon Salmon Fillets

Poached Cod with Mango Salsa

Taco Salad

Baked Italian Chicken Breast

SIDE DISHES AND SALADS   281

Cauliflower Rice

Lemony Brussels Sprouts

Cucumber and Tomato Salad

South-of-the-Border Slaw

Strawberry-Bacon-Avocado Salad

Black Sesame Seed Slaw

SNACKS AND DESSERTS   287

Topp Paleo Flatbread

Apricot Cookies

No-Pain Ice "Cream"

Banana-Almond Muffins

INTRODUCTION: *TRUE* GLUTEN-FREE COOKING

Most of the ingredients in the following recipes are found in any super-market. In cases where an ingredient may not be that familiar or not widely available, I'll provide at least one brand name and/or source to help you find it. Again, ideally all produce should be organic, as should other items such as almond flour and coconut milk. If at all possible meat should be from free-range or grass-fed animals, which means it is inherently non-GMO and organic. Poultry should be from free-range birds, as should eggs. Try to use only wild-caught fish. Feel free to sub-stitute bison or venison for beef. Several recipes have variations, but

feel free to make your own substitutions. There are very few manufactured ingredients in the recipes, but the occasional item such as salsa
should be organic and contain no added sugars or other nasty ingredients.

To make delicious meals without problematic ingredients:

- In lieu of bread crumbs or oats, use mashed cauliflower, yams,
or potatoes (potatoes in the Kickoff phase only) and a beaten egg
to hold together a meat loaf.

- Use grated zucchini (or thin slices made with a vegetable peeler
or spiral slicer) or spaghetti squash as a base for spaghetti sauce
and other sauces.

- Use tapioca, almond, coconut, banana, and arrowroot flour to
make pancakes and baked goods. Such packaged products are
still processed foods and may contain additives to preserve them.

- Keep nut and other flours in the freezer or refrigerator to avoid
rancidity. Better yet, grind your own nut flours in a high-powered
blender such as a Vitamix.

- Each flour has a slightly different flavor and texture. Nut flours
are heavier than grain flours and absorb more liquid. When
adapting recipes, you may have to experiment to get the right
proportion of liquids to dry ingredients.

- Using some arrowroot or tapioca flour with nut flours helps
keep baked goods from being too dense.

- You may also need more eggs than conventional recipes that use
baking powder or baking soda.

BREAKFAST AND BRUNCH DISHES

KANE'S ULTRA PURE PROTEIN SMOOTHIE

Phases: 1 and 2   Makes: 1 serving
Active time: 5 minutes
Total time: 5 minutes

My beef protein powder and vegetable-fruit blend combine to make a delicious protein- and vitamin-filled smoothie in minutes. Use another soy- and gluten-free protein powder if you prefer; however, most other fruit and vegetable powders have wheat or oat grass in them. A scoop is about 2 tablespoons. I named this smoothie for my 13-year-old son, who makes it every day after his gymnastics practice—it makes a great snack as well.

½ cup frozen strawberries
½ cup frozen blueberries
½ banana
1 cup cold water
1 scoop Ultra Pure Protein Vanilla powder*
1 scoop Ultra Food*

1. Place the strawberries, blueberries, banana, water, Ultra Pure Protein Vanilla powder, and Ultra Food in a blender and blend until smooth, scraping down the sides with a spatula to get all the powder to mix.

2. Add a few ice cubes or more water if you prefer a thinner consistency.

VARIATIONS

- Use chocolate or unflavored gluten-free protein powder instead of vanilla.

- Use fresh fruits instead of frozen ones.

- For a green protein smoothie, replace the Ultra Food with fresh or frozen spinach.

*Available at glutenfreesociety.org/shop/.

GARDEN FRITTATA

Phases: 1 and 2   Makes: 6 servings

Active time: 15 minutes

Total time: 40 minutes

This dish would also make a great lunch or dinner. For Phase 2, omit the bell pepper and replace with another zucchini or two.

1 tablespoon extra-virgin olive oil

½ pound grain-free pork or turkey breakfast sausage meat

1 medium carrot, peeled and shredded

2 cloves garlic, minced

½ medium yellow onion, diced

½ red bell pepper, seeded, stemmed, and diced (optional)

1 zucchini, shredded

2 cups chopped fresh spinach

10 eggs

Sea salt and ground black pepper

1. Heat oven to 350° F.

2. Heat the olive oil in a large iron or other ovenproof skillet over medium-high heat. Add the olive oil, and when it is shimmering, add the sausage. Break up gently with a spatula, and brown the sausage, turning as necessary.

3. Add the carrot, garlic, onion, and bell pepper and sauté until almost tender, stirring occasionally, about 5 minutes. Add the zucchini and spinach and sauté a minute more. Remove from heat and set aside.

4. In a large bowl, beat the eggs and add sea salt and black pepper to taste. Pour the eggs over the sausage and sautéed veggies. Place in the oven and bake for 20 to 25 minutes or until the eggs are puffed up and nicely browned.

5. Cut into wedges and serve.

(continued on next page)

VARIATIONS

- Instead of the vegetables above, substitute broccoli, cauliflower, or any acceptable cooked vegetable leftovers. If using leftovers, reduce sauté time.

HOMEMADE BREAKFAST SAUSAGE

Phases: 1 and 2   Makes: 6 servings
Active time: 10 minutes
Total time: 20 minutes

Although you can purchase sausage made from free-range hogs or wild boar, it always tastes better when you make it yourself, and there's no chance of any sneaky grain-based fillers finding their way in.

1 pound lean ground pork (or wild boar)
1 teaspoon mustard powder
1 teaspoon onion powder
1 teaspoon ground sage
1 teaspoon ground black pepper
½ teaspoon ground fennel
2 teaspoons extra-virgin olive oil

1. In a large bowl, mix together the pork, mustard powder, onion powder, ground sage, black pepper, and ground fennel.

2. Form into 6 patties about ½ inch thick.

3. Heat the olive oil in a large skillet (with a lid) over medium heat. When the oil shimmers, add the patties, leaving space between them. Cover and cook for about 5 minutes. Remove lid, flip the patties, replace the lid, and cook for another 5 minutes or until browned.

VARIATION

- Use ground turkey instead of pork.

SUPER SIMPLE BANANA PANCAKE

Phases: 1 and 2   Makes: 1 serving
Active time: 10 minutes
Total time: 10 minutes

Just four ingredients make this delicious grain-free pancake. Double or triple the recipe for each additional person.

1 ripe banana
1 egg
¼ teaspoon ground cinnamon
Scant teaspoon coconut oil

1. In a small bowl, mash the banana. Add the egg and cinnamon and mix until smooth.

2. Add coconut oil to a small skillet, and heat over medium heat. Add pancake batter. Cook until lightly browned on one side, about 2 minutes. Flip and cook another minute or two.

3. Serve with (real) maple syrup, if desired.

LUNCH AND DINNER DISHES

ROASTED LEMON-DILL CHICKEN
WITH CARROTS AND POTATOES

Phases: 1 and 2   Makes: 6 servings
Active time: 10 minutes
Total time: 1½ hours

To make this hearty dish suitable for Phase 2, replace the nightshade-family potatoes with white or yellow Japanese sweet potatoes, which have a similar starchy texture. This dish is just as good when reheated the next day.

2 medium potatoes, peeled and quartered
1 (2½–3½-pound) whole broiler/fryer chicken
1 pound baby carrots
¾ cup fresh lemon juice
2–3 tablespoons dried dill weed

1. Heat oven to 350° F.

2. Peel the potatoes and cut into cubes.

3. Pat the chicken dry and place in a cast-iron casserole or a chicken roaster with a tight lid. Arrange the potatoes and carrots around the sides of the chicken. Pour the lemon juice over the chicken and vegetables and sprinkle with dill.

4. Cover the roaster and bake for about 90 minutes or until the chicken is cooked through and carrots and potatoes are tender. (The chicken juices should run clear or an instant-read thermometer should read 165°F.)

VARIATIONS

• Use other root vegetables such as white turnips, winter squash, or parsnips instead of potatoes.

CHICKEN-APPLE-AVOCADO SALAD

Phases: 1 and 2   Makes: 2 servings
Active time: 10 minutes
Total time: 10 minutes

Crunchy apple and buttery avocado give this simple-to-prepare dish a pleasing contrast in textures.

1 cup cooked chicken, cut in small chunks
1 ripe Hass avocado, chopped
1 unpeeled green apple, diced
Juice of 1 lemon
Mixed greens (optional)

1. Place the chicken, avocado, and apple in a medium bowl.

2. Add the lemon juice and toss gently. Serve over mixed greens, if you wish.

VARIATION

• Substitute a not-too-ripe pear for the apple.

CHICKEN "UNWICHES"

Phases: 1 and 2   Makes: 4 servings
Active time: 10 minutes
Total time: 10 minutes

Be sure to use mustard made with apple cider or wine vinegar to avoid the grain in most mustard. Eden Foods' organic Yellow Mustard comes in a glass jar. I use Applegate organic deli meats (found in the deli section of most supermarkets) and bacon. To make this easy-to-prepare lunch suitable for Phase 2, simply omit the tomatoes, which are members of the nightshade family.

(continued on next page)

8 iceberg lettuce leaves, rinsed and patted dry
1 pound sliced cooked chicken breast
Mustard made with cider or wine vinegar
4 slices bacon, cooked
1 ripe Hass avocado, sliced
1 large tomato, thinly sliced
Organic dill pickles

1. To assemble, overlap 2 pieces of lettuce on each of 4 plates. Place several slices of chicken on each lettuce layer, and add mustard to taste, followed by a slice of bacon.

2. Divide the slices of avocado and tomato into 4 portions and top each bacon slice with them.

3. Roll up the lettuce leaves around each "unwich" like a burrito. Serve with pickles on the side.

VARIATIONS

- Replace the sliced chicken breast with turkey breast, also made by Applegate.

- Use leftover chicken or meat instead of deli chicken.

SOUTH-OF-THE-BORDER TURKEY BURGERS

Phases: 1 and 2   Makes: 4 servings
Active time: 15 minutes
Total time: 25 minutes

To make this dish suitable for Phase 2, omit both the poblano and bell peppers and the chile powder. If you like your burgers milder, do so in Phase 1 as well.

1 pound ground turkey thigh
½ medium yellow onion, roughly chopped
1 poblano pepper, seeded, stemmed, and roughly chopped
1 red bell pepper, seeded, stemmed, and roughly chopped
1 teaspoon ground cumin

1 teaspoon chile powder
1 teaspoon garlic powder
Sea salt and ground black pepper
1 tablespoon extra-virgin olive oil or bacon grease

1. Place the ground turkey in a large bowl.

2. Place the chopped onion, poblano pepper, and bell pepper in a food processor fitted with an S blade. Process until minced. Add to the ground turkey.

3. Add the cumin, chile powder, and garlic powder. Season to taste with sea salt and black pepper. Mix well and pat into 4 burgers.

4. Heat a large skillet with olive oil or bacon grease and cook the burgers for about 5 minutes on either side, or until cooked through.

5. Serve with South-of-the-Border Slaw (page 283).

VARIATIONS

• Replace the chopped turkey with grass-fed ground beef or bison.

CHICKEN CURRY SOUP

Phase: 1   Makes: 10 servings
Active time: 30 minutes
Total time: 2 hours

This main-dish soup owes its creamy texture to canned coconut milk, not to be confused with coconut milk beverage or coconut cream, which is full of added sugar. The curry flavor comes from curry paste. Thai Kitchen is one brand readily available in most supermarkets.

1 whole (3–5-pound) roaster chicken
1 large yellow onion, chopped
5 large carrots, peeled and chopped
5 stalks celery, trimmed and chopped
4 cloves garlic, minced
1 (4-ounce) jar red curry paste

(continued on next page)

1 (14-ounce) can coconut milk
1 large head cauliflower, chopped
2 tablespoons peeled and grated fresh ginger
Juice of 1 lemon

1. Place the chicken, onion, carrots, celery, and garlic in a large stock-pot. Cover with water and a lid. Bring to a boil, and then reduce heat to a low boil until the chicken is cooked through, about 60 to 90 minutes.

2. Let the chicken cool in the pot for about an hour. Debone the chicken, picking off the meat. Discard the skin and bone. Place the meat back into the pot with the broth and veggies.

3. Add the curry paste and coconut milk, stir, and then add the cauli-flower and enough water if necessary to cover. Return to a slow boil. Reduce heat and simmer for 20 minutes. Add the ginger and continue to simmer for 15 minutes more.

4. Remove from the cooktop and add lemon juice before serving.

CHICKEN NOODLE SOUP WITH A SURPRISE

Phases: 1 and 2   Makes: 10 servings
Active time: 25 minutes
Total time: 2 hours

This gluten-free version of a (almost) classic soup uses zucchini "noodles" made with a spiral slicer. If you don't have one, simply grate the zucchini.

1 whole (3–5-pound) roaster chicken
1 large yellow onion, chopped
5 large carrots, peeled and chopped
5 stalks celery, trimmed and chopped
4 cloves garlic, minced
2 pounds zucchini, trimmed
Sea salt and ground black pepper

1. Place the chicken, onion, carrots, celery, and garlic in a large stock-pot. Cover with water. Bring to a boil, and then reduce heat to a low boil until the chicken is cooked through, about 60 to 90 minutes.

2. Let the chicken cool in the pot for about an hour. Debone the chicken, picking off the meat. Discard the skin and bone. Reserve the broth. Place the meat back into the pot with the broth, onion, carrots, celery, and garlic. Add water if necessary to cover. Return to a slow boil.

3. Meanwhile, using a spiral slicer, make the zucchini into "noodles." Add to the pot when it is at a slow boil and cook until they are tender, about 4 or 5 minutes. Season to taste with sea salt and black pepper.

CHICKEN FAJITAS

Phase: 1   Makes: 4 servings
Active time: 20 minutes
Total time: 45 minutes plus 4 to 6 hours marinating time

This Mexican-inspired dish is sure to please the whole family. You might want to serve it on Topp Paleo Flatbread (page 287) instead of lettuce leaves. Be sure to use salsa with no added sugar.

1 pound boneless, skinless raw chicken breast, cut into strips

1 red bell pepper, stemmed, seeded, and sliced

1 medium yellow onion, sliced

4 cloves garlic, minced

Juice of 1 lemon

Juice of 1 lime

1 teaspoon chile powder

1 teaspoon ground cumin

1 teaspoon ground coriander

1 teaspoon oregano

2 tablespoons extra-virgin olive oil

1 ripe Hass avocado

Juice of 1 lemon or lime

1 head butterhead lettuce

1 (16-ounce) jar salsa

(continued on next page)

1. In a large bowl, combine the chicken, red pepper, onion, garlic, lemon and lime juice, chile powder, ground cumin, ground coriander, and oregano. Cover and refrigerate for 4 to 6 hours.

2. Remove the chicken and vegetables.

3. In a large skillet, heat the olive oil over medium-high heat until it shimmers. Place the chicken and vegetables with the juices in the skillet and cook until the chicken is cooked through and the vegetables are tender, about 10 to 15 minutes.

4. Meanwhile, mash the avocado with lemon or lime juice.

5. Serve the fajitas on butterhead lettuce leaves with salsa and mashed avocado.

VARIATION

- Replace the chicken breast with sliced sirloin or flank steak.

BAKED ALMOND-DUSTED PORK CHOPS

Phases: 1 and 2   Makes: 4 servings
Active time: 10 minutes
Total time: 40 to 55 minutes

Instead of gluten-filled bread crumbs, this hearty dish calls for ground almonds. An alternative way to coat the chops is to place the almond flour in a paper bag and add one chop at a time, close securely, and shake.

4 bone-in thin cut pork chops (about 1 pound)
1 cup almond flour
1 tablespoon Italian herb mix
1 tablespoon garlic powder
1 tablespoon onion powder
1 teaspoon sea salt

1. Heat oven to 350° F.

2. Pat the chops dry.

3. Mix almond flour, Italian herb mix, garlic powder, onion powder, and sea salt in a bowl. Coat both sides of the pork chops with the mixture and pat gently.

4. Place the coated chops on a rimmed baking sheet. Bake for 30 to 45 minutes until cooked through. Juices should run clear or the internal temperature read at least 145° F on an instant thermometer.

HERB-SEASONED SHEPHERD'S PIE

Phases: 1 and 2   Makes: 8–10 servings
Active time: 20 minutes
Total time: 80 to 120 minutes

To make this classic dish suitable for Phase 2, omit the tomato paste and add slightly more beef broth. Penzeys herb and spice mixes (penzeys.com /shop/spices/) are free of gluten, and eliminate the need to buy dozens of herbs and spices you rarely use. Mural of Flavor seasoning includes shallots, onion, garlic, lemon peel, chives, and orange peel; Fox Point seasoning is made with salt, shallots, chives, garlic, onion, and green peppercorns. Use your own preferred herbs and spices if you prefer.

    3 medium white-fleshed Japanese sweet potatoes, peeled and cut into chunks
    2 tablespoons extra-virgin olive oil
    1 medium yellow onion, chopped
    3 cloves garlic, minced
    2 large carrots, diced
    2 stalks celery, trimmed and diced
    1 pound ground grass-fed beef
    1 teaspoon Penzeys Mural of Flavor herb mix
    ½ teaspoon sea salt
    1–2 cups organic beef broth, divided
    4 ounces tomato paste
    3 tablespoons Penzeys Fox Point herb mix
    Sea salt and ground black pepper

(continued on next page)

1. Steam the Japanese sweet potatoes over boiling water in a covered pot until tender, about 15 to 20 minutes. Remove and drain; set aside.

2. To make the meat filling, heat the olive oil in a large skillet over medium-high heat. When the oil is shimmering, add the onion, garlic, carrots, and celery and sauté for about 10 minutes, stirring occasionally.

3. Add the ground beef, Mural of Flavor herb mix, and ½ teaspoon of sea salt. Sauté, gently breaking up the meat and turning, until it is browned. Add 1 cup of beef broth and the tomato paste. Stir until well combined and transfer the mixture into a 9-by-13-inch casserole dish.

4. Heat oven to 350° F.

5. To prepare the potato topping, add the Fox Point herb blend and ½ cup of beef broth. Using a hand mixer, mash until smooth, adding more broth as needed. The potatoes should not be too dry. Add sea salt and pepper to taste.

6. Spoon the potato mixture over the meat mixture and bake uncovered for 45 to 60 minutes. The potatoes should be nicely browned.

VARIATIONS

• Use ground lamb, venison, or bison instead of beef.

PANCIT WITH GLASS NOODLES

Phases: 1 and 2   Makes: 4 servings
Active time: 20 minutes
Total time: 35 minutes

Pancit is a staple Filipino stir-fried noodle dish, but our version subs out the grain-based noodles for glass noodles, which are gluten free. Buy the kind made from Japanese yam or sweet potato flour, which you'll find in Asian markets or a well-stocked supermarket in the international food section. Don't overcook glass noodles, which can quickly become gummy. Check the texture after 5 minutes. Once the texture pleases you, drain immediately and rinse with cold water several times. Coconut Secret Coconut Aminos are available at Amazon.com.

1 pound package of sweet potato glass noodles
2 tablespoons extra-virgin olive oil, divided
1 pound boneless, skinless chicken thighs, cubed
2 cloves crushed garlic
½ medium head cabbage, shredded
4 to 6 carrots, peeled and shredded
1 bunch green onions, trimmed and chopped
½–1 cup Coconut Aminos, divided

1. Bring a large pot of water to boil and add sweet potato glass noodles. Cook at a slow boil for 5 minutes. Check to make sure they are tender but not mushy. Cook slightly longer if necessary. Drain in a colander. Rinse with cold water and drain several more times. Set aside.

2. Heat a large, deep pan or wok over medium-high heat. Add 1 table-spoon of olive oil; when it shimmers, add the cubed chicken and garlic. Stir-fry just until the chicken is cooked. Remove the chicken and garlic from the pan and place it and the juices in a bowl. Set aside.

3. Add the remaining tablespoon of oil to the pan and stir-fry the cab-bage and carrots, until tender, 7 to 10 minutes, adding the green onions for the last 2 or 3 minutes. Return the chicken and juices to the pan. Add ½ cup of Coconut Aminos and stir together.

4. Add the noodles, along with more Coconut Aminos to taste, and heat for another minute or two before serving.

VARIATIONS

- Use cubed lean pork in lieu of chicken thighs.

- Replace the cabbage and carrots with any other acceptable vegeta-bles, such as snow peas and asparagus.

SAUSAGE WITH CABBAGE "NOODLES"

Phases: 1 and 2　　　　　　　　　　　Makes: 6 servings
Active time: 15 minutes
Total time: 15 minutes

You can have this five-ingredient, one-dish meal on the table in 15 minutes, and it tastes even better the next day! Read the label on the sausages carefully, as Italian sausage may contain grain-fed pork or seasonings with gluten. For Phase 2, use only unspiced Italian sausage.

1 tablespoon extra-virgin olive oil
1 pound bulk Italian sausage
½ pound bulk spicy Italian sausage
1 large yellow onion, thinly sliced
1 2-pound green cabbage, thinly sliced

1. Heat the olive oil in a large skillet over medium-high heat. When the oil shimmers, add the sausage. Gently turn it with a spatula for about 5 minutes or until browned. Remove with a slotted spoon, drain, and place in a bowl. Set aside.

2. Return the skillet to the burner. Add a little more olive oil (if needed) and the onion and cook until the slices start to brown, about 7 minutes. Add the cabbage and cook until it becomes as soft as noodles. Return the sausage to the skillet, mix together, and heat for a minute or two.

VARIATION

- Use drained prepared sauerkraut instead of cabbage and cook for 30 minutes before returning the sausage to the pan.

PINEAPPLE-CHICKEN KABOBS

Phases: 1 and 2   Makes: 4 servings

Active time: 25 minutes

Total time: 45 minutes plus 6 to 8 hours marinating time

To make this dish suitable for Phase 2, eliminate the red peppers (a night-shade vegetable). Tropical Traditions (tropicaltraditions.com) is one brand of organic coconut water vinegar. Do not use the marinade as a sauce. If you don't make your own pineapple juice—you'll need another pineapple for this—use juice from a glass container, not a can. You can make the sauce ahead and reheat if you wish. Coconut Secret Coconut Aminos are available at Amazon.com. In lieu of grilling, you can broil the kabobs in the oven.

Marinade

¼ cup pineapple juice

3 tablespoons Coconut Aminos

3 tablespoons raw honey

2 tablespoons coconut water vinegar

½ teaspoons fresh ginger, peeled and finely grated

½ teaspoon garlic powder

2 tablespoons extra-virgin olive oil

Sauce

½ cup pineapple juice

2 tablespoons raw honey

1 tablespoon extra-virgin olive oil

1 tablespoon Coconut Aminos

1 pound boneless, skinless chicken breast, cut into 1-inch cubes

2 red bell peppers, seeded, stemmed, and cut into 1-inch squares

1 red onion, cut in 1-inch pieces

1 pineapple, skin removed, cored, and cut into 1-inch cubes

8 wooden skewers

1. Make the marinade: Mix the pineapple juice, Coconut Aminos, raw honey, coconut water vinegar, ginger, garlic powder, and olive oil in a glass bowl. Add the chicken cubes. Cover and refrigerate for 6 to 8 hours.

(continued on next page)

2. Soak the wooden skewers in water for 20 minutes.

3. Heat the grill to medium and oil the grate.

4. Meanwhile, make the sauce: In a small saucepan, combine the pineapple juice, raw honey, olive oil, and Coconut Aminos. Bring to a boil, then reduce heat to a simmer. Simmer for 8 to 10 minutes.

5. Remove chicken from the marinade and discard the marinade. Alternate pieces of bell pepper, onion, and pineapple with the chicken cubes on the skewers. Cook the kabobs, turning and brushing with the sauce often. Grill for 15 to 20 minutes or until the chicken is cooked through.

VARIATION

• Use cubed lean pork in lieu of chicken.

SPEEDY SALMON CAKES

Phases: 1 and 2   Makes: 4 servings
Active time: 15 minutes
Total time: 15 minutes

This is a great entrée for nights when there's no protein source in the fridge or freezer. All Alaska salmon is wild caught. Avoid Atlantic salmon, which may be farmed. Grey Poupon is made with white wine vinegar, making it an acceptable seasoning, unlike most mustard made with rice vinegar.

12 ounces drained canned (or vacuum packed) wild-caught salmon
2 tablespoons finely chopped yellow onion
1 clove garlic, finely minced
1 egg, beaten
1 tablespoon Dijon mustard
3 tablespoons extra-virgin olive oil

1. In a medium bowl, mix together the salmon, onion, garlic, egg, and mustard, then form into 4 patties.

2. In a large skillet over medium heat, heat the oil until it shimmers. Add the patties, being careful that they don't touch one another. Cook for about 3 minutes per side until lightly browned.

VARIATION

- Use leftover salmon or another mild fish in lieu of canned or vacuum-packed salmon.

DIJON SALMON FILLETS

Phases: 1 and 2   Makes: 4 servings
Active time: 10 minutes
Total time: 30 minutes

Be sure to use Dijon mustard made with cider or white wine vinegar to avoid grains. And use only Alaska or Pacific Ocean wild-caught salmon. Atlantic Ocean salmon is often farmed.

4 tablespoons Dijon mustard
2 tablespoons pure maple syrup
4 (6-ounce) salmon fillets

1. Heat oven to 400° F.

2. Mix the mustard and maple syrup in a small bowl.

3. Place the salmon on a rimmed baking sheet and spread the mixture on the salmon. Bake for 12 to 15 minutes or until cooked through.

POACHED COD WITH MANGO SALSA

Phases: 1 and 2   Makes: 4 servings

Active time: 20 minutes

Total time: 30 minutes plus 30 minutes marinating time

This mild white fish takes well to the complex flavors of the salsa, which can also be used with any baked or broiled fish, poultry, or meat. Be careful not to overcook the fish. Eliminate the jalapeño for Phase 2.

1 ripe mango, diced

½ red onion, diced

1 jalapeño pepper, finely diced

2 tablespoons chopped fresh cilantro

Juice of 1 lemon

Juice of 1 lime

4 (6-ounce) cod fillets

Sea salt and ground black pepper

1. In a medium bowl, mix the mango, red onion, jalapeño, cilantro, and lemon and lime juices. Add sea salt and black pepper to taste. Let sit at room temperature for 30 minutes for the flavors to marry.

2. In a pot large enough to hold the fillets and with a well-fitting lid, place enough water to come half way up the fillets. Once the water begins to simmer, place the fillets in the pan and cover. Cook for 6 to 8 minutes or until the fish just begins to flake.

3. Gently remove each fillet with a slotted spatula to a paper towel to remove excess water. Place the fillets on four plates and top with salsa.

TACO SALAD

Phase: 1   Makes: 4 servings

Active time: 20 minutes

Total time: 30 minutes

Forget about the taco "bowl"! Here's another family-favorite meal with a Southwest flavor. Again, be sure to use salsa without added sugar. You'll find pitted black olives at the olive bar in most supermarkets, which are more flavorful than the canned kind.

1 teaspoon medium chile powder

1 teaspoon cumin

1 teaspoon garlic powder

½ teaspoon dried oregano

½ teaspoon onion powder

½ teaspoon sea salt

1 teaspoon extra-virgin olive oil

1 small yellow onion, diced

1 pound ground beef (or bison)

1 head iceberg lettuce, shredded

2 medium tomatoes, diced

1 ripe Hass avocado, cubed

1 (16-ounce) jar salsa

1 cup black olives, sliced

1. Mix the chile powder, cumin, garlic powder, oregano, onion powder, and sea salt.

2. Heat the oil in a skillet and cook the onion and beef until browned, stirring gently. Once browned, add the herb/spice mixture and ¼ cup of water. Stir well and continue to simmer until the liquid has evaporated.

3. Divide the lettuce and place in four bowls. Add the meat and then the tomatoes, the avocado, a scoop of salsa, and lastly the black olives.

BAKED ITALIAN CHICKEN BREAST

Phases: 1 and 2   Makes: 4 servings
Active time: 5 minutes
Total time: 50 minutes

This basic dish uses a minimum of ingredients and takes a minimum of effort, but delivers maximum flavor. Serve with your favorite vegetable or a side salad.

    4 chicken breasts (skin on and bone in)
    ⅓–½ cup extra-virgin olive oil
    1 teaspoon garlic powder
    1½ tablespoons Italian herb mix
    Sea salt and black ground pepper

1. Heat oven to 425° F.

2. Place the chicken breasts in an ovenproof glass dish. Cover evenly and liberally with the oil, turning to coat both sides, and using your hands to cover all the edges.

3. Sprinkle with the garlic powder, Italian herbs, and sea salt and black pepper to taste.

4. Bake for 30 to 45 minutes or until cooked through (165° F on an instant-read thermometer). The juices should run clear.

SIDE DISHES AND SALADS

CAULIFLOWER RICE

Phases: 1 and 2   Makes: 4 servings
Active time: 15 minutes
Total time: 25 minutes

This dish looks remarkably similar to white rice, but has far more flavor and personality minus the grain full of pain.

4 tablespoons extra-virgin olive oil
1 medium onion, diced small
1 clove garlic, minced
3 stalks celery, trimmed and cut in small dice
1 medium head cauliflower, trimmed and cut into pieces
Sea salt and ground black pepper

1. In a large skillet, heat the olive oil over medium heat until it shimmers. Add onion, garlic, and celery and sauté until soft, about 5 minutes.

2. Place the cauliflower in a food processor with the S blade and pulse until the cauliflower has the consistency of rice, being careful not to overprocess.

3. Remove cauliflower to the skillet and cover. Cook over medium heat until soft, about 10 minutes. Season to taste with sea salt and black pepper.

LEMONY BRUSSELS SPROUTS

Phases: 1 and 2   Makes: 4 servings
Active time: 15 minutes
Total time: 20 minutes

Brussels sprouts often get a bad rap because they have been boiled too long, but this dish will change hearts and minds! A Microplane makes fast work of zesting without any scraped knuckles.

Zest and juice of 1 lemon
1 tablespoon raw honey
2 tablespoons extra-virgin olive oil
1 pound Brussels sprouts, trimmed and halved
⅔ cup water
Sea salt and ground black pepper

1. In a small bowl mix the lemon juice, lemon zest, and honey. Set aside.

2. In a large skillet, heat the olive oil over medium-high heat. Place the sprouts in a single layer, cut side down, in the skillet and cook until the cut sides brown, about 8 to 10 minutes. Add the water and cover. Lower the heat to medium. Cook until the spouts are tender when pierced with a fork.

3. Remove the lid and pour the lemon and honey mixture on the sprouts. Stir, raise the heat to medium-high and cook until all the liquid has evaporated, stirring frequently.

4. Season with sea salt and black pepper and serve.

CUCUMBER AND TOMATO SALAD

Phase: 1   Makes: 4 servings
Active time: 10 minutes
Total time: 10 minutes

This simple salad is perfection itself in late summer, when local tomatoes are ripe. Substitute a cup of sliced cherry tomatoes if heirlooms are not available. To partially peel the cucumbers, run a vegetable peeler lengthwise, leaving some of the peel to create a striped effect.

¼ cup white wine vinegar
¼ cup extra-virgin olive oil
¼ teaspoon garlic powder
2 seedless cucumbers, partially peeled, then sliced
1 large heirloom tomato, chopped
1 small yellow onion, sliced
1 ripe Hass avocado, chopped
Sea salt and ground black pepper

1. Combine the vinegar, olive oil, and garlic powder, and set aside.

2. In a large bowl place the cucumbers, tomato, onion, and avocado. Pour the oil and vinegar mixture over the veggies and mix well but gently, adding sea salt to taste.

SOUTH-OF-THE-BORDER SLAW

Phases: 1 and 2   Makes: 4 servings
Active time: 15 minutes
Total time: 20 minutes

A food processor allows you to make this slaw in minutes. Eliminate the chile powder to make it suitable for Phase 2. It is the perfect complement to any grilled or baked or roasted meat dish, including South-of-the-Border Turkey Burgers (page 266).

(continued on next page)

1 small head of cabbage

2 ripe Hass avocados

Juice of 1 lime

Juice of 1 lemon

1 teaspoon ground cumin

1 teaspoon chile powder

½ teaspoon garlic powder

Sea salt and ground black pepper

1. Shred the cabbage in a food processor, using the shredder blade. Place cabbage in a large bowl and set aside. Wipe out food processor bowl.

2. Place the avocados, lime and lemon juice, cumin, chile powder, and garlic powder in the food processor. With the S blade, process until the mixture is creamy.

3. Stir the avocado cream into the cabbage. Serve immediately or refrigerate, covered, for up to 24 hours.

VARIATIONS

- Use ½ head of purple cabbage and ½ head of green cabbage.

- Add some grated carrots.

STRAWBERRY-BACON-AVOCADO SALAD

Phases: 1 and 2   Makes: 4 servings

Active time: 15 minutes

Total time: 15 minutes

The unusual combination of bacon, avocado, and strawberries is unexpectedly delicious and textured. Add some leftover cooked chicken slices to make this a main-course salad.

2 cups of fresh strawberries, stemmed (divided)

¼ cup extra-virgin olive oil

2 tablespoons apple cider vinegar

2 tablespoons raw honey

1 10-ounce bag baby spinach

4 slices of organic bacon, cooked and crumbled

1 ripe Hass avocado, chopped

Sea salt and ground black pepper

1. Place 1 cup of the strawberries and the olive oil, apple cider vinegar, and honey in a blender. Blend at medium power until smooth. Set aside.

2. Slice the remaining strawberries.

3. Place the spinach in a bowl and pour some of the dressing. Top with sliced strawberries, bacon, and avocado. Add the remaining dressing and season to taste with sea salt and black pepper.

BLACK SESAME SEED SLAW

Phases: 1 and 2   Makes: 4 servings

Active time: 10 minutes

Total time: 10 minutes

To make this crunchy slaw suitable for Phase 2, just omit the sesame seeds. The almonds will still supply a satisfying crunch. You'll find black sesame seeds in Asian groceries as well as in the international foods section of well-stocked supermarkets.

¼ cup extra-virgin olive oil

¼ cup apple cider vinegar

1 tablespoon raw honey

¾ teaspoon sea salt

½ medium head cabbage, shredded

3 green onions, trimmed and chopped

⅓ cup slivered almonds

1½ tablespoons black sesame seeds

(continued on next page)

1. Whisk together the olive oil, apple cider vinegar, raw honey, and sea salt. Set aside.

2. Place the cabbage in a bowl and pour the dressing over it, stirring to evenly coat the cabbage. Sprinkle the green onions, slivered almonds, and sesame seeds on top.

VARIATIONS

- Use red cabbage instead of green, or mix the two. Or use Chinese cabbage.

- Swap cabbage for slivered raw Brussels sprouts.

SNACKS AND DESSERTS

TOPP PALEO FLATBREAD

Phases: 1 and 2   Makes: 4 servings

Active time: 20 minutes

Total time: 20 minutes

Honeyville blanched almond flour (shop.honeyville.com), also available at Amazon.com, is ultra-fine, non-GMO (meaning it's also organic), and certified gluten free. Rhonda Topping, who identifies herself as a Gluten-Free Warrior, developed this recipe. Visit her blog to learn more about cooking these flatbreads and other gluten-free goodies: ajourneytoembrace.blog spot.com/2013/04/quick-and-easy-flatbread.html.

½ cup blanched almond flour

½ cup arrowroot

3 large or 4 medium egg whites, lightly whisked

Dash of sea salt

¼ cup water (or more)

1 tablespoon coconut oil

1. Mix together the almond flour, arrowroot, egg whites, sea salt, and water. The batter should be thin. If necessary, thin with more water, adding a tablespoon at a time

2. Heat the coconut oil in a 10-inch or larger skillet at medium-high heat. Remove the skillet from the cooktop and add the batter to the skillet, spreading it out in a roughly circular shape with a spoon before returning it to the heat.

3. Cook for 3 to 5 minutes. Flip and cook the other side for another 3 to 5 minutes.

4. Remove from the heat and cut in 4 wedges.

VARIATION

- Replace the almond flour with ¼ cup coconut flour and increase the water to ½ to ¾ cup.

APRICOT COOKIES

Phases: 1 and 2   Makes: 12 cookies
Active time: 10 minutes
Total time: 30 minutes

The combination of apricots, coconut, and ground almonds is delectable. Who needs flour and sugar when grain-free tastes so great?

1 cup dried unsulfured apricots
¾ cup almond flour
½ cup unsweetened finely shredded coconut
1 tablespoon coconut oil
1 egg, beaten

1. Heat oven to 350° F.

2. Place the apricots in a food processor and pulse several times, adding some of the almond flour if they stick to the blade. Add the remaining almond flour, shredded coconut, and coconut oil. Pulse until the mixture is crumbly.

3. Remove from the processor. Place in a bowl and stir in the egg. Using your fingers and a tablespoon, roll into balls and place on a parchment-lined cookie sheet. Press the balls to flatten them a bit.

4. Bake for 18 minutes. Cool on a wire rack.

VARIATION

• Swap dried peaches for the apricots.

NO-PAIN ICE "CREAM"

Phases: 1 and 2   Makes: 4 servings
Active time: 10 minutes
Total time: 10 minutes

Be sure to use canned coconut milk, not coconut milk beverage, and the full-fat version. I like to use equal portions of banana, strawberries, and blueberries, but you can experiment with other mixtures. Once your bananas ripen, pop them into the freezer for use in this dessert or a breakfast smoothie.

    3 cups unsweetened frozen fruit and/or berries
    1 cup full-fat coconut milk
    Pure liquid stevia (optional)

1. Place berries and chopped fruit in a high power blender, such as a Vitamix. Add the coconut milk. Blend on high until thoroughly mixed. If too thick, add more coconut milk.

2. Taste, and if not sweet enough add a small amount of stevia.

3. Serve immediately or place in the freezer.

VARIATION

• For a more sorbet-like texture, add a few ice cubes to the blender.

BANANA-ALMOND MUFFINS

Phases: 1 and 2   Makes: 10 muffins
Active time: 25 minutes
Total time: 50 minutes

One yummy muffin makes a nice snack or serve with sausage and eggs for breakfast. Almond flour lends a lovely texture. Make sure your bananas are nice and ripe. Use a brand of baking powder, such as Hain Pure Foods, made with potato starch instead of the usual corn starch.

    1½ cups almond flour
    1 teaspoon baking soda
    1 teaspoon baking powder
    2 teaspoons ground cinnamon
    ½ teaspoon sea salt
    3 ripe bananas
    2 eggs, whisked
    ¼ cup coconut oil, melted

(continued on next page)

1 teaspoon pure vanilla extract

1 teaspoon raw honey

1. Heat oven to 350° F.

2. In a large bowl, mix the almond flour, baking soda, baking powder, ground cinnamon, and sea salt. Set aside.

3. In a small bowl, mash the bananas with a spatula. Add the eggs, coconut oil, vanilla extract, and raw honey, and mix with a hand mixer until well combined.

4. Pour the wet ingredients into the dry ingredients and mix well with the hand mixer.

5. Pour batter into a muffin tin (2½-inch diameter cups) lined with 10 baking cups. Bake for 25 to 30 minutes until a tester comes out clean.

ACKNOWLEDGMENTS

No man is an island. As much as I have personally pushed to educate the world about grain and its deleterious effects on human health, my work and contributions on this topic are minimal in comparison to—and would not have been possible without—the people who came before me, those who came with me, and those who picked up the proverbial torch and joined me. To all of you I owe a great deal of gratitude. There aren't enough pages to thank everyone who played a role, so kindly grant me latitude if your name is not listed below.

THOSE WHO CAME BEFORE ME

I would like to recognize the work of Jacopo Bartolomeo Beccari, the Italian chemist who first isolated gluten in 1745. The English chemist with whom I share a last name, Thomas Burr Osborne, sometimes referred to as the father of plant protein chemistry, originally isolated and classified the different types of gluten (prolamins and glutelins). Thanks to the father of functional medicine, Dr. Linus Pauling; the father of functional medicine in psychiatry, Dr. Abram Hoffer; Dr. Bruce Ames for his eloquence in describing genetic mutations and the ability to improve them with nutrition; Dr. Roger Williams for fundamentally shedding light on biochemical individualism; Dr. Jeffrey Bland for bringing the brightest minds in functional medicine together to share their knowledge; Dr. Weston Price for his work on the effects of processed foods on human health; and Dr. Francis Pottenger, whose cats helped me understand the fundamentals of real food.

Special thanks to my uncle, Dr. Eddie Stephenson, who inspired me to pursue a higher education; Dr. Marios Hadjivassiliou, whose work has connected gluten to brain and nerve damage; Dr. Rodney

Ford, whose tireless efforts bring knowledge of gluten to the parents of very sick children; Dr. Kenneth Fine for challenging the diagnostic status quo; Dr. Michael Marsh, whose research on celiac disease has been invaluable; Dr. Alessio Fasano for his research on leaky gut; Dr. William Davis for being brave enough to stand up to and challenge the propaganda put forth by the grain industry; Dr. Loren Cordain for shedding more light on the toxicity of grains; and Dr. Umberto Volta for his work into non-celiac gluten sensitivity. I am also grateful to Dr. Aristo Vojdani for his commitment to improving lab accuracy; Dr. David Perlmutter for shining light on gluten-induced brain damage; Juan P. Ortiz-Sánchez, Francisco Cabrera Chávez, and Ana M. Calderón de la Barca for their work on corn gluten and dairy products; Dr. Robert Anderson and his group, who discovered new forms of gluten proteins; and Dr. Melissa Arbuckle for her work in predictive autoimmunity.

THOSE WHO CAME WITH ME

My wife, Kate, has always believed in and supported my work. She deserves a medal for listening to me talk and talk and talk about gluten, biochemistry, functional medicine, and more gluten. Thank you for being my sounding board in all things, attending my talks and events, managing and putting up with my constant travels and frequent absence, for being my silent hero in the back of the room, and for always exploring new ways to lovingly create gluten-free meals. Behind every successful man, there is always a brilliant woman. Kate, you are that and so much more. My three sons, Anthony, Conan, and Kane, taught me to stand and be a man, always inspiring me to be better. Carrie and Leon Kliethermes took me in and made me a part of their family, always willing to lend a loving hand of support. Willie Vinson, you supported me like a father, and you will always be remembered. And where would I be without my patients, most of whom came to me at their wits' end? They found the courage to make meaningful changes. They listened, complied, and got better despite all the skeptical doctors they'd seen previously. They taught me more than any medical textbook or research paper ever could. Huge thanks to my wonderful staff at Origins Healthcare: Debbie German, Michelle Gilcrease, Casey Todd, and Sally Wood. Without the four of you, the cogwheels wouldn't turn, and the people who need functional medicine would be left in the dark. Without the help of my personal mentors Bedros Keuilian and Craig Ballantyne, Gluten Free Society would not have been able to help so many. I am grateful to all my undergraduate and graduate professors who helped stoke the fires of nutritional and biochemical inquisitiveness. I owe a huge debt to all of my fellow functional medicine colleagues, who like me pushed the envelope of current dogmatic beliefs, risking their livelihood and reputations: Dr. Charles Parker, Sayer Ji, Dr. Tom O'Bryan, Dr. Kelly Brogan, Chris Kresser, Dr. Sara Gottfried, Dr. Hyla Cass, Dr. Joseph Mercola, Dr. Ron Grisanti, Ron Hoggan, JJ Virgin, Dr. Stephanie Seneff, Dr. Daniel Amen, Jeffrey Smith, Mark Sisson, Dr. Sherri Tenpenny, Dr. Terry Wahls, and Dr. John Symes—this list could go on and on, but as with any acknowledgment, it would impossible to point out every single person who made an impact, so again, forgive me if I left you out.

THOSE WHO JOINED ME

Special thanks to Melissa Wilson of Fox News; and to my agents Celeste Fine and John Maas, whose unflagging commitment and support helped me to navigate the complex world of book publishing. Olivia Bell Buehl's talent for wordsmithing is unsurpassed, and her knowledge contributed greatly to putting this book together. She worked diligently through weekends and holidays to help make a very tight deadline. To all of my affiliates who helped share the mission of Gluten Free Society with the world, I so appreciate your efforts. Michelle Howry and the rest of the Simon & Schuster team took a chance on me and helped make this book a reality. You are the best. Brad Kuntz, Andrew Minion, and Sydney Osborne, I know how hard you worked as my web team to put together the technology pieces to accompany this book. You did a great job, again under a tight deadline.

A huge thanks to my Facebook supporters, my blog readers and followers, and all those who watched one of my whiteboard videos to educate themselves on nutrition. And to those of you who argued with me or challenged my positions, I appreciate you as well: debate is the spark of progress toward greater truth. Finally, to those of you who are just picking this book up, welcome.

You all helped *No Grain, No Pain* become a reality. I am in your debt.

VALUABLE RESOURCES

Gluten Free Society
GlutenFreeSociety.org
Education and resources for going grain free

The following companies offer products to help you live a grain-free, pain-free life:

FOOD AND SNACKS

Against the Grain Gourmet
againstthegraingourmet.com
Grain-free bread and pizza

Cappello's Gluten Free
cappellosglutenfree.com
Grain-free pasta and cookie dough

Hail Merry
hailmerry.com
Grain-free treats and desserts

Nick's Sticks
nicks-sticks.com
Grass-fed beef and free-range turkey jerky sticks

Pete's Paleo
petespaleo.com
Grain-free meals delivered to your home

Steve's PaleoGoods
stevespaleogoods.com
Grain-free snacks, bars, granola, and jerky

Thrive Market
thrivemarket.com
Natural and nontoxic foods (and other products) delivered to your home

US Wellness Meats
grasslandbeef.com
Grass-fed and organic food

Vital Choice Wild Seafood & Organics
vitalchoice.com
Wild seafood and organic foods

COSMETICS AND SKIN CARE

Annmarie
annmariegianni.com
Organic skin care

Red Apple Lipstick
redapplelipstick.com
Gluten-free, paraben-free lipstick and other cosmetics

AIR PURIFICATION

IQAir
iqair.com
Whole-house air purifiers

NOTES

CHAPTER 1: WHAT'S THE GRAIN-PAIN CONNECTION?
WHY "HEALTHY" FOODS MAKE US FEEL SO BAD

1. Jeanie Lerche Davis, "Joint Pain Not Inevitable with Age," WebMD, 2003, webmd.com/osteoarthritis/features/joint-pain-management-age.

2. P. R. Shewry et al., "Seed Storage Proteins: Structures and Biosynthesis," *Plant Cell* 7 (1995): 945–56, ncbi.nlm.nih.gov/pmc/articles/PMC160892/pdf /070945.pdf.

3. G. Gasbarrini et al., "When Was Celiac Disease Born? The Italian Case from the Archeologic Site of Cosa," *Journal of Clinical Gastroenterology* 44 (2010): 502–3, ncbi.nlm.nih.gov/pubmed/20631553.

4. J. H. van de Kamer et al., "Coeliac Disease: V: Some Experiments on the Cause of the Harmful Effect of Wheat Gliadin," *Acta Paediatrica* 42 (1953): 223–31, onlinelibrary.wiley.com/doi/10.1111/j.1651-2227.1955.tb04269.x/abstract.

5. Sidney Valentine Haas and Merrill Patterson Haas, *Management of Celiac Disease* (Philadelphia: Lippincott, 1951; reprinted 2011, Literary Licensing, LLC).

6. V. De Re et al., "The Versatile Role of Gliadin Peptides in Celiac Disease," *Clinical Biochemistry* 46, no. 6 (2013): 552–60, ncbi.nlm.nih.gov/pubmed/23142684.

7. Helene Arentz-Hansen et al., "The Molecular Basis for Oat Intolerance in Patients with Celiac Disease," *PLoS Medicine* 1, no. 1 (2004): e1, ncbi.nlm.nih .gov/pmc/articles/PMC523824.

8. A. Real et al., "Molecular and Immunological Characterization of Gluten Proteins Isolated from Oat Cultivars That Differ in Toxicity for Celiac Disease," *PLoS One* 7, no. 12 (2012): e48365, ncbi.nlm.nih.gov/pmc/articles /PMC3524229; I. Comino et al., "Diversity in Oat Potential Immunogenicity: Basis for the Selection of Oat Varieties with No Toxicity in Coeliac Disease," *Gut* 60, no. 7 (2011): 915–22, ncbi.nlm.nih.gov/pubmed/21317420.

9. E. Varjonen et al., "Skin-Prick Test and RAST Responses to Cereals in Children with Atopic Dermatitis. Characterization of IgE-Binding Components in Wheat and Oats by an Immunoblotting Method," *Clinical & Experimental Allergy* 25, no. 11 (1995): 1100–1107, onlinelibrary.wiley.com/doi/10.1111/j.1365 -2222.1995.tb03257.x/abstract.

10. Elaine Watson, "What's the Size of the US Gluten-Free Prize? $490M, $5BN, or $10BN?," *FoodNavigator-USA*, February 17, 2014, foodnavigator-usa.com /Markets/What-s-the-size-of-the-US-gluten-free-prize-490m-5bn-or-10bn.

11. J. R. Hollon et al., "Trace Gluten Contamination May Play a Role in Mucosal and Clinical Recovery in a Subgroup of Diet-Adherent Non-Responsive Celiac Disease Patients," *BMC Gastroenterology* 13 (2013): 40, biomedcentral .com/1471-230X/13/40.

12. A. Lanzini et al., "Complete Recovery of Intestinal Mucosa Occurs Very Rarely in Adult Coeliac Patients Despite Adherence to Gluten-Free Diet," *Alimentary Pharmacology & Therapeutics* 29, no. 12 (2009): 1299–308, ncbi.nlm.nih.gov /pubmed/19302264.

13. C. Catassi et al., "Non-Celiac Gluten Sensitivity: The New Frontier of Gluten Related Disorders," *Nutrients* 5, no. 10 (2013): 3839–53, ncbi.nlm.nih.gov /pubmed/24077239.

14. "Aspirin," *Medline Plus*, November 15, 2014, nlm.nih.gov/medlineplus/drug info/meds/a682878.html, accessed 6/9/15.

15. University of Chicago Celiac Disease Center, "Symptoms and Conditions Potentially Due to Celiac Disease," adapted from C. J. Libonati, *Recognizing Celiac Disease* (Fort Washington, PA: Gluten Free Works Publishing, 2007), cureceliacdisease.org/wp-content/uploads/2011/09/CDCFactSheets10 _SymptomList.pdf, accessed 6/9/15.

16. A. Di Sabatino et al., "Small Amounts of Gluten in Subjects with Suspected Nonceliac Gluten Sensitivity: A Randomized, Double-Blind, Placebo-Controlled, Cross-Over Trial," *Clinical Gastroenterology and Hepatology* (epub ahead of print) (2015), pii: S1542-3565(15)00153–156, ncbi.nlm.nih.gov/pub med/25701700.

17. F. G. Chirdo et al., "Presence of High Levels of Non-Degraded Gliadin in Breast Milk from Healthy Mothers," *Scandinavian Journal of Gastroenterology* 33, no. 11 (1998): 1186–92, ncbi.nlm.nih.gov/pubmed/9867098; R. Troncone et al., "Passage of Gliadin into Human Breast Milk," *Acta Paediatrica* 76, no. 3 (1987): 453–56, ncbi.nlm.nih.gov/pubmed/3300148.

18. J. A. Tye-Din et al., "Comprehensive, Quantitative Mapping of T Cell Epitopes in Gluten in Celiac Disease," *Science Translational Medicine* 2, no. 41 (2010): 41ra51, stm.sciencemag.org/content/2/41/41ra51.

19. Y. Ohtsuka et al., "Reducing Cell Membrane N-6 Fatty Acids Attenuate Mucosal Damage in Food-Sensitive Enteropathy in Mice," *Pediatric Research* 42, no. 6 (1997): 835–39, ncbi.nlm.nih.gov/pubmed/9396566.

20. G. Kristjánsson et al., "Mucosal Reactivity to Cow's Milk Protein in Coeliac Disease," *Clinical & Experimental Immunology* 147, no. 3 (2007): 449–55, wiley .com/doi/10.1111/j.1365-2249.2007.03298.x/abstract.

21. Hollon et al., "Trace Gluten Contamination."

22. C. Briani et al., "Celiac Disease: From Gluten to Autoimmunity," *Autoimmunity Reviews* 7, no. 8 (2008): 644–50, ncbi.nlm.nih.gov/pubmed/18589004;

National Foundation for Celiac Awareness, "Non-Celiac Gluten Sensitivity," celiaccentral.org/non-celiac-gluten-sensitivity.

CHAPTER 2: WHERE DOES IT HURT?
ESCAPING THE PAIN-FUTILITY CYCLE FOR GOOD

1. D. J. Frantz et al., "Current Perception of Nutrition Education in U.S. Medical Schools," *Current Gastroenterology Reports* 13, no. 4 (2011): 376–79, doi: /10.1007/s11894-011-0202-z; K. M. Adams et al., "Nutrition Education in U.S. Medical Schools: Latest Update of a National Survey," *Academic Medicine* 85, no. 9 (2010): 1537–42, ncbi.nlm.nih.gov/pmc/articles/PMC4042309.

2. A. Fasano et al., "Nonceliac Gluten Sensitivity," *Gastroenterology* 148, no. 6 (2015): 1195–204, ncbi.nlm.nih.gov/pubmed/25583468; R. Troncone and V. Discepolo, "Celiac Disease and Autoimmunity," *Journal of Pediatric Gastroenterology and Nutrition* 59 (Suppl 1) (2014): S9–S11, ncbi.nlm.nih.gov /pubmed/24979198; Fasano et al., "Nonceliac Gluten Sensitivity"; A. S. Joshi et al., "Graves' Disease and Coeliac Disease: Screening and Treatment Dilemmas," *British Medical Journal: Case Reports* (2014), pii: bcr2013201386, ncbi.nlm .nih.gov/pubmed/25342186; F. Dickerson et al., "Markers of Gluten Sensitivity and Celiac Disease in Recent-Onset Psychosis and Multi-Episode Schizophrenia," *Biological Psychiatry*, 68, no. 1, no. (2010): 100–104, ncbi.nlm.nih .gov/pubmed/20471632; L. Rodrigo et al., "Prevalence of Celiac Disease in Multiple Sclerosis," *BMC Neurology* 11 (2011): 31, biomedcentral.com/1471 -2377/11/31.

3. "Autoimmune disease," *Wikipedia*, en.wikipedia.org/wiki/Autoimmune _disease, accessed 6/8/15; American Autoimmune Related Diseases Association, "Autoimmune and Autoimmune-Related Diseases," aarda.org/auto immune-information/list-of-diseases, accessed 6/8/15.

4. R. Aguado et al., "Antiadenohypophysis Autoantibodies in Patients with Nongluten-Related Gastroenteropathies," *Journal of Clinical Laboratory Analysis* 28, no. 1 (2014): 59–62, ncbi.nlm.nih.gov/pubmed/24375500; R. Locher et al., "Tiredness, Hyperpigmentation, Weight Loss, Nausea and Vomiting. Polyglandular Autoimmune Syndrome (PAS) Type 2," *Praxis* 99, no. 20 (2010): 1223–28 (article in German), ncbi.nlm.nih.gov/pubmed/20931500; C. Lipowsky et. al., "19-Year-Old Patient with Adrenal Cortex Insufficiency—Only the Tip of the Iceberg. Polyendocrine Autoimmune Syndrome Type II (Schmidt Syndrome)," *Praxis* 97, no. 2 (2008): 77–81 (article in German), ncbi.nlm.nih .gov/pubmed/18303665.

5. C. T. Lutz and L. S. Quinn, "Sarcopenia, Obesity, and Natural Killer Cell Immune Senescence in Aging: Altered Cytokine Levels as a Common Mechanism," *Aging* 4, no. 8 (2012): 535–46, impactaging.com/papers/v4/n8/full /100482.html.

6. J. R. Jackson et al., "Neurologic and Psychiatric Manifestations of Celiac Disease and Gluten Sensitivity," *Psychiatric Quarterly* 83, no. 1 (2012): 91–102, ncbi.nlm.nih.gov/pmc/articles/PMC3641836.

7. D. Vissides et al., "A Double-Blind Gluten-Free/Gluten-Load Controlled Trial in a Secure Ward Population," *British Journal of Psychiatry* 148 (1986): 447–52, ncbi.nlm.nih.gov/pubmed/3524724.

8. J. Jackson et al., "Gluten Sensitivity and Relationship to Psychiatric Symptoms in People with Schizophrenia," *Schizophrenia Research* 159, no. 2–3 (2014): 539–42, ncbi.nlm.nih.gov/pubmed/25311778.

9. N. Cascella et al., "Prevalence of Celiac Disease and Gluten Sensitivity in the United States Clinical Antipsychotic Trials of Intervention Effectiveness Study Population," *Schizophrenia Bulletin* 37, no. 1 (2011): 94–100, schizophreniabulletin.oxfordjournals.org/content/37/1/94.long.

10. F. Dickerson et al., "Markers of Gluten Sensitivity and Celiac Disease in Recent-Onset Psychosis and Multi-Episode Schizophrenia," *Biological Psychiatry* 68, no. 1 (2010): 100–104, ncbi.nlm.nih.gov/pubmed/20471632.

11. D. Samaroo et al., "Novel Immune Response to Gluten in Individuals with Schizophrenia," *Schizophrenia Research* 118, no. 1–3 (2010): 248–55, ncbi.nlm.nih.gov/pmc/articles/PMC2856786.

12. A. Kalaydjian et al., "The Gluten Connection: The Association between Schizophrenia and Celiac Disease," *Acta Psychiatrica Scandinavica* 113, no. 2 (2006): 82–90, ncbi.nlm.nih.gov/pubmed/16423158.

13. L. Hernandez and P. H. Green, "Extraintestinal Manifestations of Celiac Disease," *Current Gastroenterology Reports* 8, no. 5 (2006): 383–89, ncbi.nlm.nih.gov/pubmed/16968605.

14. L. B. Weinstock and A. S. Walters, "Restless Legs Syndrome Is Associated with Irritable Bowel Syndrome and Small Intestinal Bacterial Overgrowth," *Sleep Medicine* 12, no. 6 (2011): 610–13, ncbi.nlm.nih.gov/pubmed/21570907.

15. R. A. Hughes, "Peripheral Neuropathy," *British Medical Journal* 324, no. 7335 (2002): 466–69, ncbi.nlm.nih.gov/pmc/articles/PMC1122393; M. Hadjivassiliou et al., "Sensory Ganglionopathy Due to Gluten Sensitivity," *Neurology* 75, no. 11 (2010): 10038, ncbi.nlm.nih.gov/pubmed/ 20837968; H. Reda and R. L. Chin, "Peripheral Neuropathies of Rheumatologic Disease and Gluten-Related Disorders," *Seminars in Neurology* 34, no. 4 (2014): 413–24, ncbi.nlm.nih.gov/pubmed/25369437; B. Anderson and A. Pitsinger, "Improvement in Chronic Muscle Fasciculations with Dietary Change: A Suspected Case of Gluten Neuropathy," *Journal of Chiropractic Medicine* 13, no. 3 (2014): 188–91, ncbi.nlm.nih.gov/pmc/articles/PMC4161713; A. Boskovic and I. Stankovic, "Axonal and Demyelinating Polyneuropathy Associated with Celiac Disease," *Indian Pediatrics* 51, no. 4 (2014): 311–12, indianpediatrics.net/apr2014/311.pdf.

16. M. Hadjivassiliou et al., "Gluten-Related Disorders: Gluten Ataxia," *Digestive Diseases* 33, no. 2 (2015): 264–68, ncbi.nlm.nih.gov/pubmed/25925933.

17. J. Finsterer and F. Leutmezer, "Celiac Disease with Cerebral and Peripheral Nerve Involvement Mimicking Multiple Sclerosis," *Journal of Medicine and Life*, no. 73 (2014): 440–44, ncbi.nlm.nih.gov/pmc/articles/PMC4233456; H. Z Batur-Caglayan et al., "A Case of Multiple Sclerosis and Celiac Disease," *Case*

Reports in Neurological Medicine (2013), 2013:576921, hindawi.com/journals /crinm/2013/576921.

18. M. Przybylska-Felus et al., "Disturbances of Autonomic Nervous System Activity and Diminished Response to Stress in Patients with Celiac Disease," *Journal of Physiology and Pharmacology* 65, no. 6 (2014): 833–41, jpp.krakow.pl/jour nal/archive/12_14/pdf/833_12_14_article.pdf; M. Barbato et al., "Autonomic Imbalance in Celiac Children," *Minerva Pediatrica* 62, no. 4 (2010): 333–38, ncbi.nlm.nih.gov/pubmed/20940666.

19. R. P. Ford, "The Gluten Syndrome: A Neurological Disease," *Medical Hypotheses* 73, no. 3 (2009): 438–40, ncbi.nlm.nih.gov/pubmed/19406584; A. Tursi et al., "Peripheral Neurological Disturbances, Autonomic Dysfunction, and Antineuronal Antibodies in Adult Celiac Disease before and after a Gluten-Free Diet," *Digestive Diseases and Sciences* 51, no. 10 (2006): 1869–74, ncbi.nlm.nih.gov /pubmed/16967315.

20. Committee on Advancing Pain Research, Care, and Education of the Board on Health Sciences Policy, Institute of Medicine, National Academies, *Relieving Pain in America: A Blueprint for Transforming Prevention, Care, Education, and Research* (Washington, DC: National Academies Press, 2011), books.nap.edu /openbook.php?record_id=13172.

21. A. Scher et al., "Prevalence of Frequent Headache in a Population Sample," *Headache* 38, no. 7 (1998): 497–506, ncbi.nlm.nih.gov/pubmed/15613165.

22. B. A. Ferrell et al., "Pain in Cognitively Impaired Nursing Home Patients," *Journal of Pain Symptom Management* 10, no. 8 (1995): 591–98, ncbi.nlm.nih.gov /pubmed/8594119.

23. R. A. Deyo et al., "Back Pain Prevalence and Visit Rates: Estimates from U.S. National Surveys, 2002," *Spine* 31, no. 23 (2006): 2724–27, ncbi.nlm.nih.gov /pubmed/17077742.

24. IMS Institute of Healthcare Informatics, *The Use of Medicines in the United States: Review of 2010* (Parsippany, NJ: IMS Institute of Healthcare Informatics, 2011), imshealth.com/deployedfiles/imshealth/Global/Content/IMS%20Institute /Static%20File/IHII_UseOfMed_report.pdf, accessed 6/9/15.

25. L. H. Chen et al., "Drug-poisoning Deaths Involving Opioid Analgesics: United States, 1999–2011," NCHS Data Brief, no. 116, September 2014, cdc.gov/nchs /data/databriefs/db166.pdf, accessed 6/9/15.

26. US Census Bureau, Quickfacts Beta, census.gov/quickfacts/table/PST045214 /00, accessed 6/9/15.

27. M. Warner et al., "Drug Poisoning Deaths in the United States, 1980–2008," NCHS Data Brief, no. 81 (December 2011): 1–8, cdc.gov/nchs/data/databriefs /db81.pdf, accessed 6/9/15.

28. J. Lazarou et al., "Incidence of Adverse Drug Reactions in Hospitalized Patients," *Journal of the American Medical Association* 279, no. 15 (1998): 1200–5, ncbi.nlm.nih.gov/pubmed/9555760.

29. S. H. Hernandez and L. S. Nelson, "Prescription Drug Abuse: Insight into the Epidemic," *Clinical Pharmacology & Therapeutics* 88, no. 3 (2010): 307–17, ncbi .nlm.nih.gov/pubmed/20686478.

30. Centers for Disease Control and Prevention, Morbidity and Mortality Weekly Report, "CDC Grand Rounds: Prescription Drug Overdoses—A U.S. Epidemic," January 13, 2012, cdc.gov/mmwr/preview/mmwrhtml/mm6101a3.htm; T. Catan et al., "Prescription for Addiction," *Wall Street Journal*, October 5, 2012, wsj.com/articles/SB10000872396390444223104578036933277566700, accessed 6/9/15.

31. J. A. Hinson et al., "Mechanisms of Acetaminophen-Induced Liver Necrosis," *Handbook of Experimental Pharmacology*, ncbi.nlm.nih.gov/pmc/articles/PMC 2836803; L. P. James et al., "Acetaminophen-Induced Hepatotoxicity," *Drug Metabolism & Disposition* 31, no. 12 (2003): 1499–506, dmd.aspetjournals.org /content/31/12/1499.long.

32. G. Mazzarella et al., "Gliadin Intake Alters the Small Intestinal Mucosa in Indomethacin-Treated HLA-DQ8 Transgenic Mice," *American Journal of Physiology: Gastrointestinal and Liver Physiology* 307, no. 3 (2014): G302–12, ajpgi.phys iology.org/content/307/3/G302.

33. J. R. Hodges and J. Sadow, "Hypothalamo-Pituitary-Adrenal Function in the Rat after Prolonged Treatment with Cortisol," *British Journal of Pharmacology* 36, no. 3 (1969): 489–95, ncbi.nlm.nih.gov/pmc/articles/PMC1703614; V. Sannarangappa and R. Jalleh, "Inhaled Corticosteroids and Secondary Adrenal Insufficiency," *Open Respiratory Medicine Journal* 8 (2014): 93–100, ncbi .nlm.nih.gov/pmc/articles/PMC4319207; P. Humbert and A. Guichard, "The Topical Corticosteroid Classification Called into Question: Towards a New Approach," *Experimental Dermatology* 24, no. 5 (2015): 393–95, ncbi.nlm.nih .gov/pubmed/25707534; D. A. Fisher, "Adverse Effects of Topical Corticosteroid Use," *Western Journal of Medicine* 162, no. 2 (1995): 123–26, ncbi.nlm.nih .gov/pmc/articles/PMC1022645.

34. G. Schmajuk et al., "Osteoporosis Screening, Prevention and Treatment in Systemic Lupus Erythematosus: Application of the Systemic Lupus Erythematosus Quality Indicators," *Arthritis Care & Research* 62, no. 7 (2010): 993–1001, ncbi.nlm.nih.gov/pmc/articles/PMC2953549; R. G. Klein et al., "Intestinal Calcium Absorption in Exogenous Hypercortisonism: Role of 25-hydroxyvitamin D and Corticosteroid Dose," *Journal of Clinical Investigation* 60, no. 1 (1977): 253–59, ncbi.nlm.nih.gov/pmc/articles/PMC372363.

35. Klein et al., "Intestinal Calcium Absorption"; A. G. Need et al., "Calcium Metabolism and Osteoporosis in Corticosteroid-Treated Postmenopausal Women," *Australian & New Zealand Journal of Medicine* 16, no. 3 (1986): 341–46, ncbi.nlm.nih.gov/pubmed/3465310; W. R. Adam et al., "Renal Potassium Adaptation in the Rat: Role of Glucocorticoids and Aldosterone," *American Journal of Physiology: Renal Physiology*, 246, no. 3 (1984): F300–08, ncbi.nlm .nih.gov/pubmed/6703064; G. M. Shenfield et al., "Potassium Supplements in Patients Treated with Corticosteroids," *British Journal of Diseases of the Chest* 69 (1975): 171–76, ncbi.nlm.nih.gov/pubmed/1201184; A. A. Yunice et al.,

"Influence of Synthetic Corticosteroids on Plasma Zinc and Copper Levels in Humans," *American Journal of the Medical Sciences* 282, no. 2 (1981): 68–74, ncbi.nlm.nih.gov/pubmed/7325187; A. Simecková et al., "Effect of Prednisolone on the Rat Bone Calcium, Phosphorus and Magnesium Concentration," *Physiologia Bohemoslovaca* 34, no. 2 (1985): 155–60, ncbi.nlm.nih.gov /pubmed/3161105; G. Rolla et al., "Hypomagnesemia in Chronic Obstructive Lung Disease: Effect of Therapy," *Magnesium and Trace Elements* 9, no. 3 (1990): 132–36, ncbi.nlm.nih.gov/pubmed/1979000; M. A. Levine and H. B. Pollard, "Hydrocortisone Inhibition of Ascorbic Acid Transport by Chromaffin Cells," *FEBS Letters* 158, no. 1 (1983): 134–38, ncbi.nlm.nih.gov/pubmed/6862031; K. S. Mehra et al., "The Effect of Vitamin A and Cortisone on Ascorbic Acid Content in the Aqueous Humor," *Annals of Ophthalmology* 14, no. 11 (1982): 1013–15, ncbi.nlm.nih.gov/pubmed/7181331; A. Peretz et al., "Selenium Status in Relation to Clinical Variables and Corticosteroid Treatment in Rheumatoid Arthritis," *Journal of Rheumatology* 14, no. 6 (1987): 1104–7, ncbi.nlm.nih .gov/pubmed/3437416.

36. D. D. Kitts and K. Weiler, "Bioactive Proteins and Peptides from Food Sources. Applications of Bioprocesses Used in Isolation and Recovery," *Current Pharmaceutical Design* 9, no. 16 (2003): 1309–23, ncbi.nlm.nih.gov/pubmed/12769739.

CHAPTER 3: PAIN CAUSED BY GRAINFLAMMATION: BUILDING STRONG MUSCLES AND AVOIDING GLUTEN-FREE WHIPLASH

1. B. Lönnerdal, "Infant Formula and Infant Nutrition: Bioactive Proteins of Human Milk and Implications for Composition of Infant Formulas," *American Journal of Clinical Nutrition* 99, no. 3 (2014): 712S–17S, ncbi.nlm.nih.gov /pubmed/24452231.

2. N. Timby et al., "Infections in Infants Fed Formula Supplemented with Bovine Milk Fat Globule Membranes," *Journal of Pediatric Gastroenterology and Nutrition* 60, no. 3 (2015): 384–89, ncbi.nlm.nih.gov/pubmed/25714582.

3. P. M. Munyaka et al., "External Influence of Early Childhood Establishment of Gut Microbiota and Subsequent Health Implications," *Frontiers in Pediatrics* 2 (2014): 109, ncbi.nlm.nih.gov/pubmed/25346925.

4. Sidney Valentine Haas and Merrill Patterson Haas, *Management of Celiac Disease* (Philadelphia: Lippincott, 1951; reprinted 2011, Literary Licensing, LLC), x.

5. J. R. Hollon et al., "Trace Gluten Contamination May Play a Role in Mucosal and Clinical Recovery in a Subgroup of Diet-Adherent Non-Responsive Celiac Disease Patients," *BMC Gastroenterology* 13 (2013): 40, biomedcentral .com/1471-230X/13/40.

6. P. Srikanthan and A. S. Karlamangla, "Muscle Mass Index as a Predictor of Longevity in Older Adults," *American Journal of Medicine* 127, no. 6 (2014): 547–53, amjmed.com/article/S0002-9343(14)00138-7/abstract.

7. U. Lindqvist et al., "IgA Antibodies to Gliadin and Coeliac Disease in Psoriatic Arthritis," *Rheumatology* 41, no. 1 (2002): 31–37, rheumatology.oxford journals.org/content/41/1/31.long.

8. R. E. Toğrol et al., "The Significance of Coeliac Disease Antibodies in Patients with Ankylosing Spondylitis: A Case-Controlled Study," *Journal of International Medical Research* 37, no. 1 (2009): 220–26, ncbi.nlm.nih.gov/pubmed/19215694.

9. A. Orlando et al., "Gastrointestinal Lesions Associated with Spondyloarthropathies," *World Journal of Gastroenterology* 15, no. 20 (2009): 2443–48, wjgnet .com/1007-9327/full/v15/i20/2443.htm; J. Teichmann et al., "Antibodies to Human Tissue Transglutaminase and Alterations of Vitamin D Metabolism in Ankylosing Spondylitis and Psoriatic Arthritis," *Rheumatology International* 30, no. 12 (2010): 1559–63, springer.com/article/10.1007/s00296-009-1186-y.

10. M. S. Song et al., "Dermatomyositis Associated with Celiac Disease: Response to a Gluten-Free Diet," *Canadian Journal of Gastroenterology & Hepatology* 20, no. 6 (2006): 433–35, pulsus.com/journals/abstract.jsp?sCurrPg=journal&jnl Ky=2&atlKy=830&isuKy=269&isArt=t.

11. M. Slim et al., "The Effects of Gluten-Free Diet versus Hypocaloric Diet among Patients with Fibromyalgia Experiencing Gluten Sensitivity Symptoms: Protocol for a Pilot, Open-Label, Randomized Clinical Trial," *Contemporary Clinical Trials* 40 (2015): 193–98, ncbi.nlm.nih.gov/pubmed/25485857; U. Volta, "Gluten-Free Diet in the Management of Patients with Irritable Bowel Syndrome, Fibromyalgia and Lymphocytic Enteritis," *Arthritis Research & Therapy* 16, no. 6 (2014): 505, arthritis-research.com/content/16/6/505; A. Rossi et al., "Fibromyalgia and Nutrition: What News?", *Clinical and Experimental Rheumatology* 33, 1 Suppl 88 (2015): S117–25, ncbi.nlm.nih.gov/pubmed/25786053; C. Isasi et al., "Non-Celiac Gluten Sensitivity and Rheumatologic Diseases," *Reumatología Clínica* (epub ahead of print) (2015), pii: S1699-258X(15)00032-37 (article in English, Spanish), ncbi.nlm.nih.gov/pubmed/25956352; J. M. García-Leiva et al., "Celiac Symptoms in Patients with Fibromyalgia: A Cross-Sectional Study," *Rheumatology International* 35, no. 3 (2015): 561–67, ncbi.nlm.nih.gov/pubmed/25119831.

12. H. J. Freeman, "Adult Celiac Disease Followed by Onset of Systemic Lupus Erythematosus," *Journal of Clinical Gastroenterology* 42, no. 3 (2008): 252–55, ncbi.nlm.nih.gov/pubmed/18223501.

13. M. Atteno et al., "The Enthesopathy of Celiac Patients: Effects of Gluten-Free Diet," *Clinical Rheumatology* 33, no. 4 (2014): 537–41, ncbi.nlm.nih.gov/pub med/24567238.

14. M. Hadjivassiliou et al., "Gluten Sensitivity: From Gut to Brain," *Lancet: Neurology* 9, no. 3 (2010): 318–30, ncbi.nlm.nih.gov/pubmed/20170845.

CHAPTER 4: PAIN CAUSED BY IMBALANCES IN THE GUT: THE TRUTH ABOUT "LEAKY GUT" AND HOW DIET CAN HEAL (OR AGGRAVATE) IT

1. T. Powley and R. Phillips, "Morphology and Topography of Vagal Afferents Innervating the GI Tract," *American Journal of Physiology: Gastrointestinal and Liver Physiology* 283, no. 6 (2002): G1217–25, ajpgi.physiology.org/content/283/6 /G1217; Michael Gershon, *The Second Brain: A Groundbreaking New Understand-*

ing of the Nervous Disorders of the Stomach and Intestine (New York: HarperCollins, 1998).

2. S. H. Lee, "Intestinal Permeability Regulation by Tight Junction: Implication on Inflammatory Bowel Diseases," *Intestinal Research* 13, no. 1 (2015): 11–18, irjour nal.org/journal/journal_view.html?year=2015&vol=13&num=1&page=11.

3. K. de Punder and L. Pruimboom, "The Dietary Intake of Wheat and Other Cereal Grains and Their Role in Inflammation," *Nutrients* 5, no. 3 (2013): 771–87, ncbi.nlm.nih.gov/pmc/articles/PMC3705319.

4. A. Lerner and T. Matthias, "Changes in Intestinal Tight Junction Permeability Associated with Industrial Food Additives Explain the Rising Incidence of Autoimmune Disease," *Autoimmunity Reviews* 14, no. 6 (2015): 479–89, ncbi .nlm.nih.gov/pubmed/25676324.

5. M. A. Daulatzai, "Non-Celiac Gluten Sensitivity Triggers Gut Dysbiosis, Neuroinflammation, Gut-Brain Axis Dysfunction, and Vulnerability for Dementia," *CNS & Neurological Disorders: Drug Targets* 14, no. 1 (2015): 110–31, ncbi .nlm.nih.gov/pubmed/25642988.

6. A. Vojdani et al., "Environmental Triggers and Autoimmunity," *Autoimmune Diseases* (2014): 2014:798029, hindawi.com/journals/ad/2014/798029; K. F. Csáki, "Synthetic Surfactant Food Additives Can Cause Intestinal Barrier Dysfunction," *Medical Hypotheses* 76, no. 5 (2011): 676–81, ncbi.nlm.nih .gov/pubmed/21300443; R. K. Cady et al., "The Bowel and Migraine: Update on Celiac Disease and Irritable Bowel Syndrome," *Current Pain and Headache Reports* 16, no. 3 (2012): 278–86, ncbi.nlm.nih.gov/pubmed/22447132.

7. N. Mitchell et al., "Randomised Controlled Trial of Food Elimination Diet Based on IgG Antibodies for the Prevention of Migraine Like Headaches," *Nutrition Journal* 10 (August 2011), nutritionj.com/content/10/1/85.

8. K. Alpay et al., "Diet Restriction in Migraine, Based on IgG against Foods: A Clinical Double-Blind, Randomised, Cross-Over Trial," *Cephalalgia* 30, no. 7 (2010): 829–37, ncbi.nlm.nih.gov/pmc/articles/PMC2899772.

9. K. Takeuchi and H. Satoh, "NSAID-Induced Small Intestinal Damage—Roles of Various Pathogenic Factors," *Digestion* 91, no. 3 (2015): 218–32, karger.com /Article/FullText/374106; P. Tsibouris et al., "Small Bowel Ulcerative Lesions Are Common in Elderly NSAIDs Users with Peptic Ulcer Bleeding," *World Journal of Gastrointestinal Endoscopy* 6, no. 12 (2014): 612–19, wjgnet.com/1948-51 90/full/v6/i12/612.htm.

10. M. Lamprecht and A. Frauwallner, "Exercise, Intestinal Barrier Dysfunction and Probiotic Supplementation," *Medicine and Sport Science: Acute Topics in Sport Nutrition* 59 (2012): 47–56, karger.com/Article/Abstract/342169; M. N. Zuhl, "Effects of Oral Glutamine Supplementation on Exercise-Induced Gastrointestinal Permeability and Tight Junction Protein Expression," *Journal of Applied Physiology* 116, no. 2 (2014): 183–91, jap.physiology.org/cgi/pmid lookup?view=long&pmid=24285149; H. J. Freeman, "Adult Celiac Disease Followed by Onset of Systemic Lupus Erythematosus," *Journal of Clinical Gastroenterology* 42, no. 3 (2008): 252–55, ncbi.nlm.nih.gov/pubmed/18223501;

K. Dokladny et al., "Physiologically Relevant Increase in Temperature Causes an Increase in Intestinal Epithelial Tight Junction Permeability," *American Journal of Physiology: Gastrointestinal and Liver Physiology* 290, no. 2 (2006): G204–12, ajpgi.physiology.org/content/290/2/G204.long.

11. E. J. Kuipers, "*Helicobacter pylori* and the Risk and Management of Associated Diseases: Gastritis, Ulcer Disease, Atrophic Gastritis and Gastric Cancer," *Alimentary Pharmacology & Therapeutics* 11, Suppl 1 (1997): 71–88, ncbi.nlm.nih .gov/pubmed/9146793; P. Sipponen and H. Hyvärinen, "Role of *Helicobacter pylori* in the Pathogenesis of Gastritis, Peptic Ulcer and Gastric Cancer," *Scandinavian Journal of Gastroenterology*, Suppl 196 (1993): 3–6, ncbi.nlm.nih.gov /pubmed/8341988.

12. T. Ochsenkühn et al., "Inflammatory Bowel Diseases (IBD)—Critical Discussion of Etiology, Pathogenesis, Diagnostics, and Therapy," *Radiologe* 43, no. 1 (2003): 1–8 (article in German), ncbi.nlm.nih.gov/pubmed/12552369.

13. S. Yurist-Doutsch et al., "Gastrointestinal Microbiota-Mediated Control of Enteric Pathogens," *Annual Review of Genetics* 48 (2014): 361–82, ncbi.nlm.nih .gov/pubmed/25251855.

14. M. A. Daulatzai, "Non-Celiac Gluten Sensitivity Triggers Gut Dysbiosis, Neuroinflammation, Gut-Brain Axis Dysfunction, and Vulnerability for Dementia," *CNS & Neurological Disorders: Drug Targets* 14, no. 1 (2015): 110–31, ncbi .nlm.nih.gov/pubmed/25642988.

15. N. Uy et al., "Effects of Gluten-Free, Dairy-Free Diet on Childhood Nephrotic Syndrome and Gut Microbiota," *Pediatric Research* 77, no. 1–2 (2015): 252–55, ncbi.nlm.nih.gov/pubmed/25310757; M. Olivares et al., "Double-Blind, Randomised, Placebo-Controlled Intervention Trial to Evaluate the Effects of *Bifidobacterium longum* CECT 7347 in Children with Newly Diagnosed Coeliac Disease," *British Journal of Nutrition* 112, no. 1 (2014): 30–40, ncbi.nlm .nih.gov/pubmed/24774670; L. F. de Sousa Moraes et al., "Intestinal Microbiota and Probiotics in Celiac Disease," *Clinical Microbiology Reviews* 27, no. 3 (2014): 482–89, cmr.asm.org/content/27/3/482.long; Y. Sanz, "Effects of a Gluten-Free Diet on Gut Microbiota and Immune Function in Healthy Adult Humans," *Gut Microbes* 1, no. 3 (2010): 135–37, tandfonline.com/doi /full/10.4161/gmic.1.3.11868#abstract; Y. Sanz, "Unraveling the Ties between Celiac Disease and Intestinal Microbiota," *International Reviews of Immunology* 30, no. 4 (2011): 207–18, ncbi.nlm.nih.gov/pubmed/21787226; L. R. Ferguson et al., "Nutrigenomics and Gut Health," *Nutrigenomics* 622, no. 1–2 (2007): 1–6, ncbi.nlm.nih.gov/pubmed/17568628; G. Dahlqvist and H. Piessevaux, "Irritable Bowel Syndrome: The Role of the Intestinal Microbiota, Pathogenesis and Therapeutic Targets," *Acta Gastro-Enterologica Belgica* 74, no. 3 (2011): 375–80 (cf. article 10), ncbi.nlm.nih.gov/pubmed/22103040.

16. L. Ohman and M. Simrén, "Intestinal Microbiota and Its Role in Irritable Bowel Syndrome (IBS)," *Current Gastroenterology Reports* 15, no. 5 (2013): 323, ncbi .nlm.nih.gov/pubmed/23580243.

17. I. G. Moraru et al., "Small Intestinal Bacterial Overgrowth Is Associated to Symptoms in Irritable Bowel Syndrome. Evidence from a Multicentre Study in

Romania," *Romanian Journal of Internal Medicine* 52, no. 3 (2014): 143–50, ncbi .nlm.nih.gov/pubmed/25509557.

18. J. R. Brestoff and D. Artis, "Commensal Bacteria at the Interface of Host Metabolism and the Immune System," *Nature Immunology* 14 (2013): 676–84, nature.com/ni/journal/v14/n7/abs/ni.2640.html.

19. R. E. Ley et al., "Microbial Ecology: Human Gut Microbes Associated with Obesity," *Nature* 444, no. 7122 (2006): 1022–23, ncbi.nlm.nih.gov/pubmed /17183309.

20. Georgia State University, "Healthy Gut Microbiota Can Prevent Metabolic Syndrome, Researchers Say," November 24, 2014, *ScienceDaily*, sciencedaily.com /releases/2014/11/141124081036.htm.

21. Centers for Medicare & Medicaid Services, "CMS Releases Prescriber-Level Medicare Data for First Time," cms.gov/Newsroom/MediaReleaseDatabase /Fact-sheets/2015-Fact-sheets-items/2015-04-30.html.

22. J. R. Lam, "Proton Pump Inhibitor and Histamine 2 Receptor Antagonist Use and Vitamin B$_{12}$ Deficiency," *Journal of the American Medical Association* 310, no. 22 (2013): 2435–42, ncbi.nlm.nih.gov/pubmed/24327038; A. Dahele and S. Ghosh, "Vitamin B$_{12}$ Deficiency in Untreated Celiac Disease," *American Journal of Gastroenterology* 96, no. 3 (2001): 745–50, ncbi.nlm.nih.gov/pub med/11280545.

23. F. Nachman et al., "Gastroesophageal Reflux Symptoms in Patients with Celiac Disease and the Effects of a Gluten-Free Diet," *Clinical Gastroenterology and Hepatology* 9, no. 3 (2011): 214–19, ncbi.nlm.nih.gov/pubmed/20601132; T. G. Theethira et al., "Nutritional Consequences of Celiac Disease and the Gluten-Free Diet," *Expert Review of Gastroenterology & Hepatology* 8, no. 2 (2014): 123–29, ncbi.nlm.nih.gov/pubmed/24417260; R. Caruso et al., "Appropriate Nutrient Supplementation in Celiac Disease," *Annals of Medicine* 45, no. 8 (2013): 522–31, ncbi.nlm.nih.gov/pubmed/24195595.

24. L. de Magistris et al., "Alterations of the Intestinal Barrier in Patients with Autism Spectrum Disorders and in Their First-Degree Relatives," *Journal of Pediatric Gastroenterology and Nutrition* 51, no. 4 (2010): 418–24, ncbi.nlm.nih. gov/pubmed/20683204; A. Fasano, "Regulation of Intercellular Tight Junctions by Zonula Occludens Toxin and Its Eukaryotic Analogue Zonulin," *Annals of the New York Academy of Sciences* 915 (2000): 214–22, ncbi.nlm.nih .gov/pubmed/11193578.

25. K. L. Reichelt and J. Landmark, "Specific IgA Antibody Increases in Schizophrenia," *Biological Psychiatry* 37, no. 6 (1995): 410–13, ncbi.nlm.nih.gov/pub med/7772650.

26. C. Briani et al., "Neurological Complications of Celiac Disease and Autoimmune Mechanisms: A Prospective Study," *Journal of Neuroimmunology* 195, no. 1–2 (2008): 171–75, ncbi.nlm.nih.gov/pubmed/18343508; F. Dickerson et al., "Markers of Gluten Sensitivity and Celiac Disease in Bipolar Disorder," *Bipolar Disorders* 13, no. 1 (2011): 52–58, ncbi.nlm.nih.gov/pubmed/21320252.

27. N. Marchi et al., "Blood-Brain Barrier Damage, but Not Parenchymal White Blood Cells, Is a Hallmark of Seizure Activity," *Brain Research* 1353 (2010): 176–86, ncbi.nlm.nih.gov/pmc/articles/PMC2933328; F. S. Sallem et al., "Gluten Sensitivity Presenting as Myoclonic Epilepsy with Cerebellar Syndrome," *Movement Disorders* 24, no. 14 (2009): 2162–63, ncbi.nlm.nih.gov/pubmed/19705357.

28. F. Capone et al., "Gluten-Related Recurrent Peripheral Facial Palsy," *Journal of Neurology, Neurosurgery, & Psychiatry* 83, no. 6 (2012): 667–68, ncbi.nlm.nih.gov/pubmed/22383733.

29. H. Niederhofer, "Association of Attention-Deficit/Hyperactivity Disorder and Celiac Disease: A Brief Report," *Primary Care Companion for CNS Disorders* 13, no. 3 (2011): PCC.10br01104, ncbi.nlm.nih.gov/pmc/articles/PMC3184556.

30. S. J. Genius and T. P. Bouchard, "Celiac Disease Presenting as Autism," *Journal of Child Neurology* 25, no. 1 (2010): 114–19, ncbi.nlm.nih.gov/pubmed/19564647; L. de Magistris et al., "Alterations of the Intestinal Barrier in Patients with Autism Spectrum Disorders and in Their First-Degree Relatives," *Journal of Pediatric Gastroenterology and Nutrition* 51, no. 4 (2010): 418–24, ncbi.nlm.nih.gov/pubmed/20683204.

31. F. Muñoz et al., "Enamel Defects Associated with Coeliac Disease: Putative Role of Antibodies against Gliadin in Pathogenesis," *European Journal of Oral Sciences* 120, no. 2 (2012): 104–12, pubfacts.com/detail/22409216/Enamel-defects-associated-with-coeliac-disease:-putative-role-of-antibodies-against-gliadin-in-patho; M. Rashid et al., "Oral Manifestations of Celiac Disease: A Clinical Guide for Dentists," *Journal of the Canadian Dental Association* (2011): 77:b39, ncbi.nlm.nih.gov/pubmed/21507289.

32. R. Shakeri et al., "Gluten Sensitivity Enteropathy in Patients with Recurrent Aphthous Stomatitis," *BMC Gastroenterology* 9 (2009): 44, biomedcentral.com/1471-230X/9/44.

33. A. J. Lucendo, "Esophageal Manifestations of Celiac Disease," *Diseases of the Esophagus* 24, no. 7 (2011): 470–75, ncbi.nlm.nih.gov/pubmed/21438963.

34. O. Pickett-Blakely, "Obesity and Irritable Bowel Syndrome: A Comprehensive Review," *Gastroenterology & Hepatology* 10, no. 7 (2014): 411–16, ncbi.nlm.nih.gov/pmc/articles/PMC4302488.

35. M. El-Salhy and D. Gundersen, "Diet in Irritable Bowel Syndrome," *Nutrition Journal* 14 (2015): 36, nutritionj.com/content/14/1/36.

36. M. I. Vazquez-Roque et al., "A Controlled Trial of Gluten-Free Diet in Patients with Irritable Bowel Syndrome-Diarrhea: Effects on Bowel Frequency and Intestinal Function," *Gastroenterology* 144, no. 5 (2013): 903–911.e3, ncbi.nlm.nih.gov/pmc/articles/PMC3633663.

37. M. B. Zanchetta et al., "Significant Bone Microarchitecture Impairment in Premenopausal Women with Active Celiac Disease," *Bone* 76 (2015): 149–57, ncbi.nlm.nih.gov/pubmed/25779933; G. Malamut and C. Cellier, "Refractory Celiac Disease: Epidemiology and Clinical Manifestations," *Digestive Diseases* 33, no. 2 (2015): 221–26, ncbi.nlm.nih.gov/pubmed/25925926.

38. K. Kurppa et al., "Celiac Disease without Villous Atrophy in Children: A Prospective Study," *Journal of Pediatrics* 157, no. 3 (2010): 373–80, 380.e1, ncbi .nlm.nih.gov/pubmed/20400102; G. J. Kahaly and D. Schuppan, "Celiac Disease and Endocrine Autoimmunity," *Digestive Diseases* 33, no. 2 (2015): 155–61, ncbi.nlm.nih.gov/pubmed/25925917.

39. K. Kurppa et al., "Diagnosing Mild Enteropathy Celiac Disease: A Randomized, Controlled Clinical Study," *Gastroenterology* 136, no. 3 (2009): 816–23, ncbi.nlm.nih.gov/pubmed/19111551; S. R. Vavricka et al., "Chronological Order of Appearance of Extraintestinal Manifestations Relative to the Time of IBD Diagnosis in the Swiss Inflammatory Bowel Disease Cohort," *Inflammatory Bowel Diseases* 21, no. 8 (2015), ncbi.nlm.nih.gov/pubmed/26020601.

40. C. C. Lanna et al., "A Cross-Sectional Study of 130 Brazilian Patients with Crohn's Disease and Ulcerative Colitis: Analysis of Articular and Ophthalmologic Manifestations," *Clinical Rheumatology* 27, no. 4 (2008): 503–9, ncbi.nlm .nih.gov/pubmed/18097711.

41. I. W. Davidson et al., "Antibodies to Maize in Patients with Crohn's Disease, Ulcerative Colitis and Coeliac Disease," *Clinical & Experimental Immunology* 35, no. 1 (1979): 147–48, ncbi.nlm.nih.gov/pmc/articles/PMC1537589; C. M. Triggs et al., "Dietary Factors in Chronic Inflammation: Food Tolerances and Intolerances of a New Zealand Caucasian Crohn's Disease Population," *Mutation Research/Fundamental and Molecular Mechanisms of Mutagenesis* 690, no. 1–2 (2010): 123–38, ncbi.nlm.nih.gov/pubmed/20144628; T. J. Green et al., "Patients' Diets and Preferences in a Pediatric Population with Inflammatory Bowel Disease," *Canadian Journal of Gastroenterology & Hepatology* 12, no. 8 (1998): 544–49, ncbi.nlm.nih.gov/pubmed/9926264.

42. J. Van Den Bogaerde et al., "Gut Mucosal Response to Food Antigens in Crohn's Disease," *Alimentary Pharmacology & Therapeutics* 16, no. 11 (2002): 1903–15, onlinelibrary.wiley.com/doi/10.1046/j.1365-2036.2002.01360.x /full; S. Huebener et al., "Specific Nongluten Proteins of Wheat Are Novel Target Antigens in Celiac Disease Humoral Response," *Journal of Proteome Research* 14, no. 1 (2015): 503–11, pubs.acs.org/doi/abs/10.1021/pr500809b.

43. V. Zevallos et al., "Purifikation, Charakterisierung und biologische Wirkungen von alpha-Amylase-/Trypsininhibitoren aus Pflanzen, Effektoren von intestinalen TLR4 bei Zöliakie," *Zeitschrift für Gastroenterologie* 7 (2012): 50 (article in German), thieme-connect.com/products/ejournals/abstract/10.1055/s-0032 -1323857; Y. Junker et al., "Wheat Amylase Trypsin Inhibitors Drive Intestinal Inflammation via Activation of Toll-Like Receptor 4," *Journal of Experimental Medicine* 209, no. 13 (2012): 2395–408, ncbi.nlm.nih.gov/pmc/articles /PMC3526354.

44. D. Schuppan and V. Zevallos, "Wheat Amylase Trypsin Inhibitors as Nutritional Activators of Innate Immunity," *Digestive Diseases* 33, no. 2 (2015): 260–63, ncbi.nlm.nih.gov/pubmed/25925932.

45. Huebener et al., "Specific Nongluten Proteins."

CHAPTER 5: PAIN CAUSED BY OBESITY: BLAME IT ON "GRAINBESITY"

1. Division of Nutrition, Physical Activity, and Obesity, "Adult Obesity Facts," Centers for Disease Control and Prevention, June 16, 2015, cdc.gov/obesity /data/adult.html, accessed 6/11/15.

2. W. Dickey and N. Kearney, "Overweight in Celiac Disease: Prevalence, Clinical Characteristics, and Effect of a Gluten-Free Diet," *American Journal of Gastroenterology* 101, no. 10 (2006): 2356–59, ncbi.nlm.nih.gov/pubmed/17032202; N. R. Reilly et al., "Celiac Disease in Normal-Weight and Overweight Children: Clinical Features and Growth Outcomes Following a Gluten-Free Diet," *Journal of Pediatric Gastroenterology and Nutrition* 53, no. 5 (2011): 528–31, ncbi .nlm.nih.gov/pubmed/21670710.

3. "Proposed Changes to the Nutrition Facts Label," U.S. Food and Drug Administration, July 27, 2015, fda.gov/Food/GuidanceRegulation/GuidanceDocu mentsRegulatoryInformation/LabelingNutrition/ucm385663.htm, accessed 6/11/15.

4. S. Song et al., "Metabolic Syndrome Risk Factors Are Associated with White Rice Intake in Korean Adolescent Girls and Boys," *British Journal of Nutrition* 113, no. 3 (2015): 479–87, ncbi.nlm.nih.gov/pubmed/25572175; S. Castellaneta et al., "High Rate of Spontaneous Normalization of Celiac Serology in a Cohort of 446 Children with Type 1 Diabetes: A Prospective Study." *Diabetes Care* 38, no. 5 (2015): 760–66, ncbi.nlm.nih.gov/pubmed/25784659; J. Larsen et al., "Effect of Dietary Gluten on Dendritic Cells and Innate Immune Subsets in BALB/c and NOD Mice," *PLoS One* 10, no. 3 (2015): e0118618, journals. plos.org/plosone/article?id=10.1371/journal.pone.0118618; Y. L. Zuñiga et al., "Rice and Noodle Consumption Is Associated with Insulin Resistance and Hyperglycaemia in an Asian Population," *British Journal of Nutrition* 111, no. 6 (2014): 1118–28, ncbi.nlm.nih.gov/pubmed/24229726; S. Song et al., "Carbohydrate Intake and Refined-Grain Consumption Are Associated with Metabolic Syndrome in the Korean Adult Population," *Journal of the Academy of Nutrition and Dietetics* 114, no. 1 (2014): 54–62, ncbi.nlm.nih.gov/pub med/24200655; A. Esmaillzadeh et al., "Whole-Grain Consumption and the Metabolic Syndrome: A Favorable Association in Tehranian Adults," *European Journal of Clinical Nutrition* 59, no. 3 (2005): 353–62, ncbi.nlm.nih.gov/pub med/15536473; S. Clemens, "Zn and Fe Biofortification: The Right Chemical Environment for Human Bioavailability," *Plant Science* 225 (2014): 52–57, ncbi .nlm.nih.gov/pubmed/25017159.

5. D. Moretti et al., "Bioavailability of Iron, Zinc, Folic Acid, and Vitamin A from Fortified Maize," *Annals of the New York Academy of Sciences* 1312 (2014): 54–65, onlinelibrary.wiley.com/doi/10.1111/nyas.12297/full; H. H. Sandstead and J. H. Freeland-Graves, "Dietary Phytate, Zinc and Hidden Zinc Deficiency," *Journal of Trace Elements in Medicine and Biology* 28, no. 4 (2014): 414–17, ncbi.nlm.nih.gov/pubmed/25439135; R. S. Gibson et al., "A Review of Phytate, Iron, Zinc, and Calcium Concentrations in Plant-Based Complementary Foods Used in Low-Income Countries and Implications for Bioavailability," *Food and Nutrition Bulletin* 31(2 Suppl) (2010):

S134–46, ncbi.nlm.nih.gov/pubmed/20715598; I. Robertson et al., "The Role of Cereals in the Aetiology of Nutritional Rickets: The Lesson of the Irish National Nutrition Survey 1943–8," *British Journal of Nutrition* 45, no. 1 (1981): 17–22, ncbi.nlm.nih.gov/pubmed/6970590; D. A. Roth-Maier et al., "Availability of Vitamin B_6 from Different Food Sources," *International Journal of Food Sciences and Nutrition* 53, no. 2 (2002): 171–79, ncbi.nlm.nih .gov/pubmed/11939111; R. D. Reynolds, "Bioavailability of Vitamin B-6 from Plant Foods," *American Journal of Clinical Nutrition* 48, 3 Suppl (1988): 863–67, ajcn.nutrition.org/content/48/3/863.long; K. Rajakumar, "Pellagra in the United States: A Historical Perspective," *Southern Medical Journal* 93, no. 3 (2000): 272–77, ncbi.nlm.nih.gov/pubmed/10728513; K. J. Carpenter, "The Relationship of Pellagra to Corn and the Low Availability of Niacin in Cereals," *Experientia Supplementum* 44 (1983): 197–222, ncbi.nlm.nih.gov /pubmed/6357846.

6. R. R. Williams, "The World Beriberi Problem Today," *American Journal of Nutrition* 1, no. 7 (1953): 513–16, ajcn.nutrition.org/content/1/7/513.full.pdf.

7. S. C. Schimpff, "The Dramatic Changes in the Causes of Death," KevinMD .com, July 26, 2012, kevinmd.com/blog/2012/07/dramatic-change-death .html.

8. P. C. Calder, "n-3 Polyunsaturated Fatty Acids, Inflammation, and Inflammatory Diseases," *American Journal of Clinical Nutrition* 83, no. 6 (2006): S1505–19S. ajcn.nutrition.org/content/83/6/S1505.full.

9. A. P. Simopoulos, "Evolutionary Aspects of Diet, the Omega-6/Omega-3 Ratio and Genetic Variation: Nutritional Implications for Chronic Diseases," *Biomedicine & Pharmacotherapy* 60, no. 9 (2006): 502–7, sciencedirect.com/science /article/pii/S0753332206002435.

10. C. L. Ogden et al., "Prevalence of Overweight and Obesity in the United States, 1999–2004," *Journal of the American Medical Association* 295, no. 13 (2006):1549–55, ncbi.nlm.nih.gov/pubmed/16595758; C. L. Ogden et al., "High Body Mass Index for Age among US Children and Adolescents, 2003–2006," *Journal of the American Medical Association* 299, no. 20 (2008): 2401–5, ncbi.nlm.nih.gov/ pubmed/18505949.

11. U.S. Department of Agriculture. "Dietary Guidelines for Americans," January 31, 2011, cnpp.usda.gov/dietaryguidelines.htm.

12. S. J. Olshansky et al., "A Potential Decline in Life Expectancy in the United States in the 21st Century," *New England Journal of Medicine* 352, no. 11 (2005): 1138–45, nejm.org/doi/full/10.1056/NEJMsr043743#t=article.

13. H. L. Walls et al., "Obesity and Trends in Life Expectancy," *Journal of Obesity* 2012, 107989, hindawi.com/journals/jobe/2012/107989.

14. S. Danielzik et al., "Parental Overweight, Socioeconomic Status and High Birth Weight Are the Major Determinants of Overweight and Obesity in 5–7 Y-Old Children: Baseline Data of the Kiel Obesity Prevention Study (KOPS)," *Int Journal of Obesity and Related Metabolic Disorders* 28, no. 11 (2004): 1494–502, ncbi .nlm.nih.gov/pubmed/15326465.

15. W. S. Agras et al., "Risk Factors for Childhood Overweight: A Prospective Study from Birth to 9.5 Years," *Journal of Pediatrics* 145 (2004): 20–25, ncbi.nlm .nih.gov/pubmed/15238901; K. F. Ferraro et al., "The Life Course of Severe Obesity: Does Childhood Overweight Matter?" *Journals of Gerontology: Series B: Psychological Sciences and Social Sciences* 58 (2003): 110–19, ncbi.nlm.nih.gov /pmc/articles/PMC3358723; M. K. Perdula et al., "Do Obese Children Become Obese Adults? A Review of the Literature," *Preventive Medicine* 22, no. 2 (1993): 167–77, ncbi.nlm.nih.gov/pubmed/8483856; F. M. Biro and M. Wien, "Childhood Obesity and Adult Morbidities," *American Journal of Clinical Nutrition* 91, no. 5 (2010): 1499S–1505S, ncbi.nlm.nih.gov/pubmed/20335542; R. C. Whitaker et al., "Predicting Obesity in Young Adulthood from Childhood and Parental Obesity," *New England Journal of Medicine* 37, no. 13 (1997): 869–73, nejm .org/doi/full/10.1056/NEJM199709253371301.

16. Paul R. Sackett and Anne S. Mavor, eds., *Assessing Fitness for Military Enlistment: Physical, Medical, and Mental Health Standards* (Washington, DC: National Academies Press, 2006), nap.edu/openbook.php?isbn=0309100798.

17. R. R. Pate et al., "Cardiorespiratory Fitness Levels among US Youth 12 to 19 Years of Age: Findings from the 1999–2002 National Health and Nutrition Examination Survey," *Archives of Pediatrics & Adolescent Medicine* 160, no. 10 (2006): 1005–12, ncbi.nlm.nih.gov/pubmed/17018458.

18. R. H. Sanders et al., "Childhood Obesity and Its Physical and Psychological Co-Morbidities: A Systematic Review of Australian Children and Adolescents," *European Journal of Pediatrics* 174, no. 6 (2015): 715–46, ncbi.nlm .nih.gov/pubmed/25922141; M. Rosenbaum, "Special Considerations Relative to Pediatric Obesity," *Endotext*, April 8, 2013, ncbi.nlm.nih.gov/books /NBK279060.

19. Hallie Kaplan, "How Do School Nutrition Policies Contribute to Childhood Obesity and Diabetes?," *Examiner*, April 26, 2011, examiner.com/article/how -do-school-nutrition-policies-contribute-to-childhood-obesity-and-diabetes; Karen Kaplan, "Is the National School Lunch Program to Blame (in Part) for the Rise of Childhood Obesity?," *Los Angeles Times*, April 6, 2011, arti cles.latimes.com/2011/apr/06/news/la-heb-school-lunch-program-obesity -20110406, accessed 6/11/15.

20. H. Vlassara and J. Uribarri, "Advanced Glycation End Products (AGE) and Diabetes: Cause, Effect, Or Both?," *Current Diabetes Reports* 14, no. 1 (2014): 453, ncbi.nlm.nih.gov/pmc/articles/PMC3903318; N. C. Chilelli et al., "AGEs, Rather than Hyperglycemia, Are Responsible for Microvascular Complications in Diabetes: A 'Glycoxidation-Centric' Point of View," *Nutrition, Metabolism, & Cardiovascular Diseases* 23, no. 10 (2013): 913–19, ncbi.nlm.nih.gov/pubmed /23786818.

21. A. Soni, "Use and Expenditures Related to Thyroid Disease among Women Age 18 and Older, U.S. Noninstitutionalized Population, 2008," Agency for Heathcare Research and Quality, U.S. Department of Health & Human Services, Statistical Brief 348, November 2011, meps.ahrq.gov/mepsweb/data _files/publications/st348/stat348.shtml, accessed 6/11/15.

22. N. Nigro and M. Christ-Crain, "Testosterone Treatment in the Aging Male: Myth or Reality?," *Swiss Medical Weekly* 142 (2012): w13539, smw.ch/content /smw-2012-13539.

23. C. Sultan et al., "Environmental Xenoestrogens, Antiandrogens and Disorders of Male Sexual Differentiation," *Molecular and Cellular Endocrinology* 178, no. 1–2 (2001): 99–105, ncbi.nlm.nih.gov/pubmed/11403899; D. Roy et al., "Biochemical and Molecular Changes at the Cellular Level in Response to Exposure to Environmental Estrogen-Like Chemicals," *Journal of Toxicology and Environmental Health* 50, no. 1 (1997): 1–29, ncbi.nlm.nih.gov /pubmed/9015129; D. Teixeira et al., "Inflammatory and Cardiometabolic Risk on Obesity: Role of Environmental Xenoestrogens," *Journal of Clinical Endocrinology & Metabolism* 100, no. 5 (2015): 1792–801, ncbi.nlm.nih .gov/pubmed/25853792; C. S. Watson et al., "Rapid Actions of Xenoestrogens Disrupt Normal Estrogenic Signaling," *Steroids* 81 (2014): 36–42, ncbi .nlm.nih.gov/pmc/articles/PMC3947648; T. J. Walsh et al., "Recent Trends in Testosterone Testing, Low Testosterone Levels, and Testosterone Treatment among Veterans," *Andrology* 3, no. 2 (2015): 287–92, ncbi.nlm.nih.gov /pubmed/25684636.

24. O. Mehrpour et al., "Occupational Exposure to Pesticides and Consequences on Male Semen and Fertility: A Review," *Toxicology Letters* 230, no. 2 (2014): 146–56, ncbi.nlm.nih.gov/pubmed/24487096.

25. M. Carruthers, "Time for International Action on Treating Testosterone Deficiency Syndrome," *Aging Male* 12, no. 1 (2009): 21–28, ncbi.nlm.nih.gov/pmc /articles/PMC2670553; J. Wendlova, "Progression of the Erectile Dysfunction in the Population and the Possibilities of its Regression with Bioregeneration," *Neuroendocrinology Letters* 34, no. 6 (2013): 482–97, ncbi.nlm.nih.gov /pubmed/24378458.

26. J. V. Neel, "Diabetes Mellitus: A 'Thrifty' Genotype Rendered Detrimental by 'Progress'?," Department of Human Genetics, University of Michigan Medical School, Ann Arbor, Mich., ncbi.nlm.nih.gov/pmc/articles/PMC1932342/pdf /ajhg00558-0047.pdf, accessed 8/7/15.

27. E. Ravussin et al., "Effects of a Traditional Lifestyle on Obesity in Pima Indians," *Diabetes Care* 17, no. 9 (1994): 1067–74, ncbi.nlm.nih.gov/pubmed/7988310; L. O. Schulz and L. S. Chaudhari, "High-Risk Populations: The Pimas of Arizona and Mexico," *Current Obesity Reports* 4, no. 1 (2015): 92–98, ncbi.nlm.nih .gov/pubmed/25954599.

28. M. Daniel and D. Gamble, "Diabetes and Canada's Aboriginal Peoples: The Need for Primary Prevention," *International Journal of Nursing Studies* 32, no. 3 (1995): 243–59, ncbi.nlm.nih.gov/pubmed/7665313.

CHAPTER 6: WHAT TO EAT—AND NOT TO EAT:
CHANGE YOUR DIET AND BANISH YOUR PAIN

1. "Guidelines for Avoiding Gluten (Unsafe Ingedients for Gluten Sensitivity)," glutenfreesociety.org/guidelines-for-avoiding-gluten-unsafe-ingredients -for-gluten-sensitivity.

2. "Labeling around the World," Just Label It!, justlabelit.org/right-to-know -center/labeling-around-the-world.

3. D. U. Himmelstein et al., "Medical Bankruptcy in the United States, 2007: Results of a National Study," *American Journal of Medicine* 122, no. 8 (2009): 741–46, amjmed.com/article/S0002-9343(09)00404-5/pdf.

4. S. Gorman et al., "Can Skin Exposure to Sunlight Prevent Liver Inflammation?," *Nutrients* 7, no. 5 (2015): 3219–39, ncbi.nlm.nih.gov/pmc/articles/PMC 4446748.

5. S. Straube et al., "Vitamin D for the Treatment of Chronic Painful Conditions in Adults," *Cochrane Database of Systematic Reviews* 5 (2015): CD007771, ncbi .nlm.nih.gov/pubmed/25946084.

6. U. Gröber et al., "Live Longer with Vitamin D?," *Nutrients* 7, no. 3 (2015): 1871–80, ncbi.nlm.nih.gov/pmc/articles/PMC4377887.

CHAPTER 7: WHICH SUPPLEMENTS HELP ELIMINATE PAIN?
SPEED HEALING BY REPLACING MEDS WITH VITAMINS,
MINERALS, AND OTHER NUTRIENTS

1. Ross Pelton et al., *Drug-Induced Nutrient Depletion Handbook* (Cincinnati: Lexi-Comp, 2001); Daphne A. Roe, *Drug-Induced Nutritional Deficiencies*, 2nd ed. (Westport, CT: AVI Publishing, 1985).

2. Anahad O'Connor, "New York Attorney General Targets Supplements at Major Retailers," "Well" (blog), *New York Times*, February 3, 2015, well.blogs .nytimes.com/2015/02/03/new-york-attorney-general-targets-supplements -at-major-retailers.

3. S. Oancea et al., "Gluten Screening of Several Dietary Supplements by Immunochromatographic Assay," *Roumanian Archives of Microbiology and Immunology* 70, no. 4 (2011): 174–77, ncbi.nlm.nih.gov/pubmed/22568265.

4. S. G. Wannamethee et al., "Associations of Vitamin C Status, Fruit and Vegetable Intakes, and Markers of Inflammation and Hemostasis," *American Journal of Clinical Nutrition* 83, no. 3 (2006): 567–74, ajcn.nutrition.org/content /83/3/567.long; G. Block et al., "Plasma C-Reactive Protein Concentrations in Active and Passive Smokers: Influence of Antioxidant Supplementation," *Journal of the American College of Nutrition* 23, no. 2 (2004): 141–47, ncbi.nlm .nih.gov/pubmed/15047680; C. Antoniades et al., "Vascular Endothelium and Inflammatory Process, in Patients with Combined Type 2 Diabetes Mellitus and Coronary Atherosclerosis: The Effects of Vitamin C," *Diabetic Medicine* 21, no. 6 (2004): 552–58, ncbi.nlm.nih.gov/pubmed/15154938; S. Goya Wannamethee et al., "Associations of Vitamin C Status, Fruit and Vegetable Intakes, and Markers of Inflammation and Hemostasis," *American Journal of*

Clinical Nutrition 83(3) (2006): 567–74, ajcn.nutrition.org/content/83/3/567. full; G. Paolisso et al., "Metabolic Benefits Deriving from Chronic Vitamin C Supplementation in Aged Non-Insulin Dependent Diabetics," *Journal of the American College of Nutrition* 14, no. 4 (1995): 387–92, ncbi.nlm.nih.gov/pub med/8568117.

5. D. Bernardo et al., "Ascorbate-Dependent Decrease of the Mucosal Immune Inflammatory Response to Gliadin in Coeliac Disease Patients," *Allergologia et Immunopathologia* 40, no. 1 (2012): 3–8, ncbi.nlm.nih.gov/pubmed/21420224.

6. Sayer Ji, "Opening Pandora's Bread Box: The Critical Role of Wheat Lectin in Human Disease," GreenMedInfo, greenmedinfo.com/page/opening-pan doras-bread-box-critical-role-wheat-lectin-human-disease, accessed 6/12/15; J. Ohno et al., "Binding of Wheat Germ Agglutinin in the Matrix of Rat Tracheal Cartilage," *Histochemical Journal* 18, no. 10 (1986): 537–40, ncbi.nlm .nih.gov/pubmed/3804790; H. E. Carlsson et al., "The Interaction of Wheat Germ Agglutinin with Keratan from Cornea and Nasal Cartilage," *FEBS* Letters 62, no. 1 (1976), 38–40. febsletters.org/article/0014-5793(76)80011-7 /abstract.

7. "The Cholesterol Myths: The Benefits of High Cholesterol," ravnskov.nu /myth9.htm, accessed 6/16/15.

8. Q. Shu et al., "Antinociceptive Effects of Curcumin in a Rat Model of Postoperative Pain," *Scientific Reports* 4 (2014): 4932, ncbi.nlm.nih.gov/pmc/arti cles/PMC4017214; P. Sahbaie et al., "Curcumin Treatment Attenuates Pain and Enhances Functional Recovery after Incision," *Anesthesia and Analgesia* 118, no. 6 (2014): 1336–44, ncbi.nlm.nih.gov/pubmed/24755847; T. Conrozier et al., "A Complex of Three Natural Anti-Inflammatory Agents Provides Relief of Osteoarthritis Pain," *Alternative Therapies in Health and Medicine* 20, Suppl 1 (2014): 32–37, ncbi.nlm.nih.gov/pubmed/24473984; H. R. Banafshe et al., "Effect of Curcumin on Diabetic Peripheral Neuropathic Pain: Possible Involvement of Opioid System," *European Journal of Pharmacology* 723 (2014): 202–6, ncbi.nlm.nih.gov/pubmed/24315931; Y. Panahi et al., "Antioxidant and Anti-Inflammatory Effects of Curcuminoid-Piperine Combination in Subjects with Metabolic Syndrome: A Randomized Controlled Trial and an Updated Meta-Analysis," *Clinical Nutrition* (epub ahead of print) (2015), pii: S0261-5614(15)00002-3, ncbi.nlm.nih.gov/pubmed/25618800; A. Sahebkar, "Are Curcuminoids Effective C-Reactive Protein-Lowering Agents in Clinical Practice? Evidence from a Meta-Analysis," *Phytotherapy Research* 28, no. 5 (2014): 633–42, ncbi.nlm.nih.gov/pubmed/23922235; Y. Panahi et al., "Adjuvant Therapy with Bioavailability-Boosted Curcuminoids Suppresses Systemic Inflammation and Improves Quality of Life in Patients with Solid Tumors: A Randomized Double-Blind Placebo-Controlled Trial," *Phytotherapy Research* 28, no. 10 (2014): 1461–67, ncbi.nlm.nih.gov/pubmed/24648302; S. Ganjali et al., "Investigation of the Effects of Curcumin on Serum Cytokines in Obese Individuals: A Randomized Controlled Trial," *Scientific World Journal* (2014), 898361, hindawi.com/journals/tswj/2014/898361; S. Kumar et al., "Curcumin for Maintenance of Remission in Ulcerative Colitis," *Cochrane Database of Systematic*

Reviews 10 (2012), CD008424, ncbi.nlm.nih.gov/pmc/articles/PMC4001731; G. C. Jagetia and B. B. Aggarwal, " 'Spicing Up' of the Immune System by Curcumin," *Journal of Clinical Immunology* 27, no. 1 (2007): 19–35, ncbi.nlm.nih.gov /pubmed/17211725.

9. S. K. Totsch et al., "Dietary Influence on Pain via the Immune System," *Progress in Molecular Biology and Translational Science* 131 (2015): 435–69, ncbi.nlm .nih.gov/pubmed/25744682; A. Al-Nahain et al., *"Zingiber officinale*: A Potential Plant against Rheumatoid Arthritis," *Arthritis* (2014): 159089, ncbi.nlm .nih.gov/pmc/articles/PMC4058601; S. M. Zick et al., "Pilot Clinical Study of the Effects of Ginger Root Extract on Eicosanoids in Colonic Mucosa of Subjects at Increased Risk for Colorectal Cancer," *Molecular Carcinogenesis* (2014), ncbi.nlm.nih.gov/pubmed/24760534; K. Jeena et al., "Antioxidant, Anti-Inflammatory and Antinociceptive Activities of Essential Oil from Ginger," *Indian Journal of Physiology and Pharmacology* 57, no. 1 (2013): 51–62, ncbi.nlm .nih.gov/pubmed/24020099.

10. S. You et al., "Inhibitory Effects and Molecular Mechanisms of Garlic Organosulfur Compounds on the Production of Inflammatory Mediators," *Molecular Nutrition & Food Research* 57, no. 11 (2013): 2049–60, ncbi.nlm.nih.gov /pubmed/23766070; C. Chen et al., "Induction of Detoxifying Enzymes by Garlic Organosulfur Compounds through Transcription Factor Nrf2: Effect of Chemical Structure and Stress Signals," *Free Radical Biology and Medicine* 37, no. 10 (2004): 1578–90, ncbi.nlm.nih.gov/pubmed/15477009; Y. J. Choi et al., "Protective Effects of Garlic Extract, PMK-S005, against Nonsteroidal Anti-Inflammatory Drugs-Induced Acute Gastric Damage in Rats," *Digestive Diseases and Sciences* 59, no. 12 (2014): 2927–34, ncbi.nlm.nih.gov/pubmed/25283375; S. Quintero-Fabián et al., "Alliin, a Garlic (*Allium sativum*) Compound, Prevents LPS-Induced Inflammation in 3T3-L1 Adipocytes," *Mediators of Inflammation* (2013), 381815, hindawi.com/journals/mi/2013/381815; J. S. Kwak et al., "Garlic Powder Intake and Cardiovascular Risk Factors: A Meta-Analysis of Randomized Controlled Clinical Trials," *Nutrition Research and Practice* 8, no. 6 (2014): 644–54, e-nrp.org/DOIx.php?id=10.4162/nrp.2014.8.6.644.

11. E. Kowalczyk et al., "Pharmacological Effects of Flavonoids from *Scutellaria baicalensis*," *Przeglad Lekarski* 63, no. 2 (2006): 95–86 (article in Polish), ncbi.nlm .nih.gov/pubmed/16967717; X. Shang et al., "The genus *Scutellaria* an Ethnopharmacological and Phytochemical Review," *Journal of Ethnopharmacology* 128, no. 2 (2010): 279–313, ncbi.nlm.nih.gov/pubmed/20064593; G. X. Shi et al., "New Advance in Studies on Antimicrobal Activity of *Scutellaria baicalensis* and Its Effective Ingredients," *Zhongguo Zhong Yao Za Zhi* 39, no. 19 (2014): 3713–18 (article in Chinese), ncbi.nlm.nih.gov/pubmed/25612426.

12. "Oral Enzyme Therapy in Osteoarthritis of the Knee. Proteolytic Enzyme Are Effective with Few Risks," *MMW Fortschritte der Medizin* 143, no. 23 (2001): 44–46 (article in German), ncbi.nlm.nih.gov/pubmed/11460424; G. Klein and W. Kullich, "Reducing Pain by Oral Enzyme Therapy in Rheumatic Diseases," *Wiener Medizinische Wochenschrift* 149, no. 21–22 (1999): 577–80 (article in German), ncbi.nlm.nih.gov/pubmed/10666820; G. H. Tilwe et al., "Efficacy

and Tolerability of Oral Enzyme Therapy as Compared to Diclofenac in Active
Osteoarthrosis of Knee Joint: An Open Randomized Controlled Clinical Trial,"
Journal of the Association of Physicians of India 49 (2001): 617–21, ncbi.nlm.nih
.gov/pubmed/11584936; G. Klein et al., "Efficacy and Tolerance of an Oral
Enzyme Combination in Painful Osteoarthritis of the Hip. A Double-Blind,
Randomised Study Comparing Oral Enzymes with Non-Steroidal Anti-
Inflammatory Drugs," *Clinical and Experimental Rheumatology* 24, no. 1 (2006):
25–30, ncbi.nlm.nih.gov/pubmed/16539815; H. M. Viswanatha Swamy and
P. A. Patil, "Effect of Some Clinically Used Proteolytic Enzymes on Inflammation in Rats," *Indian Journal of Pharmacological Sciences* 70, no. 1 (2008): 114–17,
ncbi.nlm.nih.gov/pmc/articles/PMC2852049; K. N. Veremeenko, "Use of Proteolytic Enzymes in Surgical Practice. (Review of the Soviet and Foreign Literature):" *Klinichna khirurhiia* 177 (1965): 53–59 (article in Russian), ncbi.nlm
.nih.gov/pubmed/14296999.

13. M. J. Lorenzo Pisarello et al., "Decrease in Lactobacilli in the Intestinal Microbiota of Celiac Children with a Gluten-Free Diet, and Selection of Potentially
Probiotic Strains," *Canadian Journal of Microbiology* 61, no. 1 (2015): 32, nrcre
searchpress.com/doi/abs/10.1139/cjm-2014-0472; L. F. de Sousa Moraes et
al., "Intestinal Microbiota and Probiotics in Celiac Disease," *Clinical Microbiology Reviews* 27, no. 3 (2014): 482–89, cmr.asm.org/content/27/3/482.long;
K. J. Rhee et al., "Role of Commensal Bacteria in Development of Gut-Associ-
ated Lymphoid Tissues and Preimmune Antibody Repertoire," *Journal of Immunology* 172, no. 2 (2004): 1118–24, jimmunol.org/content/172/2/1118.long;
L. Golfetto et al., "Lower Bifidobacteria Counts in Adult Patients with Celiac
Disease on a Gluten-Free Diet," *Arquivos de Gastroenterolgia* 51, no. 2 (2014): 139–
43, scielo.br/scielo.php?script=sci_arttext&pid=S0004-28032014000200139;
T. Pozo-Rubio et al., "Immune Development and Intestinal Microbiota in
Celiac Disease," *Journal of Immunology Research* (2012): 654143, hindawi.com
/journals/jir/2012/654143; Y. Sanz et al., "Unraveling the Ties between Celiac
Disease and Intestinal Microbiota," *International Reviews of Immunology* 30,
no. 4 (2011): 207–18, ncbi.nlm.nih.gov/pubmed/21787226; Y. Sanz, "Effects
of a Gluten-Free Diet on Gut Microbiota and Immune Function in Healthy
Adult Humans," *Gut Microbes* 1, no. 3 (2010): 135–37, tandfonline.com/doi
/abs/10.4161/gmic.1.3.11868; Anahad O'Connor, "Many Probiotics Taken for
Celiac Disease Contain Gluten," "Well" (blog), *New York Times*, May 19, 2015,
well.blogs.nytimes.com/2015/05/19/many-probiotics-taken-for-celiac-dis
ease-contain-gluten.

14. Robert Preidt, "Probiotic Supplements May Contain Traces of Gluten," Health-
Day News, *WebMD*, May 15, 2015, webmd.com/digestive-disorders/news
/20150515/probiotic-supplements-may-contain-traces-of-gluten, accessed 6/12
/15; L. M. Bustos Fernandez et al., "Intestinal Microbiota: Its Role in Digestive Diseases," *Journal of Clinical Gastroenterology* 48, no. 8 (2014): 657–66, ncbi
.nlm.nih.gov/pubmed/24921207.

15. S. Nazareth et al. "Dietary Supplement Use in Patients with Celiac Disease in
the United States," *Journal of Clinical Gastroenterology* 49, no. 7 (2014): 577–81,
ncbi.nlm.nih.gov/pubmed/25203364.

CHAPTER 8: DAYS 1 TO 15: KICK OFF YOUR PLAN BY ELIMINATING ALL GRAINS

1. A. Vojdani and I. Tarash, "Cross-Reaction between Gliadin and Different Food and Tissue Antigens," *Food and Nutrition Sciences* 4, no. 1 (2013): 20–32, scirp .org/Journal/PaperInformation.aspx?paperID=26626.

2. A. Glenn et al., "Fungal and Mycotoxin Contamination of Coffee Beans in Benguet Province, Philippines," *Food Additives & Contaminants: Part A* 32, no. 2 (2015): ncbi.nlm.nih.gov/pubmed/25534333; J. Cui et al., "Oxidative DNA damage Is Involved in Ochratoxin A-Induced G2 Arrest through Ataxia Telangiectasia-Mutated (ATM) Pathways in Human Gastric Epithelium GES-1 Cells in Vitro," *Archives of Toxicology* 87, no. 10 (2013): 1829–40, ncbi .nlm.nih.gov/pubmed/23515941; "Plants Poisonous to Livestock: Aflatoxins: Occurrence and Health Risks," Department of Animal Science, College of Agriculture and Life Sciences, Cornell University, ansci.cornell.edu/plants /toxicagents/aflatoxin/aflatoxin.html; M. E. Zain, "Impact of Mycotoxins on Humans and Animals," *Journal of Saudi Chemical Society* 15, no. 2 (2011): 129–44, sciencedirect.com/science/article/pii/S1319610310000827.

3. R. W. Bretveld et al., "Pesticide Exposure: The Hormonal Function of the Female Reproductive System Disrupted?," *Reproductive Biology and Endocrinology* 4 (2006): 30, biomedcentral.com/content/pdf/1477-7827-4-30.pdf.

4. S. Lohsiriwat et al., "Effect of Caffeine on Lower Esophageal Sphincter Pressure in Thai Healthy Volunteers," *Diseases of the Esophagus* 19, no. 3 (2006): 183–88, ncbi.nlm.nih.gov/pubmed/16722996; C. Hoecker et al., "Caffeine Impairs Cerebral and Intestinal Blood Flow Velocity in Preterm Infants," *Pediatrics* 109, no. 5 (2002): 784–87, ncbi.nlm.nih.gov/pubmed/11986437; Y. S. Cho et al., "Caffeine Enhances Micturition through Neuronal Activation in Micturition Centers," *Molecular Medicine Reports* 10, no. 6 (2014): 2931–36, ncbi.nlm.nih.gov/pubmed/25323389.

5. Z. Ming et al., "Caffeine-Induced Natriuresis and Diuresis via Blockade of Hepatic Adenosine-Mediated Sensory Nerves and a Hepatorenal Reflex," *Canadian Journal of Physiology and Pharmacology* 88, no. 11 (2010): 1115–21, ncbi .nlm.nih.gov/pubmed/21076499; Y. Tajima, "Coffee-induced Hypokalaemia," *Clinical Medicine Insights: Case Reports* 3 (2010): 9–13, la-press.com/coffee-in duced-hypokalaemia-article-a1995-abstract.

6. J. K. Yeh et al., "Influence of Injected Caffeine on the Metabolism of Calcium and the Retention and Excretion of Sodium, Potassium, Phosphorus, Magnesium, Zinc and Copper in Rats," *Journal of Nutrition* 116, no. 2 (1986): 273–80, jn.nutrition.org/content/116/2/273.long.

7. A. Coscia et al., "Cow's Milk Proteins in Human Milk," *Journal of Biological Regulators and Homeostatic Agents* 26, 3 Suppl (2012): 39–42, ncbi.nlm.nih.gov/pub med/23158513.

8. F. Cabrera-Chávez et al., "Bovine Milk Caseins and Transglutaminase-Treated Cereal Prolamins Are Differentially Recognized by IgA of Celiac Disease Patients According to Their Age," *Journal of Agriculture and Food Chemistry* 57, no. 9 (2009): 3754–59, ncbi.nlm.nih.gov/pubmed/19290628; F. Cabrera-

Chávez and A. M. de la Barca, "Bovine Milk Intolerance in Celiac Disease Is Related to IgA Reactivity to Alpha- and Beta-Caseins," *Nutrition* 25, no. 6 (2009): 715–16, ncbi.nlm.nih.gov/pubmed/19268534; G. Kristjánsson et al., "Mucosal Reactivity to Cow's Milk Protein in Coeliac Disease," *Clinical & Experimental Immunology* 147, no. 3 (2007): 449–55, onlinelibrary.wiley.com /doi/10.1111/j.1365-2249.2007.03298.x/full.

9. M. Perkkiö et al., "Morphometric and Immunohistochemical Study of Jejunal Biopsies from Children with Intestinal Soy Allergy," *European Journal of Pediatrics* 137, no. 1 (1981): 63–69, ncbi.nlm.nih.gov/pubmed/7196837.

10. A. Real et al., "Molecular And Immunological Characterization of Gluten Proteins Isolated from Oat Cultivars That Differ in Toxicity for Celiac Disease," *PLoS One* 7, no. 12 (2012): journals.plos.org/plosone/article?id=10.1371 /journal.pone.0048365; P. Fric et al., "Celiac Disease, Gluten-Free Diet, and Oats," *Nutrition Reviews* 69, no. 2 (2011): 107–15, ncbi.nlm.nih.gov/pubmed /21294744.

11. M. Silano et al., "Diversity of Oat Varieties in Eliciting the Early Inflammatory Events in Celiac Disease," *European Journal of Nutrition* 53, no. 5 (2014): 1177–86, ncbi.nlm.nih.gov/pmc/articles/PMC4119590.

12. M. Maglio et al., "Immunogenicity of Two Oat Varieties, in Relation to Their Safety for Celiac Patients," *Scandinavian Journal of Gastroenterology* 46, no. 10 (2011): 1194–205, ncbi.nlm.nih.gov/pubmed/21843037.

13. T. Thompson et al., "Gluten Contamination of Grains, Seeds, and Flours in the United States: A Pilot Study," *Journal of the Academy of Nutrition and Dietetics* 110, no. 6 (2010): 937–40, ncbi.nlm.nih.gov/pubmed/20497786.

14. F. Cabrera-Chávez et al., "Maize Prolamins Resistant to Peptic-Tryptic Digestion Maintain Immune-Recognition by IgA from Some Celiac Disease Patients," *Plant Foods for Human Nutrition* 67, no. 1 (2012): 24, 30, ncbi.nlm.nih.gov/pub med/22298027; J. H. Skerritt et al., "Cellular and Humoral Responses in Coeliac Disease. 2. Protein Extracts from Different Cereals," *Clinica Chimica Acta* 204, no. 1–3 (1991): 109–22, ncbi.nlm.nih.gov/pubmed/1819454.

15. I. W. Davidson et al., "Antibodies to Maize in Patients with Crohn's Disease, Ulcerative Colitis and Coeliac Disease," *Clinical & Experimental Immunology* 35, no. 1 (1979): 147–48, ncbi.nlm.nih.gov/pmc/articles/PMC1537589.

16. F. Cabrera-Chávez et al., "Transglutaminase Treatment of Wheat and Maize Prolamins of Bread Increases the Serum IgA Reactivity of Celiac Disease Patients," *Journal of Agricultural and Food Chemistry* 56, no. 4 (2008): 1387–91, ncbi.nlm.nih.gov/pubmed/18193828.

17. G. Kristjánsson et al., "Gut Mucosal Granulocyte Activation Precedes Nitric Oxide Production: Studies in Coeliac Patients Challenged with Gluten and Corn," *Gut* 54 (2005): 769–74, gut.bmj.com/content/54/6/769.long.

18. Y. Ohtsuka et al., "Reducing Cell Membrane n-6 Fatty Acids Attenuate Mucosal Damage in Food-Sensitive Enteropathy in Mice," *Pediatric Research* 42, no. 6 (1997): 835–39, ncbi.nlm.nih.gov/pubmed/9396566.

19. L. B. Bullerman, "Occurrence of *Fusarium* and Fumonisins on Food Grains and in Foods," *Advances in Experimental Medicine and Biology* 392 (1996): 27–38, ncbi .nlm.nih.gov/pubmed/8850603; G. Sun et al., "Co-Contamination of Aflatoxin B_1 and Fumonisin B_1 in Food and Human Dietary Exposure in Three Areas of China," *Food Additives & Contaminants: Part A* 28, no. 4 (2011): 461–70, ncbi .nlm.nih.gov/pubmed/21259142; P. M. Scott, "Recent Research on Fumonisins: A Review," *Food Additives & Contaminants: Part A* 29, no. 2 (2012): 242–48, ncbi.nlm.nih.gov/pubmed/21337235.

20. C. Dall'Asta et al., "Dietary Exposure to Fumonisins and Evaluation of Nutrient Intake in a Group of Adult Celiac Patients on a Gluten-Free Diet," *Molecular Nutrition & Food Research* 56, no. 4 (2012): 632–40, ncbi.nlm.nih.gov/pubmed /22495987.

21. "Statistics About Diabetes," May 18, 2015, American Diabetes Association, diabetes.org/diabetes-basics/statistics, accessed 6/12/15; "Diabetes," fact sheet no. 312, January 2015, World Health Organization, who.int/mediacen tre/factsheets/fs312/en, accessed 6/12/15.

22. "IDF Diabetes Atlas," 6th ed., International Diabetes Federation, 2014, idf.org /diabetesatlas.

23. E. A. Hu et al., "White Rice Consumption and Risk of Type 2 Diabetes: Meta-Analysis and Systematic Review," *British Medical Journal* (2012): 344:e1454, bmj.com/content/344/bmj.e1454.

24. S. H. Yun et al., "The Association of Carbohydrate Intake, Glycemic Load, Glycemic Index, and Selected Rice Foods with Breast Cancer Risk: A Case-Control Study in South Korea," *Asia Pacific Journal of Clinical Nutrition* 19 (2010): 383–92, apjcn.nhri.org.tw/server/APJCN/19/3/383.pdf.

25. I. Hojsak et al., "Arsenic in Rice: a Cause for Concern," *Journal of Pediatric Gastroenterology and Nutrition* 60, no. 1 (2015): 142–45, ncbi.nlm.nih.gov/pub med/25536328; B. P. Jackson et al., "Arsenic Concentration and Speciation in Infant Formulas and First Foods," *Pure and Applied Chemistry* 84, no. 2 (2012): 215–23, ncbi.nlm.nih.gov/pmc/articles/PMC3371583; S. Munera-Picazo et al., "Inorganic and Total Arsenic Contents in Rice-Based Foods for Children with Celiac Disease," *Journal of Food Science* 79, no. 1 (2014): T122–28, ncbi.nlm.nih .gov/pubmed/24313911.

26. M. Kaneta et al., "Chemical Form of Cadmium (and Other Heavy Metals) in Rice and Wheat Plants," *Environmental Health Perspectives* 65 (1986): 33–37, ncbi.nlm.nih.gov/pmc/articles/PMC1474683; M. C. Jung and I. Thornton, "Environmental Contamination and Seasonal Variation of Metals in Soils, Plants and Waters in the Paddy Fields around a Pb-Zn Mine in Korea," *Science of the Total Environment* 198, no. 2 (1997): 105–21, ncbi.nlm.nih.gov/pub med/9167264; C. Xu, "Speciation and Bioavailability of Heavy Metals in Paddy Soil Irrigated by Acid Mine Drainage," *Huan Jing Ke Xue* 30, no. 3 (2009): 900–906 (article in Chinese), ncbi.nlm.nih.gov/pubmed/19432348.

27. L. Caminiti et al., "Food Protein Induced Enterocolitis Syndrome Caused by Rice Beverage," *Italian Journal of Pediatrics* 39 (2013): 31, ncbi.nlm.nih.gov

/pmc/articles/PMC3667091; I. Hojsak et al., "Rice Protein-Induced Enterocolitis Syndrome," *Clinical Nutrition* 25, no. 3 (2006): 533–36, ncbi.nlm.nih.
gov/pubmed/16697497; A. Nowak-Węgrzyn, "Food Protein-Induced Enterocolitis Syndrome and Allergic Proctocolitis," *Allergy and Asthma Proceedings*
36, no. 3 (2015): 172–84, ncbi.nlm.nih.gov/pmc/articles/PMC4405595;
A. Nowak-Węgrzyn et al., "Non-IgE-Mediated Gastrointestinal Food Allergy,"
Journal of Allergy and Clinical Immunology 135, no. 5 (2015): 1114–24, ncbi.nlm
.nih.gov/pubmed/25956013; M. A. Ruffner et al., "Food Protein-Induced
Enterocolitis Syndrome: Insights from Review of a Large Referral Population,"
Journal of Allergy and Clinical Immunology: In Practice 1, no. 4 (2013): 343–49,
ncbi.nlm.nih.gov/pubmed/24565539.

28. V. F. Zevallos et al., "Variable Activation of Immune Response by Quinoa (*Che-
nopodium quinoa Willd.*) Prolamins in Celiac Disease," *American Journal of Clinical
Nutrition* 6, no. 2 (2012): 337–44, ajcn.nutrition.org/content/96/2/337.long.

29. P. Collin et al., "The Safe Threshold for Gluten Contamination in Gluten-
Free Products. Can Trace Amounts Be Accepted in the Treatment of Coeliac
Disease?," *Alimentary Pharmacology & Therapeutics* 19, no. 12 (2004): 1277–83,
onlinelibrary.wiley.com/doi/10.1111/j.1365-2036.2004.01961.x/full; A. D. Cor-
rea et al., "Chemical Constituents, in Vitro Protein Digestibility, and Presence
of Antinutritional Substances in Amaranth Grains," *Archivos Latinoamericanos de
Nutrición* 36, no. 2 (1986): 319–26, ncbi.nlm.nih.gov/pubmed/3632210; T. B.
Koerner et al., "Gluten Contamination of Naturally Gluten-Free Flours and
Starches Used by Canadians with Celiac Disease," *Food Additives & Contaminants: Part A* 30, no. 12 (2013): 2017–21, ncbi.nlm.nih.gov/pubmed/24124879.

30. T. Thompson et al. "Gluten Contamination of Grains, Seeds, and Flours in the
United States: A Pilot Study," *Journal of the Academy of Nutrition and Dietetics*
110, no. 6 (2010): 937–40, ncbi.nlm.nih.gov/pubmed/20497786.

CHAPTER 9: DAYS 16 TO 30:
BANISH THE LAST OF YOUR PAIN IN THE CHALLENGE PHASE

1. I. Marković et al., "Gluten-Sensitive Enteropathy: A Disease to Take into
Consideration—A Case Report," *Reumatizam* 60, no. 1 (2013): 32–36 (article
in Croatian), ncbi.nlm.nih.gov/pubmed/24003682.

2. B. Patel et al., "Potato Glycoalkaloids Adversely Affect Intestinal Permeability and Aggravate Inflammatory Bowel Disease," *Inflammatory Bowel Diseases*
8, no. 5 (2002): 340–46, ncbi.nlm.nih.gov/pubmed/12479649; V. Iablokov
et al., "Naturally Occurring Glycoalkaloids in Potatoes Aggravate Intestinal
Inflammation in Two Mouse Models of Inflammatory Bowel Disease," *Digestive Diseases and Sciences* 55, no. 11 (2010): 3078–85, ncbi.nlm.nih.gov/pub
med/20198430; P. Robertson and P. Roberts, "The Solanaceae and Their Para-
doxical Effects on Arthritis and Other Degenerative Disease States," *Australian
Journal of Medical Herbalism* 15, no. 4 (2003): 114, search.informit.com.au/docu
mentSummary;dn=407770610818604;res=IELHEA; N. F. Childers and M. S.
Margoles, "An Apparent Relation of Nightshades (Solanaceae) to Arthritis,"
Journal of Neurological and Orthopedic Medical Surgery 12 (1993): 227–31, noarthri

tis.com/research.htm; Norman F. Childers and Gerald M. Russo, *Nightshades and Health* (New Brunswick, NJ: Norman F. Childers, 1977); *Arthritis: Childers' Diet to Stop It! The Nightshades, Ill Health, Aging, and Shorter Life,* 4th ed. (New Brunswick, NJ: Norman F. Childers, 1993): 19–21; T. Kuiper-Goodman and P. S. Nawrot, "Solanine and Chaconine," unpublished first draft, n.d., Bureau of Chemical Safety, Health and Welfare Canada, inchem.org/documents/jecfa /jecmono/v30je19.htm; G. Smith, "Nightshades: Problems from These Popular Foods Exposed to the Light of Day," Health Topics, Weston A. Price Foundation, March 30, 2010, westonaprice.org/health-topics/nightshades.

3. R. F. Hurrell, "Influence of Vegetable Protein Sources on Trace Element and Mineral Bioavailability," *Journal of Nutrition* 133, no. 9 (2003): 2973S-77S, jn.nutrition.org/content/133/9/2973S.long; N. Roos et al., "Screening for Anti-Nutritional Compounds in Complementary Foods and Food Aid Products for Infants and Young Children," *Maternal & Child Nutrition* 9 (Suppl 1) (2013): 47–71, ncbi.nlm.nih.gov/pubmed/23167584; R. S. Gibson et al., "A Review of Phytate, Iron, Zinc, and Calcium Concentrations in Plant-Based Complementary Foods Used in Low-Income Countries and Implications for Bioavailability," *Food and Nutrition Bulletin* 31, 2 Suppl (2010): S134–46, ncbi.nlm.nih .gov/pubmed/20715598.

4. J. W. Dorner, "Management and Prevention of Mycotoxins in Peanuts," *Food Additives & Contaminants: Part A* 25, no. 2 (2008): 203–8, ncbi.nlm.nih.gov/pub med/18286410.

5. Loren Cordain, *The Paleo Answer: 7 Days to Lose Weight, Feel Great, Stay Young* (Hoboken, NJ: John Wiley & Sons, 2012).

6. Mark Sisson, "Nuts and Phytic Acid. Should You Be Concerned?," Mark's Daily Apple, May 16, 2012, marksdailyapple.com/nuts-and-phytic-acid/#axzz 3ajIZkF4L, accessed 6/12/15.

7. K. L. Stanhope et al., "Adverse Metabolic Effects of Dietary Fructose: Results from the Recent Epidemiological, Clinical, and Mechanistic Studies," *Current Opinion in Lipidology* 24, no. 3 (2013): 198–206, ncbi.nlm.nih.gov/pmc/articles /PMC4251462; G. A. Bray, "Energy and Fructose from Beverages Sweetened with Sugar or High-Fructose Corn Syrup Pose a Health Risk for Some People," *Advances in Nutrition* 4 (2013): 220–25, advances.nutrition.org/content /4/2/220.full.

8. M. B. Vos and J. E. Levine, "Dietary Fructose in Nonalcoholic Fatty Liver Disease," *Hepatology* 57, no. 6 (2013): 2525–31, ncbi.nlm.nih.gov/pubmed /23390127; M. Basaranoglu et al., "Fructose as a Key Player in the Development of Fatty Liver Disease," *World Journal of Gastroenterology* 19, no. 8 (2013): 1166–72, wjgnet.com/1007-9327/full/v19/i8/1166.htm; J. J. DiNicolantonio, "Added Fructose: A Principal Driver of Type 2 Diabetes Mellitus and its Consequences," *Mayo Clinic Proceedings* 90, no. 3 (2015): 372–81, ncbi.nlm.nih.gov /pubmed/25639270; M. Saygin et al., "The Impact of High Fructose on Cardiovascular System: Role of α-lipoic Acid," *Human and Experimental Toxicology* (epub ahead of print) (2015): pii: 0960327115579431, het.sagepub.com /content/early/2015/03/27/0960327115579431.full.pdf

9. G. A. Bray, "Energy and Fructose from Beverages Sweetened with Sugar or High-Fructose Corn Syrup Pose a Health Risk for Some People," *Advances in Nutrition* 4, no. 2 (2013): 220–25, advances.nutrition.org/content/4/2/220 .long; C. M. Brown et al., "Sugary Drinks in the Pathogenesis of Obesity and Cardiovascular Diseases," *International Journal of Obesity* 32, Suppl 6 (2008): S28–34, ncbi.nlm.nih.gov/pubmed/19079277; B. Charrez et al., "The Role of Fructose in Metabolism and Cancer," *Hormone Molecular Biology and Clinical Investigation* 22, no. 2 (2015): 79–89, ncbi.nlm.nih.gov/pubmed/25965509.

10. L. Fontana and L. Partridge, "Promoting Health and Longevity through Diet: From Model Organisms to Humans," *Cell* 161, no. 1 (2015): 106–18, ncbi.nlm .nih.gov/pubmed/25815989.

11. A. Michalsen and C. Li, "Fasting Therapy for Treating and Preventing Disease— Current State of Evidence," *Forschende Komplementärmedizin* 20, no. 6 (2013): 444–53, ncbi.nlm.nih.gov/pubmed/24434759; A. Michalsen et al., "The Short-Term Effects of Fasting on the Neuroendocrine System in Patients with Chronic Pain Syndromes," *Nutritional Neuroscience* 6, no. 1 (2003): 11–18, ncbi.nlm.nih .gov/pubmed/12608732; F. Wilhemi de Toledo et al., "Fasting Therapy—An Expert Panel Update of the 2002 Consensus Guidelines," *Forschende Komplementärmedizin* 20, no. 6 (2013): 434–43, karger.com/Article/FullText/357602; C. Li et al., "Metabolic and Psychological Response to 7-Day Fasting in Obese Patients with and Without Metabolic Syndrome," *Forschende Komplementärmedizin* 20, no. 6 (2013): 413–20, karger.com/?DOI=10.1159/000353672; H. Müller et al., "Fasting Followed by Vegetarian Diet in Patients with Rheumatoid Arthritis: A Systematic Review," *Scandinavian Journal of Rheumatology* 30, no. 1 (2001): 1–10, ncbi.nlm.nih.gov/pubmed/11252685.

CHAPTER 10: BEYOND FOOD: HOW TO MINIMIZE DAMAGE FROM TOXINS THAT CAN COMPOUND THE EFFECTS OF GRAIN

1. K. F. Csáki, "Synthetic Surfactant Food Additives Can Cause Intestinal Barrier Dysfunction," *Medical Hypotheses* 76, no. 5 (2011): 676–81, ncbi.nlm.nih.gov/ pubmed/21300443; A. Lerner and T. Matthias, "Changes in Intestinal Tight Junction Permeability Associated with Industrial Food Additives Explain the Rising Incidence of Autoimmune Disease," *Autoimmunity Reviews* 14, no. 6 (2015): 479–89, sciencedirect.com/science/article/pii/S1568997215000245; L. Vasiluk et al., "Oral Bioavailability of Glyphosate: Studies Using Two Intestinal Cell Lines," *Environmental Toxicology and Chemistry* 24, no. 1 (2005): 153–60, ncbi.nlm.nih.gov/pubmed/15683179; H. Isoda et al., "Effects of Organophosphorous Pesticides Used in China on Various Mammalian Cells," *Environmental Sciences* 12, no. 1 (2005): 9–19, ncbi.nlm.nih.gov/pubmed/15793557; A. Samsel and S. Seneff, "Glyphosate, Pathways to Modern Diseases II: Celiac Sprue and Gluten Intolerance," *Interdisciplinary Toxicology* 6, no. 4 (2013): 159–84, ncbi.nlm.nih.gov/pmc/articles/PMC3945755; V. Braniste et al., "Impact of Oral Bisphenol A at Reference Doses on Intestinal Barrier Function and Sex Differences after Perinatal Exposure in Rats," *Proceedings of the National Academy of Sciences* 107, no. 1 (2010): 448–53, ncbi.nlm.nih.gov/pmc/articles/PMC 2806743; J. Visser et al., "Tight Junctions, Intestinal Permeability, and Auto-

immunity: Celiac Disease and Type 1 Diabetes Paradigms," *Annals of the New York Academy of Sciences* 1165 (2009): 195–205, ncbi.nlm.nih.gov/pmc/articles/PMC2886850.

2. R. Dufault et al., "Mercury from Chlor-Alkali Plants: Measured Concentrations in Food Product Sugar," *Environmental Health* 8 (2009): 2, ehjournal.net/content/8/1/2; R. Dufault et al., "Mercury Exposure, Nutritional Deficiencies and Metabolic Disruptions May Affect Learning in Children," *Behavioral and Brain Functions* 5 (2009): 44, behavioralandbrainfunctions.com/content/5/1/44.

3. M. Valko et al., "Metals, Toxicity and Oxidative Stress," *Current Medical Chemistry* 12, no. 10 (2005): 1161–208, ncbi.nlm.nih.gov/pubmed/15892631.

4. H. I. Afridi et al., "Estimation of Toxic Elements in the Samples of Different Cigarettes and Their Effect on the Essential Elemental Status in the Biological Samples of Irish Smoker Rheumatoid Arthritis Consumers," *Environmental Monitoring and Assessment* 187, no. 4 (2015): 157, ncbi.nlm.nih.gov/pubmed/25736830; M. Abdulla and J. Chmielnicka, "New Aspects on the Distribution and Metabolism of Essential Trace Elements after Dietary Exposure to Toxic Metals," *Biological Trace Element Research* 23 (1989–1990): 25–53, ncbi.nlm.nih.gov/pubmed/2484425; O. A. Levander, "Metabolic Interactions between Metals and Metalloids," *Environmental Health Perspectives* 25 (1978): 77–80, ncbi.nlm.nih.gov/pmc/articles/PMC1637173/; B. A. Chowdhury and R. K. Chandra, "Biological and Health Implications of Toxic Heavy Metal and Essential Trace Element Interactions," *Progress in Food & Nutrition Science* 11, no. 1 (1987): 55–113, ncbi.nlm.nih.gov/pubmed/3303135.

5. B. Sharma et al., "Biomedical Implications of Heavy Metals Induced Imbalances in Redox Systems," *Biomedical Research International* (2014), 640754, hindawi.com/journals/bmri/2014/640754.

6. B. S. Gillis et al., "Analysis of Lead Toxicity in Human Cells," *BMC Genomics* 13 (2012): 344, biomedcentral.com/1471-2164/13/344; Agency for Toxic Substances and Disease Registry, "Lead Toxicity: What is the Biological Fate of Lead?," Centers for Disease Control and Prevention, Department of Health and Human Services, August 20, 2007, atsdr.cdc.gov/csem/csem.asp?csem=7&po=9, accessed 6/13/15.

7. Y. C. Hong et al., "Postnatal Growth Following Prenatal Lead Exposure and Calcium Intake," *Pediatrics* 134, no. 6 (2014): 1151–59, ncbi.nlm.nih.gov/pubmed/25422017; C. M. Taylor et al., "Adverse Effects of Maternal Lead Levels on Birth Outcomes in the ALSPAC Study: A Prospective Birth Cohort Study," *British Journal of Obstetrics and Gynaecology* 122, no. 3 (2015): 322–28, onlinelibrary.wiley.com/doi/10.1111/1471-0528.12756/full.

8. State of Connecticut Department of Public Health, "Consumer Products Safety Commission Recalls," ct.gov/dph/cwp/view.asp?a=3140&q=387514, accessed 6/13/15.

9. P. Suksabye et al., "Effect of Biochars and Microorganisms on Cadmium Accumulation in Rice Grains Grown in Cd-Contaminated Soil," *Environmental Science and Pollution Research* (epub ahead of print) (2015), ncbi.nlm.nih.gov/pub

med/25943511; M. A. Davis et al., "A Dietary-Wide Association Study (DWAS) of Environmental Metal Exposure in US Children and Adults," *PLoS One* 9, no. 9 (2014): e104768, journals.plos.org/plosone/article?id=10.1371/journal .pone.0104768.

10. A. Chen et al., "Thyroid Hormones in Relation to Lead, Mercury, and Cadmium Exposure in the National Health and Nutrition Examination Survey, 2007–2008," *Environmental Health Perspectives* 121, no. 2 (2013): 181–86, ehp .niehs.nih.gov/1205239.

11. R. Nath et al., "Molecular Basis of Cadmium Toxicity," *Progress in Food & Nutrition Science* 8, no. 1–2 (1984): 109–63, ncbi.nlm.nih.gov/pubmed/6385135; L. Järup, "Hazards of Heavy Metal Contamination," *British Medical Bulletin* 68 (2003):167–82, bmb.oxfordjournals.org/content/68/1/167.long.

12. S. Kapaj et al., "Human Health Effects from Chronic Arsenic Poisoning—A Review," *Journal of Environmental Science and Health, Part A: Toxic/Hazardous Substances and Environmental Engineering* 41, no. 10 (2006): 2399–428, ncbi.nlm.nih .gov/pubmed/17018421.

13. M. S. Rahman et al., "Bisphenol-A Affects Male Fertility via Fertility-Related Proteins in Spermatozoa," *Scientific Reports* 5 (2015): 9169, ncbi.nlm.nih.gov /pmc/articles/PMC4360475; H. A. Jeng, "Exposure to Endocrine Disrupting Chemicals and Male Reproductive Health," *Front Public Health* 2 (2014): 55, ncbi.nlm.nih.gov/pmc/articles/PMC4046332.

14. V. Braniste et al., "Impact of Oral Bisphenol A at Reference Doses on Intestinal Barrier Function and Sex Differences after Perinatal Exposure in Rats," *Proceedings of the National Academy of Sciences* 107, no. 1 (2010): 448–53, pnas.org/con tent/107/1/448.full.

15. K. H. Al-Gubory, "Environmental Pollutants and Lifestyle Factors Induce Oxidative Stress and Poor Prenatal Development," *Reproductive Biomedicine Online* 29, no. 1 (2014): 17–31, ncbi.nlm.nih.gov/pubmed/24813750; F. Rancière et al., "Bisphenol A and the Risk of Cardiometabolic Disorders: A Systematic Review with Meta-Analysis of the Epidemiological Evidence," *Environmental Health* 14, no. 1 (2015): 46, ehjournal.net/content/14/1/46; W. Holtcamp, "Obesogens: An Environmental Link to Obesity," *Environmental Health Perspectives* 120, no. 2 (2012): a62–a68, ncbi.nlm.nih.gov/pmc/articles/PMC3279464.

16. M. de Bastos et al., "Combined Oral Contraceptives: Venous Thrombosis," *Cochrane Database of Systematic Reviews* 3 (2014), CD010813, ncbi.nlm.nih.gov /pubmed/24590565.

17. T. B. Hayes et al., "Atrazine Induces Complete Feminization and Chemical Castration in Male African Clawed Frogs (*Xenopus laevis*)," *Proceedings of the National Academy of Sciences* 107, no. 10 (2010): 4612–17, pnas.org/content /107/10/4612.full.pdf.

18. A. Samsel and S. Seneff, "Glyphosate, Pathways to Modern Diseases II: Celiac Sprue and Gluten Intolerance," *Interdisciplinary Toxicology* 6, no. 4 (2013): 159–84, ncbi.nlm.nih.gov/pmc/articles/PMC3945755.

19. W. Holtcamp, "Obesogens: An Environmental Link to Obesity," *Environmental Health Perspectives* 120, no. 2 (2012): a62, ncbi.nlm.nih.gov/pmc/articles/PMC 3279464.

20. A. P. Pereira-Fernandes et al., "Evaluation of a Screening System for Obesogenic Compounds: Screening of Endocrine Disrupting Compounds and Evaluation of the PPAR Dependency of the Effect," *PLoS One* 8, no. 10 (2013): e77481, ncbi.nlm.nih.gov/pmc/articles/PMC3796469.

21. G. Spinucci et al., "Endogenous Ethanol Production in a Patient with Chronic Intestinal Pseudo-Obstruction and Small Intestinal Bacterial Overgrowth," *European Journal of Gastroenterology & Hepatology* 18, no. 7 (2006): 799–802, ncbi.nlm.nih.gov/pubmed/16772842.

22. Y. M. Shevchuk and J. M. Conly, "Antibiotic-Associated Hypoprothrombinemia: A Review of Prospective Studies, 1966–1988," *Clinical Infectious Diseases* 12, no. 6 (1990): 1109–26, ncbi.nlm.nih.gov/pubmed/2267487; S. Kikuchi et al., "Acquired Coagulopathy Caused by Administration of Parenteral Broad-Spectrum Antibiotics," *Rinsho Byori* 39, no. 1 (1991): 83–90 (article in Japanese), ncbi.nlm.nih.gov/pubmed/1901116.

23. J. Zempleni et al., "Biotin and Biotinidase Deficiency," *Expert Review of Endocrinology and Metabolism* 3, no. 6 (2008): 715–24, ncbi.nlm.nih.gov/pmc/articles /PMC2726758.

24. "CMS Releases Prescriber-Level Medicare Data for First Time," Centers for Medicare & Medicaid Services, April 30, 2015, cms.gov/Newsroom/Media ReleaseDatabase/Fact-sheets/2015-Fact-sheets-items/2015-04-30.html, accessed 6/13/15.

25. D. A. Gorard et al., "Effect of a Tricyclic Antidepressant on Small Intestinal Motility in Health and Diarrhea-Predominant Irritable Bowel Syndrome," *Digestive Diseases and Sciences*, 40, no. 1 (1995): 86–95, link.springer.com/arti cle/10.1007/BF02063948; J. L. Jackson et al., "Treatment of Functional Gastrointestinal Disorders with Antidepressant Medications: A Meta-Analysis," *American Journal of Medicine* 108, no. 1 (2000): 65–72, sciencedirect.com/sci ence/article/pii/S0002934399002995.

26. C. A. Heyneman, "Zinc Deficiency and Taste Disorders," *Annals of Pharmacotherapy* 30, no. 2 (1996): 186–87, ncbi.nlm.nih.gov/pubmed/8835055.

27. Sayer Ji, "Mycotoxins: The Hidden Hormone Danger in Our Food Supply," GreenMedInfo, December 2, 2012, greenmedinfo.com/blog/mycotoxins-hid den-hormone-danger-our-food-supply, accessed 6/13/15.

28. F. Berthiller et al., "Masked Mycotoxins: A Review," *Molecular Nutrition & Food Research* 57, no. 1 (2013): 165–86, ncbi.nlm.nih.gov/pmc/articles/PMC 3561696; S. Marin et al., "Mycotoxins: Occurrence, Toxicology, and Exposure Assessment," *Food and Chemical Toxicology* 60 (2013): 218–37, ncbi.nlm .nih.gov/pubmed/23907020; "Overview of IAQ," Indoor Air Quality Scientific Findings Resource Bank, Lawrence Berkeley National Laboratory, iaqscience .lbl.gov/overview.html, accessed 6/13/15.

29. "Care for Your Air: A Guide to Indoor Air Quality," April 4, 2013, Environmental Protection Agency, epa.gov/iaq/pubs/careforyourair.html, accessed 6/13/15.

30. "Facts on Air," Canadian Water Filter, 2009, canadianwaterfilter.com/Facts_on_air.htm, accessed 6/13/15.

31. "FDA Taking Closer Look at 'Antibacterial' Soap," Food and Drug Administration, December 16, 2013, fda.gov/ForConsumers/ConsumerUpdates/ucm 378393.htm, accessed 6/13/15.

32. B. M. Kuehn, "Triclosan Concerns," *Journal of the American Medical Association* 303, no. 20 (2010): 2022, jama.jamanetwork.com/article.aspx?articleid =185932.

33. H. Okada et al., "The 'Hygiene Hypothesis' for Autoimmune and Allergic Diseases: An Update," *Clinical & Experimental Immunology* 160, no. 1 (2010): 1–9, ncbi.nlm.nih.gov/pmc/articles/PMC2841828.

CHAPTER 11: BEYOND SELF-HELP:
FUNCTIONAL MEDICINE IS THE FUTURE OF MEDICINE

1. R. N. Moynihan et al., "Expanding Disease Definitions in Guidelines and Expert Panel Ties to Industry: A Cross-sectional Study of Common Conditions in the United States," *PLoS Medicine* 10, no. 8 (2013): e1001500, journals.plos .org/plosmedicine/article?id=10.1371/journal.pmed.1001500; Jerome P. Kassirer, "Why Should We Swallow What These Studies Say?," *Washington Post*, August 1, 2004, B03, washingtonpost.com/wp-dyn/articles/A29456-2004Jul 31.html.

2. G. Jones and A. Barker, "Reference Intervals," *Clinical Biochemist Reviews* 29, Suppl 1 (2008): S93–S97, ncbi.nlm.nih.gov/pmc/articles/PMC2556592.

3. Roger Williams, *Biochemical Individuality* (New Canaan, CT: Keats Publishing, 1956).

4. "Clinical Solutions for Advanced Health and Wellness," SpectraCell Laboratories, spectracell.com/about-spectracell/about-our-lab.

5. Avik Roy, "Why the American Medical Association Had 72 Million Reasons to Shrink Doctors' Pay," *Forbes*, November 28, 2011, forbes.com/sites/theapothe cary/2011/11/28/why-the-american-medical-association-had-72-million-rea sons-to-help-shrink-doctors-pay.

6. D. J. Frantz et al., "Current Perception of Nutrition Education in U.S. Medical Schools," *Current Gastroenterology Reports* 13, no. 4 (2011): 376–79, ncbi.nlm .nih.gov/pubmed/21597916; K. M. Adams et al., "Nutrition Education in U.S. Medical Schools: Latest Update of a National Survey," *Academic Medicine* 85, no. 9 (2010): 1537–42, ncbi.nlm.nih.gov/pmc/articles/PMC4042309.

GLOSSARY

ACE inhibitors. A group of drugs that blocks or slows the action of certain enzymes by dilating blood vessels, thereby reducing blood pressure.

Acid reflux. Tightness in the chest and burning in the stomach or throat area, and indigestion; also known as heartburn.

Aflatoxin. A form of mold found in corn, peanuts, and other plants that has been linked to a greater risk for cancer, hepatitis B, and other diseases.

AGEs. An acronym for advanced glycation end products, formed when blood sugar binds with proteins, making cells more likely to age prematurely.

Allergy. An immune response to a food or another factor that produces excessive inflammation.

Analgesic. A medication such as acetaminophen that blocks pain but doesn't address inflammation.

Antibody. A chemical the body produces as an immune system response to a toxin or other substance.

Antibody response. A chemical reaction to a provoking agent, such as wheat or another grain.

Antinutrients. Chemicals in certain foods, including grains and legumes, that block the body's absorption of nutrients in other foods.

ATIs. An acronym for amylase trypsin inhibitors, proteins that are natural pesticides found in seeds that dissuade predators from eating a food; ATIs impede digestion and cause inflammation and gut pain.

Atrazine. One of the most common herbicides used on conventionally grown GMO corn, wheat, soy, and other crops; a known hormone disruptor.

Autoimmune disease. Any condition resulting from chronic inflammation that causes the immune system to go rogue and attack the body.

Bacteroidetes. One form of "good" gut bacteria.

Basal metabolism. The rate at which the body burns calories (energy) even at rest; also known as resting metabolism.

Bioaccumulation. Buildup of heavy metals or other toxins in the body over years, as opposed to recent exposure.

Blood-brain barrier. A protective "wall" designed to keep blood from leaking into the brain, causing all sorts of problems. Certain foods, including grains, can weaken the walls of the capillaries in the brain that comprise this barrier.

Blood glucose. The amount of sugar in the bloodstream, which is transported to cells for use as energy; also known as blood sugar.

BMI (body-mass index). A rough gauge of underweight, normal weight, overweight, and obesity based on the ratio of weight to height, although since it does not distinguish between body fat and muscle, it is inexact.

BPA (bisphenol). A phthalate, a petrochemical found in plastics, that mimics estrogen and has been linked to cancer, intestinal permeability, and obesity.

BROW. An acronym for barley, rye, oats, and wheat, the four "classic" gluten grains.

Carbohydrate. One of the three macronutrients in foods; effectively, anything not fat or protein is considered carbohydrate.

Casein. A protein found in milk.

Catabolism. The breakdown of muscle, bone, and other tissues.

Celiac disease. An autoimmune disease characterized by the inability to absorb nutrients as a result of intestinal damage caused by consuming gluten-containing foods; once considered the only form of gluten sensitivity.

Collagen. The protein used to make muscles, tendons, ligaments, cartilage, and joints.

Cortisol. A hormone made by the adrenal glands that downregulates inflammation.

COX inhibitors. A class of drugs used to treat inflammation from autoimmune conditions by blocking the production of enzymes known as COX-1 and COX-2.

Dysbiosis. A bacterial imbalance or overgrowth that can cause the immune system to attack the body.

Environmental medicine. A field of practice that deals with the health implications of exposure to provoking agents in air, food, water, drugs, furnishings, buildings, etc.

Enzyme. A protein that can produce biochemical changes in the body.

Esophagus. The tube that leads from the throat to the stomach.

Estrogen dominance. Hormonal imbalance in men or women, which can be caused by exposure to estrogen mimics such as grain, environmental toxins, and certain medications.

Firmicutes. A form of gut bacteria.

Functional medicine. The practice of medicine that involves the patient as a partner with the doctor and focuses on identifying the *causes* of disease rather than simply treating the symptoms.

Folate. A B vitamin that helps make the components of energy and enables the formation of cartilage essential for joint integrity.

Food Guide Pyramid. A graphic representation used until 2011 meant to explain how much of certain foods supposedly made up a healthy diet.

Frood. My word for junk food devoid of nutrients.

GALT. The acronym for gastro-associated lymphoid tissue, the first line of defense in the gut wall, comprising a significant portion of the immune system.

Genetically modified organism (GMO). An animal or plant that has had a gene or genes inserted into its DNA to produce certain desirable features.

Genetic testing. A mouth swab test to ascertain whether a person has a genetic predisposition to develop certain diseases under certain circumstances.

GERD. The acronym for gastroesophageal reflux disease, the backup of stomach acid and stomach contents into the esophagus when the sphincter between them relaxes.

Ghrelin. The hunger hormone.

Gluten. A storage protein found in all grains.

Gluten-free whiplash. The return of pain and inflammation after eliminating "traditional" gluten sources (barley, rye, oats, and wheat) from the diet and replacing them with "gluten-free" products made with other grains.

Gluten intolerance. Difficulty in digesting grain due to insufficient enzymes, producing bloating and pain.

Glutenology. My term for the study of grains and our reactions to them.

Gluten sensitivity. A combination of an allergic reaction to and an intolerance of gluten.

Glycation. The process in which blood glucose bonds to protein, producing AGEs.

Glycemic index (GI). A measure of how quickly a carb food converts to glucose in the body.

Glyphosate. The chemical in the pesticide Roundup used by conventional growers of GMO corn, sorghum, and sugarcane; a hormone disruptor.

GMO. See **Genetically modified organism.**

Grainbesity. My name for grain-induced obesity.

Grainflammation. My name for grain-induced inflammation.

Hashimoto's disease. An autoimmune disease characterized by an underactive thyroid gland.

Hemoglobin. A protein in the blood that carries oxygen to cells.

H. pylori. The abbreviation for *Helicobacter pylori*, a bacterium that can pierce the mucosal wall of the GI tract

High-fructose corn syrup (HFCS). A manufactured sugar made from cornstarch that is sweeter and higher in fructose than sugar; linked to the rise in obesity and diabetes.

High-intensity interval training (HIIT). A form of exercise that alternates extremely intense activity and short periods of rest, producing results comparable to longer periods of less intense activity.

Homocysteine. A marker for inflammation associated with heart disease.

Hormone disruptors. Substances that mimic the effects of natural hormones, interfering with their balance.

Humoral immune system. The individualized portion of the immune system adapted to produce specific antibodies.

Hypothalmus. The part of the brain that controls the autonomous nervous system, which regulates sleep, digestion, blood pressure, and other such processes.

Hypothyroidism. See **Hashimoto's disease.**

Immunoglobulin. An antibody used by the immune system to identify and neutralize bacteria and viruses.

Inflammation. The outcome of an immune reaction and the natural process that breaks down damaged tissue so it can be replaced with healthy tissue.

Innate immune system. The natural immunity passed from mother to infant that becomes fully functional by age 3; nonspecific immunity.

Insulin. A hormone produced by the pancreas used to ferry blood glucose to the cells so they can produce energy.

Intermittent fasting. A modified form of fasting, comprising a single day or a number of hours within a day.

Lactose. A sugar found in milk and other dairy products.

Leaky brain. A breach of the blood-brain barrier that keeps toxic compounds out of the brain's blood supply, which leads to neurological and mental problems.

Leaky gut. Damage to the mucosal wall, which allows bacteria, food, and viral proteins to leak from the intestine into surrounding tissues.

Lectin. Gluten-like proteins and chemical compounds found in legumes and certain other seeds, which can create inflammation and GI problems.

Legumes. The family of beans, peas, lentils, coffee, and other plants that grow in pods.

Lymphatic system. A complex of tubes responsible for removing waste products and toxins and distributing antibodies and immune cells to the different tissues in the body.

Melatonin. A hormone the body produces that helps modulate sleep. Exposure to sunlight aids in its production.

Metabolic syndrome. The confluence of truncal obesity in combination with at least two of the following factors: high blood sugar, high blood pressure (hypertension), and high triglycerides or high cholesterol; can be a precursor to heart disease and type 2 diabetes.

Metabolism. The body's burning of energy (calories from food) to fuel its processes.

Microvilli. Minute, cone-shaped tendrils found on the villi in the surface of the gut's mucosal lining.

Monounsaturated fats. A group of "healthy" fats known to minimize inflammation; especially the omega-3 fats found in cold-water fish and other sources.

Mucosal layer. The first of five barriers that separate the gut from the rest of the body.

Mycotoxin. A mold toxin often found in corn, coffee, and other crops.

Myelin. A fatty substance that wraps around and protects nerve endings and enables signal transmission throughout the body.

My Plate. The FDA's recent replacement for the Food Guide Pyramid.

Neuropathy. Nerve pain and lack of feeling in the extremities.

Nightshade family. A family of New World vegetables, including white potatoes, tomatoes, peppers, eggplant, and tobacco, which often cause joint inflammation.

Non-celiac gluten sensitivity (NCGS). Sensitivity to gluten absent celiac disease. Also known simply as gluten sensitivity.

NSAIDs. The acronym for nonsteroidal anti-inflammatory drugs such as salicylates (aspirin) that temporarily block the perception of pain and reduce fever.

Obesitis. My word for the combination of obesity and inflammation, aggravated by eating sugar and grain.

Omega fatty acids. Essential (meaning the body cannot make them) fats that must be derived from food (or supplements).

Peptide. A short chain of two or more types of amino acids (proteins).

Peristalsis. The contractions and relaxations that force along the contents of the GI tract.

Phthalates. Hormone-disrupting compounds found in plastic water bottles, cosmetics, and other petrochemical-based products.

Phytic acid. A chemical in legumes that prevents the seed from sprouting until conditions are suitable for germination, but that also binds to minerals, interfering with absorption and causing deficiencies.

Polycystic ovary syndrome (PCOS). A hormonal imbalance in which a woman experiences irregular periods, infertility, weight grain, high blood sugar, and excessive hair growth.

Polyunsaturated fats. Fats found in grains and associated with poor health.

Probiotic. A live culture of *Lactobacillus* and *Bifidobacterium* strains, which help restore healthy bacteria.

Protein. Along with fat and carbohydrate, one of the three macronutrients in food; chains of amino acids.

Pseudo-grains. Buckwheat, amaranth, and quinoa, all of which look like grains but are botanically vegetables.

Rheumatology. The medical specialty devoted to autoimmune diseases that cause chronic pain.

Sarcorpenia. Age-related muscle loss.

Serotonin. A chemical produced primarily in the gut brain that is a natural pain reliever.

SIBO. The acronym for small intestinal bacteria overgrowth.

Statins. Drugs such as Lipitor and many others that block an enzyme called HMG-CoA reductase to lower total and LDL cholesterol, but also block production of CoQ10 and vitamin D.

Steroids. Drugs such as prednisone that mimic the action of cortisol, which naturally fights stress and inflammation and reduces pain.

Sugar alcohols. Natural sugar-free sweeteners such as mannitol and sorbitol that have minimal impact on blood sugar levels; FODMAPs (fermentable oligosaccharides, disaccharides, monosaccharides, and polyols).

Tight junctions. Minute, anchor-like proteins, which "snap" intestinal cells together; the second of five protective barriers in the GI tract.

Tricolsan. An antibacterial agent used in soaps and other products that is a hormone disruptor.

Triglycerides. Fats that circulate in the bloodstream and are stored as body fat.

Truncal obesity. Excess weight carried around the middle of the body.

Type 1 diabetes. High blood sugar resulting from destruction of certain cells in the pancreas; an autoimmune disease.

Type 2 diabetes. High blood sugar resulting from an inability to use insulin to ferry sugar into cells.

Vagus nerve. A nerve that runs from the brain to the colon, carrying signals between the brain and the gut brain.

Villi. Tiny tendrils on the surface of the gut's mucosal lining.

Villous atrophy. Flattening or destruction of villi when the gut becomes inflamed, reducing the gut's ability to absorb nutrients; also known as villous flattening, an indication of celiac disease.

Yeast overgrowth. When antibiotics destroy good gut bacteria, yeast proliferates, creating inflammation and infection in the GI tract. Yeast also converts sugar into alcohol, which can damage the liver.

INDEX

blood pressure (*cont.*)
supplements and, 152, 153, 154; toxins
and, 226
blood sugar, 60, 99, 102, 106–7, 113,
121, 135, 151, 154, 203, 211
bones, 42, 75, 151, 153, 154, 225,
226
bowels; and benefits of No-Grain, No-Pain
program, 119; diseases and, 88, 89, 211;
GI tract and, 70, 79, 87, 88, 91; gluten
sensitivity and, 20; sugar substitutes
and, 199; and testing of poop, 253–54;
zinc and, 151; *See also* irritable bowel
syndrome
brain; and benefits of gluten-free diet,
5; and breakfast, 203; calories and,
134–35; diet and, 123; GI tract
interactions with, 69, 70–72, 86, 90–91,
92; gluten sensitivity and, 20, 86; leaky,
86; nerves and, 36–37; and pain, 45–46,
70; stress and, 72; supplements and,
152, 153, 155, 156; toxins and, 225,
226; *See also* head/headaches
Bread Madness: history of, 35–36
breakfast; in Challenge Phase,
203–4, 208–10; fast food for, 122;
grains for, 121–23, 185–86; history of,
122–23; and Kickoff Phase, 187–89;
meal plans for, 187–89, 204, 208–10;
myth about, 203–4; and No-Grain,
No-Pain program, 121–23; and reasons
for elimination of all grains, 185–86;
recipes for, 186, 257, 260–63; and
standard American diet, 121–22;
"traditional," 121–22, 204
Brillat-Savarin, Jean Anthelme,
115
BROW (barley, rice, oats, wheat); and
definition of gluten, 10; elimination of,
138; GI tract and, 87, 88; and gluten-
free whiplash, 55; and hidden sources
of gluten, 11, 13; and myths about
gluten, 15, 16; reasons for elimination
of, 181–86; as sources of gluten, 12;
and symptoms of celiac disease, 23; and
testing for gluten sensitivity, 16; weight
and, 109
brunch: recipes for, 257, 260–63
buckwheat, 56, 138, 161, 173, 185
Burt (patient), 221

cadmium, 184, 225–26
caffeine, 153, 171–72

calcium, 42, 193, 195, 196, 224, 225, 232,
238
calories, 99, 103, 106, 107, 134–36, 178,
180, 207
cancer, 104, 124, 146, 151, 157, 184, 196,
197, 226, 227, 231
Candra (patient), 158–59, 180
canola oil, 30–31, 130–31
carbohydrates, 98, 106, 123, 125, 126,
153, 178–80, 195, 204
cardiovascular system, 151, 152, 225,
227
carnitine, 18, 146, 211
Cauliflower Rice (recipe), 188, 208, 258,
281
celiac disease, 89, 151, 157, 162, 175;
cause of, 11–13, 14, 16; cure for, 56;
diagnosis of, 23, 91; genetics and,
88; GI tract and, 31, 35, 78, 87, 88,
91, 92; gluten and, 11, 13–15, 16, 23,
31, 53; in history, 11; and identifying
root cause of pain, 6; immune system
and, 53; NSAIDs and, 41; and other
autoimmune diseases, 31, 35, 64;
prevalence of, 11, 14, 36; psychiatric
disorders and, 35, 36; and reasons for
elimination of all grains, 182, 184;
research about, 11–12; "safe" grains
and, 12; symptoms of, 11, 88; testing
for, 6, 53, 85, 88, 92; weight and, 97,
98, 112
cereals, 121–23, 165, 177, 185, 203,
204
Challenge Phase; basics of, 136–37;
breakfast in, 203–4, 208–10; cooking
during, 207; dinner in, 208–10; and
eating out, 128, 212; elimination of
foods in, 162, 167, 172, 191–92,
193–96; fasting during, 162, 178, 191,
200–203, 206, 207; follow-up to, 212;
and food variety, 205–6; hydration in,
192; initiation of, 162; legumes and,
194–96; lunch in, 208–10; meal plans
for, 204, 207–10; and nightshades,
193–94; nuts and seeds in, 192,
196–97; overview about, 120,
191–92; as phase of No-Grain, No-Pain
program, 136–37; physical activity in,
191, 192, 210, 216; portion control
and, 178; questions about, 212–13; and
reintroduction of certain foods, 213;
and Sheryl's illness, 211–12; smoothies
in, 204–5; snacks in, 196, 206–7; sugar

digestion (*cont.*)
GI tract relationship, 66–67; and nuts and seeds, 196; of protein, 232; and reasons for elimination of all grains, 185; and rules of nutrition, 116; smell of food and, 116; supplements and, 158; testing and, 251, 253, 254; toxins and, 226
Dijon Salmon Fillets (recipe), 188, 258, 277
dining out. *See* eating out
dinner; and Challenge Phase, 208–10; and grains, 124–25; and Kickoff Phase, 187–89; meal plans for, 187–89, 208–10; No-Grain, No-Pain program and, 124–25; recipes for, 257–58, 264–80; and standard American diet, 124–25
dizziness, 37, 152, 226, 238. *See also* balance; vertigo
doctors; and diagnosis versus cause, 247–48; and doctor-patient relationship, 2, 117, 241, 247–49; experience of, 255–56; good versus great, 241; labeling of diseases by, 248; lack of acceptance about gluten sensitivity by, 13; motivation of, 255; questions to ask functional medicine, 256; role of functional medicine, 241, 242; traditional treatments prescribed by, 27; training of, 2, 27–28, 255, 256
drugs, 121, 162, 192, 211-12; and acute versus chronic conditions, 242; changing/stopping, 117, 212–13; cycles with, 145; functional medicine and, 242; GI tract and, 81; and gluten sensitivity, 28–29; and limits of lab testing, 243; over-the-counter, 6, 39, 81, 117; and pain, 6, 28–29, 39, 41, 231–33; side effects of, 192, 221; supplements and, 144, 145, 150, 152, 233; when to use conventional, 242; *See also* painkillers; prescription drugs; *type of drug or disease*
Drushel, Henry, 122
Dukan, Pierre, 95

ears, 152, 211. *See also* vertigo
eating out, 126–29, 180–81, 212, 222–23
eczema, 8, 22, 31, 33, 34, 51, 52, 72–73, 151, 174

eggs; and acceptable foods, 166; and breakfast, 185, 203–4; and Challenge Phase, 207; duck, 125, 166; elimination of, 162; and Kickoff Phase, 162, 166, 186; meal plans and, 186; No-Grain, No-Pain program and, 125, 136; and reasons for elimination of all grains, 185; and recipes, 258, 259
energy, 97, 121, 139, 158, 211, 223, 255; and benefits of Kickoff Phase, 161; and benefits of No-Grain, No-Pain program, 119; GI tract and, 72, 73, 90, 91; supplements and, 152, 153, 154; toxins and, 223; weight and, 106, 113; *See also* fatigue
environmental medicine, 224–29
Environmental Protection Agency (EPA), 235
environmental toxins, 220, 222–23, 235–36, 251. *See also* air; water
Environmental Working Group, 237, 239
estrogen, 108–9, 113, 171, 227, 230, 231
exercise. *See* physical activity
eyes, 17, 38, 89, 107, 153, 162–63

Fallon, Sally, 169
family meals, 180–81
Fasano, Alessio, 93
fast food, 122, 124–25, 127, 130. *See also* junk food
fasting, 7, 26, 67, 117, 120, 162, 178, 191, 200–203, 206, 207
fatigue, 96, 120, 193, 211, 223, 238, 254–55; and benefits of No-Grain, No-Pain program, 119; and brain-pain relationship, 46; fibromyalgia and, 63; GI tract and, 72–73, 81; gluten sensitivity and, 17, 21; supplements and, 150, 151, 152, 153; toxins and, 224, 225, 226, 230; weight and, 108, 112; *See also* energy
fats; acceptable, 180; as bad, 98; in dairy products, 174; diet and, 98; impact of grains on, 113; importance of, 100; and Kickoff Phase, 174, 178–80; muscles and, 60; NAS guidelines for, 179; No-Grain, No-Pain program and, 126; and nuts and seeds, 196; portion control and, 178; and rule of thirds, 178–80; and standard American diet, 100, 125; and unacceptable food, 174; weight and, 98, 106, 113

gut. *See* GI (gastrointestinal) tract; leaky
  gut
gut migraines, 31, 35, 76

head/headaches, 211, 254–55; and
  benefits of No-Grain, No-Pain program,
  120; cluster, 31, 33; common pain
  conditions in, 31, 33; GI tract and,
  72–73, 81, 90–91; gluten sensitivity
  and, 16, 20–21; and intestinal
  problems, 90–91; prevalence of, 39;
  tension, 31, 33; toxins and, 226;
  vitamin B12 and, 152; *See also* migraine
  headaches
health coach, 255–56
heart; and drugs that contribute to
  pain, 233; functions of, 58, 77;
  ginger root and, 156; and gluten, 20,
  60–61; muscles, 58; and reasons for
  elimination of all grains, 183; and
  standard American diet, 124; and
  sugar, 197; supplements and, 153, 154,
  155; toxins and, 226, 231; weight and,
  104
heavy metals, 55, 151, 184, 211,
  222–23, 224–27, 230, 251, 252–53.
  See also specific metal
Herb-Seasoned Shepherd's Pie (recipe),
  189, 257, 271–72
herbs, 156–57, 168. *See also specific herb*
high-fructose corn syrup, 124, 148, 172,
  183, 197, 198
high-intensity interval training, 210,
  216
Homemade Breakfast Sausage (recipe),
  188, 208, 257, 262
hormones; and acceptable foods, 171;
  and brain-pain relationship, 46; and
  Candra's illness, 158; diet as treatment
  for imbalance of, 27; fasting and, 203;
  gluten and, 9, 21–22; grainbesity and,
  60; and head pain, 33; impact of grains
  on, 108–9; and Kickoff Phase, 171, 174;
  and obesity, 105–6; plastic and, 128;
  testing and, 254; toxins and, 225, 227,
  228, 230–31; and unacceptable food,
  174; weight and, 105–6, 107, 108–9,
  113; *See also specific hormone*
household cleaners, 236–37
hunger, 135–36, 178, 202. *See also*
  appetite
hydration, 135, 140–41, 172, 190, 192,
  201, 202. *See also* beverages

hygiene hypothesis, 238
Hyman, Mark, 161
hypertension, 104, 153, 155, 225
hypothyroidism, 9, 16, 108, 113

ibuprofen, 42, 44–45, 111
immune system; arthritis and, 63;
  breakfast and, 203; celiac disease and,
  53; cycles and, 59, 97; functions of,
  50–51; GI tract and, 70, 72–73, 74,
  75, 76, 77, 78, 79, 80, 82, 83, 91, 92,
  93; gluten and, 16, 22, 23, 52–53,
  59, 84, 85, 93; grain and, 29, 30, 47,
  54–55; humoral, 50–51, 52, 53, 67;
  hydration and, 140; inflammation
  and, 50–55; innate, 50, 51, 52, 53,
  54, 67, 85; and Kickoff Phase, 179;
  muscles/joints and, 34, 58; as a pair,
  50–51; protein and, 58; and rule of
  thirds, 179; sunshine/vitamin D and,
  140; supplements and, 151, 156; and
  testing, 243, 250–52, 253; toxins and,
  220, 226, 234, 238
individuals: uniqueness of, 2–3, 10,
  13, 23, 52, 85, 119, 159, 241,
  245–46
infections, 22, 72–73, 78, 82, 87, 151,
  242, 251, 254–55. *See also type of
  infection*
inflammation; as bad, 30; cause of, 9,
  10, 46, 67; diet and, 26, 38; drugs
  and, 26, 41–42; functions of, 49–50,
  67; GI tract and, 75, 77; gluten and,
  10, 14, 17–18, 23, 52–55, 57, 59; as
  good, 59; grain and, 9, 29, 46, 67; as
  housekeeper, 30, 49; immune system
  and, 50–55; injuries and, 65; *itis* and,
  9, 62; muscles and, 59–60; myths
  about, 30–32; nerves and, 36; as
  normal, 67; and Pain-Futility Cycle,
  40; painkillers as blocking, 49–50, 67;
  physical activity and, 65; prevalence of,
  47; "silent," 57; supplements and, 145;
  symptoms of chronic, 68; treatment
  for, 26, 41–42; and vegetable oils,
  30–32; *See also* grainflammation; *specific
  condition*
injuries, 65, 111, 242
insulin, 46, 60, 103, 106, 113, 121, 140,
  152, 203
insurance companies, 248
iron; and aspirin side effects, 41; collagen
  and, 66; and drugs that contribute to

myths; about aging, 61–62; about breakfast, 203–4; about diet, 98; about eating small meals, 135; about food-health relationship, 96; about genetics, 246–47; about gluten, 15–17; about inflammation, 30–32; about metabolism, 62; about multi-meals-a-day, 135; about painkillers, 25; about plastics, 227–29; about standard American diet, 98–99; about vegetable oils, 30–32

Nancy (patient), 162–63
National Academy of Sciences (NAS), 28, 179
National School Lunch Program, 105
Neel, James, 112–13
nerves,; autonomic, 116; brain and, 36–37; GI tract and, 66–67, 75, 92, 116; and gluten, 9, 20–21, 66–67; and grain, 29; myelin and, 38; overview about, 36–37; pain in, 32, 36–39, 138–39; parasympathetic, 66; and rules of nutrition, 116; supplements and, 152, 153, 154, 156; sympathetic, 66; toxins and, 224, 226; weight and, 113
neurogastroenterology, 71–72
neuropathy; cause of, 146; diabetes and, 107; fasting and, 200; GI tract and, 72, 73, 81; gluten sensitivity and, 37; supplements and, 144, 152, 153; as symptom of nervous system, 21, 32, 36; weight and, 111
nightshade plants, 125, 128, 133, 136, 192, 193–94
No-Grain, No-Pain program; basics of, 136–41; benefits of, 97–98, 102, 116, 119–20, 128, 137, 180, 215; calories and, 134–36, 178; "cheating" in, 139; and cost of food, 132–34; dinner and, 124–25; drugs and, 117; and eating out, 126–29; elimination of food/grains during, 136–38, 181–86; and family meals, 180–81; fast food and, 122, 124–25, 127, 130; fasting and, 120; GMOs and, 130–32; hydration and, 140–41; initiation of, 119, 141; lifestyle and, 116, 119, 120; lunch and, 123–24; motivation for, 200; and nutrition, 144–49; organic food and, 130–32; overview of, 115–17; physical activity and, 116, 139–40; portion

control in, 178–80; and priorities, 132–34; processed food in, 131; questions about, 141–42; recipes for, 141, 257–90; and rules of nutrition, 116–17; sandwiches and, 129–30; skepticism about, 120–21; snacks and, 125–26; and social situations, 127, 180–81; and sunshine, 140; supplements and, 142, 143–59; Triangle of Health as basis for, 115; as two-phase program, 116, 119–20, 136–38; and water, 140–41; weight and, 97–98, 102; *See also* Challenge Phase; Kickoff Phase
No-Pain Ice "Cream" (recipe), 168, 258, 288–89
non-celiac gluten sensitivity (NCGS), 7–8, 13, 85, 97–98
NSAIDs (non-steroridal anti-inflammatory drugs); cycles and, 40, 97; effectiveness of, 47; functions of, 34, 41–42; garlic and, 157; GI tract and, 76, 77; ginger root and, 156; gut migraines and, 76; as inducing pain, 43; overuse of, 45; overview about, 41–42; proteolytic enzymes and, 157; side effects of, 41, 43, 44–45, 66, 156, 157; supplements and, 144, 145, 150
nutrition; complexity of, 255–56; doctors training in, 27–28; effects of drugs on, 46; GI tract and, 74, 75, 91; and GMOs, 147–49; and grains, 56–57; importance of, 28; lack of knowledge about, 27–28, 105; and No-Grain, No-Pain program, 144–49; and pain remedies, 150–56; and reasons for taking supplements, 144–47; rules of, 116–17, 119, 121; school lunches and, 104–5; testing for, 149; video about, 114
nuts; acceptable, 169–70; and breakfast, 204; and Challenge Phase, 192, 196–97; as gluten-free substitutes, 165, 169–70; and Kickoff Phase, 169–70, 177, 179, 180; No-Grain, No-Pain program and, 125, 126; and recipes, 259; and rule of thirds, 179, 180; snacks and, 207; unacceptable, 177, 197

oats, 17, 173, 181–82. *See also* BROW
obesity. *See* grainbesity; weight
oils, 170, 177, 180. *See also* type of oil
olive oil, 170, 186, 207

physical activity (*cont.*)
of, 34, 110–11, 221; inflammation and, 65; and Kickoff Phase, 190; leaky gut and, 78, 82–83; longevity and, 60; motivation for, 140; and muscles/joints, 34, 59, 60, 64–66; pain as reason for avoiding, 46; toxins and, 253; video about, 210; ways to increase, 110–11; weight and, 97, 102, 104, 106, 110–11, 113, 114

Pineapple-Chicken Kabobs (recipe), 188, 258, 275–76

plastic, 78, 128, 193, 220, 222, 223, 226, 227–29, 231, 234, 236

Poached Cod with Mango Salsa (recipe), 187, 209, 258, 278

poop: testing of, 253–54

portion control, 178–80

Post, C.W., 122–23

poultry; acceptable, 166; and basics of No-Grain, No-Pain program, 136; and Challenge Phase, 207; elimination of, 162, 177; and gluten substitutes, 166; and Kickoff Phase, 162, 166, 177, 186; meal plans and, 186; organic, 186; and recipes, 258; as snacks, 125; unacceptable, 177

pregnancy, 21, 225

prescription drugs, 60, 61, 72, 96, 97; abuse of, 2, 40; adverse effects of, 1, 2, 40; changing/stopping, 117; cycle of, 40, 43, 44; diet as substitute for, 26–27, 28–29, 47; effectiveness of, 47; and effects of No-Grain, No-Pain program, 117; functions of, 6, 25, 70; GI tract and, 81, 90; most commonly prescribed, 39; prevalence of, 39; side effects of, 26, 40, 97; supplements and, 144; as traditional treatments, 1, 27, 46; and treating symptoms and not causes, 40; weight and, 111; *See also* painkillers; *specific drug*

preservatives, 55, 123, 259

probiotics, 80, 157, 158, 216, 231

processed food; and basics of No-Grain, No-Pain program, 131, 136, 137; and cost of food, 133; elimination of, 162, 176–78, 198; and food substitutions, 164; gluten and, 8, 12, 17, 55–56, 57, 67, 163, 176–78; GMOs and, 131; healthy food and, 164; hidden grains in, 182; and identifying root cause of pain, 6, 8; and Kickoff Phase, 131, 162,

175, 176–78, 198; organic, 163; and reasons for elimination of all grains, 182, 183; recipes and, 259; and rules of nutrition, 116; sales of, 12; soy in, 175; substitutions for, 164; sugar in, 163, 197, 198; and thinking healthy, 163; toxins and, 224; as unacceptable food, 176–78; weight and, 104–5; *See also type of food*

protein; for breakfast, 186, 203–4; and Challenge Phase, 191; digestion of, 232; and digestion of grains, 73, 85; and drugs that contribute to pain, 232; GI tract and, 81, 92; gluten and, 10, 59, 91–92; gut migraines and, 76; immune system and, 58; and Kickoff Phase, 174, 176, 178–80; muscles and, 58, 59; NAS guidelines for, 179; portion control and, 178; questions about, 141; and reasons for elimination of all grains, 184, 186; and rule of thirds, 178–80; smoothies and, 204–5; and snacks in No-Grain, No-Pain program, 125, 126; sources of, 141; and standard American diet, 125; supplements and, 152, 154; and unacceptable food, 174, 176; vegetarians and, 141; weight and, 106, 112

pseudo-grains, 138, 161, 172, 173, 185–86. *See also* amaranth; buckwheat; quinoa

psoriasis, 10, 22, 31, 34, 174

psoriatic arthritis, 21, 63

questions; about Challenge Phase, 212–13; about Kickoff Phase, 189–90; about No-Grain, No-Pain program, 141–42; about recipes, 141; to ask functional medicine doctors, 256

quinoa, 138, 161, 173, 184–85

Rachel (patient), 145–47

recipes; adaptations/substitutions in, 258–59; for breakfast, 186, 257, 260–63; for brunch, 257, 260–63; for desserts, 258, 287–90; for dinner, 257–58, 264–80; for lunch, 257–58, 264–80; for No-Grain, No-Pain program, 141, 257–90; paleo, 141; questions about, 141; for salads, 258, 281–86; for side dishes, 258, 281–86; for snacks, 258, 287–90; *See also specific recipe*

ABOUT THE AUTHOR

Dr. Peter Osborne is a doctor of pastoral medicine, a doctor of chiropractic, and a board-certified nutritionist, but informally, he regards himself as the "Gluten-Free Warrior." As clinical director of Origins Healthcare in Sugar Land, Texas, he practices functional medicine, meaning his goal is to find the origin of a disease, instead of simply treating the symptoms. His current practice includes primarily patients with chronic pain. Using a combination of diet and supplementation, he has eliminated or alleviated the chronic pain of thousands of his patients.

In addition, Dr. Osborne is a leader in the gluten-free universe. His website, glutenfreesociety.org, is must reading for anyone concerned with the confluence of diet and disease. He is also devotes much of his time to mentoring, educating, and training other health professionals about functional medicine, gluten sensitivity, and the direct relationship between grain consumption and chronic pain.

Dr. Osborne is the world's leading expert on the effects of gluten on pain and on the distinctions between celiac disease and other manifestations of gluten sensitivity. He created the Glutenology Physician and Healthcare Practitioner Certification Program, a comprehensive, 10-hour postgraduate course on gluten sensitivity. He has also served as executive secretary for the American Clinical Board of Nutrition from 2006 to 2011, when he was appointed vice president. Previously, he was on the organization's examining board, which writes the questions medical students are asked to answer to ensure a minimum knowledge of nutrition before getting their degree.

Dr. Osborne is a nationally recognized and sought-after speaker. He regularly lectures on gluten sensitivity, autoimmune disease, drug-induced nutritional deficiencies, and functional medicine. He is also a regular contributor on Fox News.

In his spare time, Dr. Osborne enjoys CrossFit training, reading scientific journals, and traveling with his wife. His lifelong goal is to ensure that functional medicine becomes the preeminent form of treatment used by doctors to address chronic health issues.